The Structure of Stuttering

Marcel E. Wingate

The Structure of Stuttering

A Psycholinguistic Analysis

With 16 Illustrations

Springer-Verlag New York Berlin Heidelberg
London Paris Tokyo

Marcel E. Wingate
Department of Speech and Hearing Sciences
Washington State University
Pullman, Washington 99164-2420

Library of Congress Cataloging-in-Publication Data
Wingate, Marcel E. (Marcel Edward), 1923–
The structure of stuttering: a psycholinguistic analysis/by Marcel E. Wingate.
p. cm.
Bibliography: p.
ISBN-13: 978-1-4615-9666-0 e-ISBN-13: 978-1-4615-9664-6
DOI: 10.1007/978-1-4615-9664-6
1. Stuttering. 2. Psycholinguistics. I. Title.
RC424.W55 1988
616.85'54—dc19 88-4977

Softcover reprint of the hardcover 1st edition 1988

Typeset by Ampersand Publisher Services, Inc., Rutland, Vermont.

9 8 7 6 5 4 3 2 1

To my wife, Cicely, and to

Nancy
Amy
Jennifer
Marcel R.
Cicely A.

Preface

This book was not written for any particular audience; generally speaking, I believe its contents should be substantive for anyone who has an interest in the nature of normal language processes and their dysfunction. Nonetheless, in writing the book I have had in mind that its contents will be of special interest and value to persons in several disciplines, most notably certain areas of psychology and linguistics, and especially where those interests overlap. It should also be worthwhile to individuals involved in what has come to be known as neurolinguistics, and, of course, to persons having a particular interest in the disorder of stuttering.

More has been written about stuttering than all the other speech disorders combined, yet it has remained an enigma. In my view the major source of the continued failure to isolate the nature of stuttering lies in the matter of the questions asked about it. It is not simply that they were not the right questions, but rather that there have actually been so few bona fide questions! Too much of what has been written and said about stuttering has come in the form of declarative statement, which typically reflects some guiding concept and assumption(s). Moreover, most of what has passed as questions has been of a similar nature.

Over many years, but particularly in the 20th century, the most favored concepts of stuttering have accounted for it as a psychological problem of some kind. The attractiveness of such explanations is not difficult to appreciate in view of the many superficial observations about stuttering that suggest, or can be supposed to reflect, psychological events. Individuals representing a very wide range of familiarity with psychological concepts, from lay person to trained professional, have made such observations the basis for their assumptions and concept of the disorder. Very often the accounts have had some psychodynamic theme, but increasingly in this century the most popular explanations have borrowed paradigms from learning theory. A central feature of these learning formulations is the contention that stuttering is not essentially abnormal, that stutter events are simply a *degree* of nonfluency rather than aberrations that are unique in type.

It was primarily because of this pervasive psychological orientation to stuttering that I became interested in studying it. Educated as a clinical psychologist, and having attained my advanced degree in an era when dynamic psychology was probably at its zenith, I was led into the investigation of stuttering under an active persuasion that it was a psychological disorder. However, I soon began to have increasing doubts that stuttering was adequately explained either as basically a psychodynamic (emotional) problem or as due to faulty learning. I found the various psychological explanations of the disorder to be marked by one or more serious flaws: internal inconsistencies, in some cases amounting to outright contradictions; hypothetical frameworks only partially, or loosely, tied to reality; marked tendencies to either disregard incompatible findings, or to compromise them in some way; a readiness to offer partial explanations that were purely fabulistic; and, most serious of all, an effort to deny the reality of the disorder.

In the rush to explain the cause of stuttering, accompanied regularly by a fervid and protective devotion to the fabrications thus created, the authors of these so-called "theories" (a true misnomer) sped right by the most focal aspect of stuttering, namely (in the simplest terms) that there is something wrong about the way the individual "links up" the sounds of words. The sounds of words, and words (and whatever else a scrutiny of these dimensions might lead to) have attracted relatively little interest, and even when they were brought under observation the focus was actually centered on some psychological notion lying beyond. Results that emanated from sporadic attention to these dimensions were predestined to be shunted into some favored preconception. In effect, one can justifiably contend that, in spite of the enormous literature on the subject, "stuttering," which means an anomaly in the flow of speech, actually has been studied very little.

For some time it has seemed clear to me that investigation of stuttering must be approached in reference to the substance of which it is an evident anomaly—oral language expression. For certain reasons, which I have developed in several previous publications, I was led to infer that an important key to the nature of stuttering lay in the prosodic dimensions of language. My pursuit of this line of study has developed into a broader perspective of stuttering as a unique, subtle disorder of expressive language function that involves several levels of the language production system. This broader perspective is the major substance of this book.

In Part I of *The Structure of Stuttering* I present first a brief but (I believe) cogent statement of the conceptual looseness and theoretical weakness in extant explanations of stuttering. I then proceed to document my criticism that: 1) much of the research in stuttering has been biased, provincial, and redundant; and 2) that a central obstacle in progress toward understanding stuttering is that the literature of stuttering has remained incredibly insulated from research on nonfluency in normal speech, which should be its basic reference. Attention is directed to a breadth of evidence that stuttering is a discriminably identifiable type of disfluency, and that the observable character of the disorder contains important clues to discovering its essential nature.

Part II is addressed to a review and critical analysis of the existing research relevant to identification of language factors in stuttering. Chapters 3 and 4 cover, in developmental sequence, the pertinent research within the field of stuttering. These studies have yielded much worthwhile data, including the recurrent identification of certain language variables that are associated with stuttering (e.g., segmental, suprasegmental, and grammatical factors). However, these data are regularly confounded by the persistent interpretation that they reflect a (reactive type) psychological problem. In fact, what turn out to be the key language factors are ignored in this research.

Chapter 5 relates the language variables, identified in the stuttering research, to pertinent findings yielded by research on normal speech. These analyses lead to an understanding of the "language factors" that is considerably different from the interpretation standardly offered in the stuttering research itself. The denouement of this chapter is the emergence of the key variables of *syllable-initial position* and *linguistic stress.*

The content of Chapter 6, the last chapter in this section, is addressed to the identification, and brief discussion, of the evident correspondence between the key language factors in stuttering and the evidence regarding syllable structure that is to be found in the linguistics literature. The content of this chapter sets the stage, built on the substance of the preceding chapters, for the "new departure" to be taken in the final chapter of the book. In the interim, however, there is some important new evidence to consider, which will extend the basis for explaining stuttering as a dysfunction in the language system.

Part III contains two chapters, Chapters 7 and 8, that report an extensive comparative study of language factors and disfluency that I conducted a few years ago over a period of several years. The data were obtained from sizeable groups: 20 young adult male stutterers and matched normal speakers. Analysis centers on 10 measures selected to assess various dimensions of language function. The findings reveal a range of differences between stutterers and normal speakers, several of them quite dramatic. All of the differences are internally consistent and, as well, consistent with previously obtained relevant findings. These data enlarge the scope for understanding stuttering as a language disability.

Part IV consists of only one chapter, Chapter 9. This chapter consolidates analyses developed in the preceding chapters, focusing on the evidence regarding the critical features of a stutter event. Discussion relates the crux of these analyses to relevant dimensions of linguistic and psycholinguistic research, and to other pertinent information about stuttering. Integration of the information from these sources leads to hypotheses about the probable anomalies in linguistic function, and their neurologic substrate, that underlie what is observed, at the surface, as stuttering.

Throughout the book a recurrent theme, often stated and always implied, points up the contribution of linguistics to the understanding of stuttering. In the material of the final chapter it becomes evident that, in turn, this achievement for stuttering contains substantial implications for understanding the nature of normal language function.

MARCEL E. WINGATE

Contents

List of Tables and Figures

Tables

Figures

Part I: Background

The content of Part I is addressed to certain basic issues whose resolution is essential to the establishment of a stable foundation for the analyses to be developed in the ensuing chapters.

The two chapters of Part I bring together many dimensions of evidence from a wide range of sources, that show stuttering to be reliably and validly identified as a unique type of irregularity in the flow of speech, characterized in terms of certain core features. These core features are necessary and sufficient to define stuttering descriptively; they constitute the essential basis for identifying it observationally and for differentiating it from normal nonfluency; and they suggest leads for discovering the underlying nature of the disorder that, contrary to many convictions or assumptions, remains unknown.

1
Introduction

Stuttering remains an enigma in spite of the fact that it has been studied, at some level, for centuries. More has been written about stuttering than about any of the other disorders of speech, yet it is still less well understood than the others. In no small measure the reason stuttering is so poorly understood is *because* so much has been written about it; the intrinsic mystery of the disorder has been embellished by the many efforts to explain it.

"Theories" and "Definitions"

Stuttering is aptly described as "The Disorder of Many Theories," the pertinent title of a recent book by a lay author (and "recovered" stutterer) who, in his efforts to learn something about stuttering from the professional literature, "found a grab bag of competing and often contradictory explanations" (Jonas, 1977, p. 8).

In spite of Jonas' reference to "theories," a term widely used in professional sources as well, one should recognize that the various beliefs about stuttering are more properly described, at best, as loosely formulated hypotheses, rather than theories (Wingate, 1977c). Conjecture about the cause of stuttering has a long-standing legacy, well reflected in a summary contained in a book published late in the 19th century (Potter, 1882). Potter reviewed the contributions on stuttering of 126 different authorities whose works had appeared over a time span of almost 24 centuries, from 484 B.C. to 1878 A.D. As part of this review Potter extracted and categorized the etiologic statements made by these authorities, an endeavor that resulted in a list of 31 separate categories of etiology. Although the range of explanation has narrowed considerably in the 20th century, conjecture about the cause of stuttering has continued to be active.

Most 20th century accounts of stuttering have centered almost exclusively in some psychological explanation of the disorder. Although psychological accounts had been offered in earlier times, the 20th century focus on psychological explanations is almost certainly due to the fact that psychology emerged as a separate discipline in the years around the turn of the century, and developed rapidly thereafter. Experimental psychology, expanding from the pioneer work of Wundt, Galton, and others, gave the new discipline a scientific respectability. In many ways this image was enhanced by the development of mental testing, through the work of Binet, Cattell, and others. However, the substance from which most 20th century beliefs about stuttering were constructed came from two sources: the "dynamic" psychology that originated in the "new" psychiatry of Bleuler, Charcot, Freud, and their followers and, somewhat later, from the "behaviorism" movement generated by John B. Watson (see Wingate, 1986c).

A unique feature found in many 20th century positions on stuttering, particularly the most popular and influential ones, is the presumption to state a conjectured explanation of stuttering as the *definition* of it.[1] Moreover, were it not for the routine lead phrase of these definitions, in which the word "stuttering" appears, one would have little idea from the defining statement itself what the author of the definition was talking about. In most instances the reader would not even have reason to guess that the definition referred to a speech problem (see next paragraph).

Although most extant positions do acknowledge, in one way or another, that stuttering is a disorder of speech, there is a decided tendency to treat the speech features of stuttering as almost incidental. The term "disorder" appears to be used largely in a superficially descriptive sense, with the speech characteristics being considered simply as intermittent perturbations in the speech process that result from influences external to the process itself. The speech process is presumed to be normal, to be fundamentally the same as that for nonstuttered speech. Such positions treat the speech anomalies, the characteristics by which we identify certain speech samples as "stuttered," as simply the indirect effects of some other circumstances. This treatment of the disorder is well represented in the fact that so many of these "definitions" of stuttering are simply statements of presumed etiology, in which the speech characteristics are not even (or are hardly) mentioned. The following definitions are exemplary:

Coriat, I.H.: [Stuttering is] a psychoneurosis caused by a persistence into later life of early pregenital oral nursing, oral sadistic, and anal sadistic components (Hahn, 1956, p.28).

Fletcher, J.M.: [Stuttering] should be diagnosed and described as well as treated as a morbidity of social consciousness, a hypersensitivity of social attitude, a pathological social response (Hahn, 1956, p. 34)[2].

Gifford, M.F.: [Stuttering is] a complex, functional speech disorder that has its roots in fear, or in some deep-seated mental and emotional conflict within the self (Hahn, 1956, p. 48).

Sheehan, J.G.: [Stuttering is] the result of a conflict between opposed urges to speak and to hold back from speaking (Hahn, 1956, p.110).[3]

Brutten, G.J., and Shoemaker, D.J.: [Stuttering is] the disorganization of normally fluent speech that is a consequence of conditioned emotion.... It is the fluency failure that results when conditioned stimuli evoke a disruptive emotional response (Travis, 1971, p. 1063).[4]

Johnson, W.: [Stuttering is] an anticipatory, apprehensive, hypertonic, avoidance reaction (Johnson, Brown, Curtis, Edney, & Keaster, 1956, p. 217).[5]

Note that such definitions not only omit specific reference to the speech characteristics, they also state that the nature of the disorder lies somewhere else than in the speech process. Actually, Johnson's position, the most widely influential in the United States, at least, and represented in the last definition given above, even repudiates the idea of a disturbance in speech function; that is, it attempts to deny that stuttering is an actual disorder of speech. This position, the "evaluational" conjecture developed by Johnson (1942, 1961b; Johnson and Associates, 1959), and modified slightly by Bloodstein (1958, 1975), centers in the contention that what is *called* stuttering is really only (unnecessary) struggle and effort occurring during speech acts. The struggle and excessive effort are presumed to reflect the individual stutterer's unwarranted assumption that (normal) speech is difficult. From this position stutter events are not accepted as realities, in the sense of being events that *happen* in the course of an individual's speaking. To the contrary, "stutter" is said to be simply a label for what the individual *does*, that is, it is just a name for his (unnecessary) struggling. Advocates of this position have persistently endeavored to rationalize stuttering as being only a degree of (normal) nonfluency, not a separate kind of disfluency denotable as an actual disorder of the speech process.

Such definitions, and the positions they reflect, prejudice the study of stuttering through their presumption of known cause. The fact of the matter remains that the cause of stuttering—its essential nature—is unknown. Efforts made toward understanding the nature of stuttering are only obstructed by investigations mounted from a motivation to support conjectures. Unfortunately, a considerable amount of stuttering research bears this onus.

A second attribute of such definitions is that, in focusing on cause, they confound the study of stuttering by diverting attention from an objective analytic consideration of the stutter events themselves. Because their central explanatory notion is typically some variant of the concept of fear (with its subsidiary notions of "expectancy," or "anticipation" and "avoidance") the positions reflected in these definitions force a preoccupation with circumstances of an affective nature, circumstances that, moreover, are claimed to occur *prior to* the stutter events. Later in this chapter, and recurrently throughout the book, we will find many reasons to consider the preoccupation with such circumstances to be a misleading emphasis. Stutter events themselves should occupy our attention first; our understanding of stutter events and their contexts is still not very well developed. As Hughlings Jackson once said, "The study of the causes of things must be preceded by a study of the things caused."[6] A focus on the study of stuttering itself should lead to a more realistic appreciation of the probable cause(s).

In order to proceed effectively in a study of "the things caused" in stuttering one must be free of the constraints imposed by the pervasive 20th century positions. It will be necessary to approach stuttering at its face value, as an observable event amenable to various levels of analysis. To do so, it is first necessary to understand the major intellectual obstacles posed by the positions broadly representative of current day thought in stuttering.

As indicated earlier, the intellectual obstacles mentioned above are posed by expressions of the belief that stuttering is not basically different from normal speech. The presumption of an essential normality of the speech of stutterers finds expression in many ways. Occasionally it appears in such extreme statements as, "There is no such thing as stuttering," a claim made by Wendell Johnson in many of his professional appearances, and repeated by others on many occasions. It was reiterated as recently as 1981 by a member of the professional audience during a conference on "Contemporary Issues in Stuttering" held at Northwestern University.[7] Similarly, in the August 1983 issue of the *Journal of Speech and Hearing Disorders*, Perkins (1983, p. 247) claimed that "the more they [the speech of stutterers and the speech of normal speakers] are compared, the more similar they appear to be." Such contentions are among the more dramatic expressions of a rather broadly based and systematic effort to question, indeed to deny, the distinctiveness of stuttering; that is, to deny that stuttering is different from normal speech.

A relatively simple, but effective, tactic for confounding a differentiation of stuttering from normal speech has been the use of class terms and gloss references that ignore pertinent distinctions to be made within these general classes. In the literature of stuttering, particularly when there is a concurrent reference to normal speech, one finds frequent use of the words "repetitions" and "hesitations." For example, Johnson (1946, p. 445), speaking of "What these laymen had diagnosed as stuttering," contended that what they had observed was "indistinguishable from the *hesitations* and *repetitions*[8] known to be characteristic of the normal speech of young children." Now, repetitions and hesitations are generic terms; applying them to both stuttered and normal speech obscures, and implicitly denies, pertinent distinctions that are indicated by subclasses within these general categories; *distinctions that research has consistently revealed to be useful for descriptive and analytic differentiation of stuttered from normal speech.* (Put succinctly, the focal distinction is in terms of elemental repetitions and prolongations; an important distinction that emerges repeatedly throughout this book.) Sometimes, claims denying the distinctiveness of stuttering are made even when subclasses of a general term are specified. For instance, Darley (1955, p. 138), discussing stuttered speech samples, spoke of "repetitions of a sound, syllable, word or phrase, speech phenomena well known to characterize the speech of normal young children."

The grandest gloss term of all is "disfluency" which, being the most encompassing generic term, effectively obscures differentiation among the full range of categories includable within it. This broad reference has a certain justifiable utility when used with discretion. However, much of the use made of it has created confusion and ambiguity (see Wingate, 1984a). Unfortunately, it has been used widely as a rhetorical device employed as a way to avoid confronting the distinctions that can be made between the subcategories within its broad scope. In fact (see Chapter 2) there has been considerable effort to substitute the use of disfluency in place of stuttering.

Although "disfluency" sounds ordinary enough, composed as it is of a well-used prefix and a main word that evidently is understood by most people, it is actually a very uncommon word. The rarity of the word disfluency is clearly revealed in the fact that it does not appear as an entry in any standard reference lexicon. Of the four unabridged dictionaries consulted, including the 12-volume Oxford English Dictionary,[9] none contains an entry for disfluency. At the same time, all four sources contain many other unusual words having a "dis-" prefix, of which disbranch, discrown, disocclude, dispauper, disrelish, and disrudder are a small sample. (In contrast, each reference source did have entries for fluency—and for stuttering.)

"Disfluency," a term unique to certain literature on stuttering, is properly described as an esoteric, special-purpose word that has been promoted by advocates of the position that stuttering does not differ from normal speech. The term emerged from efforts initiated by Johnson (Johnson, 1961a; Johnson and Associates, 1959)[10] to provide a means of talking about all kinds of fluency irregularity—those that characterize stuttering as well as those typically found in normal speech—as though they are essentially all the same. Disfluency affords a normalizing vehicle by implicitly dismissing pertinent distinctions to be made within the broad range of this general, or class, term.

It is pertinent to note, additionally, that in the literature reporting investigation of fluency irregularities in normal speech *only* (i.e., literature having no comparative or other interest in stuttering), one will find that a different term, "hesitation phenomena," is used to refer to irregularities in speech fluency. This matter and its significance is addressed in Chapter 2.

Another measure employed in the effort to support the contention that stuttering is not essentially different from normal speech has been to emphasize the "overlap" in types of disfluencies found in studies comparing stuttered and normal speech samples. This argument, like the use of general, broad-category terms, diverts attention to superficialities and away from focal issues.[11] This matter, too, is considered again in Chapter 2.

Proponents of the contention that stuttering and normal speech are not essentially different believe they find support in the results of certain research that purports to show that judges cannot reliably differentiate stutters from normal nonfluencies. Perkins (1983, p. 247) grandly overstates the matter in his claim that "the best judgments of loci of stuttering are not much better than chance." His statement epitomizes the belief found among those who subscribe to this position. However, the findings of this research (that purportedly demonstrates unreliability in judgments of stutters) are highly suspect. First, there is extensive documentation from countless sources that stuttered speech is routinely and reliably differentiated from normal speech, by both lay and sophisticated individuals. Thus there is a profound contradiction here: generally, stuttered speech is readily identified, yet under special circumstances it is said to not be reliably recognized (or so it seems). The dimensions of this contradiction lead one to suspect that the problem does not lie in what is being judged, nor in the judges, but in the special circumstances themselves, that is, in the research itself. The findings of this research seem clearly to represent what Roger Brown (1973, p. 44) called "the pigeon ping-pong problem," in allusion to the pigeons that Skinner trained to peck a ball back and forth, an activity that resembled the game of Ping-Pong. The allusion illustrates the fact that often a research procedure does not preserve essential properties of the circumstances it is supposed to represent, and the findings are thus invalid. The studies purporting to show unreliability of stutter judgments are particulary vulnerable to this kind of distortion; in fact, one will find in them major faults of both design and execution, faults that reflect either oversight, or bias, or both (see Wingate, 1981, for a criticism of one such study).

At the same time, the most telling contradiction of the claims made regarding unreliability of judgments of stuttering is supplied in the many studies in which demonstration of high values of inter- and intra-judge agreement about stutters have been a routine part of the procedure.

A Clear and Certain Focus

Stuttering has been identified and discussed at length for centuries, throughout which time, there is ample reason to believe, everyone has known what everyone else has been talking about.[12] The efforts made to deny the distinctiveness of stuttering, a relatively recent preoccupation, have been a wasteful and futile pursuit. In the final analysis one is invariably confronted by the fact that whether the speech features of stuttering are minimized, ignored, taken for granted, denied, or otherwise obscured, the study of stuttering—from whatever orientation—*always* proceeds in primary reference to certain distinctive speech characteristics. And it has always done so, even in those works oriented toward denying its reality. Definitions of stuttering aside, and efforts to normalize stuttering notwithstanding, it is only because of certain notable speech characteristics that a topical focus of study exists.

The word *stuttering* denotes certain kinds of events in speech, and one cannot speak of stuttering without making at least implicit reference to these notable events. The distinctiveness of these events is attested by several impressive lines of evidence:

1. the onomatopoeic structure of words for stuttering in many different languages
2. the etymological derivation of words for stuttering
3. immediately recognizable metaphorical use of the word "stutter" in lay literature as well as in common parlance, and
4. the fact that repeated research findings consistently match up neatly with the first three lines of evidence.[13]

The speech events that characterize stuttering can be specified succinctly as *silent or audible elemental repetitions or prolongations* (see Wingate, 1964; 1976, chap. 4). This designation is more descriptive than, but essentially equivalent to, *clonic* and *tonic*, terms that were widely used for well over a century after their introduction by Serre d'Alais in 1839 (see Klingbeil, 1939; Potter, 1882). During that long time clonic and tonic were used routinely with the word "spasm" in reference to stutter events. However, because of its neurological implications, spasm became unacceptable to those who wished to explain stuttering as "learned behavior" and therefore direct steps were taken, during the 1940s, to expunge spasm from the literature of stuttering.[14] Evidently clonic and tonic fell into disfavor because of their previous association with spasm, for they came to be used less frequently thereafter. However, in spite of the fact that clonic and tonic are not presently in wide use in the literature of stuttering they still have a currency in the field; their reference is readily understood, which constitutes a direct commentary on their validity.

Much has been made in the literature of stuttering about the extent and variety of "symptoms" supposedly manifested by stutterers (for actual examples, see Froeschels, 1921, 1961; Johnson, 1944a, 1944b; Solomon, 1932). This claim is well represented in a statement by St. Onge that "stuttering, whatever it is, presents itself to us with a bewildering array of signs and symptoms" (1963, p. 195). A good example of the purported array can be found in "a brief survey of the literature" conducted some years ago by Van Riper (1937) from which he was able to draw up a list of over 100 different symptoms that had been reported in the sources he reviewed. Froeschels (1961), speaking in reference to "many thousands of cases," claimed that "no two cases ever had identical symptoms." Van Riper (1937), from his own observation of 30 adult stutterers, reported finding "an almost incredible variety of such abnormalities."

There is good reason to question whether it is appropriate to consider the acts described in this literature as "symptoms" of stuttering. The acts described are, in most instances, not discernible as central features of stutter events. For instance, in spite of the extent, and all the apparent variety, that Van Riper reported, only two features stood out as the symptoms common to all stutterers. In Van Riper's words, "all other symptoms varied; the clonic or tonic blocks alone were experienced by all" (p. 185).

The same finding has surfaced repeatedly. In fact, it has recurred with such regularity that extended reference is superfluous. The matter is well summarized in a statement by Sheehan (1974):[15]

> Of all the diverse symptoms of stuttering mentioned in the literature, involving almost every conceivable type of behavior, only two have found to be common to all stutterers: (1) tonus, the prolonging or holding of muscular posture or activity, and (2) clonus, the series of rapid repetitive movements involving the speech musculature (p. 195).

The invariant recurrence of these two features marks them as the only *true* symptoms of stuttering. All other aspects can be readily assigned to *accessory* status (see Wingate, 1964, 1976, chap. 4).

It is significant for the analysis and understanding of stuttering that these two cardinal features of stuttered speech have regularly been understood to reflect a common disorder. At certain times in the past some authorities (see Klingbeil, 1939; Potter, 1882) have used stuttering to refer essentially to the clonic features and stammering to refer to the tonic type. Nonetheless, the two types were still considered to be manifestations of the same disorder. Parker (1932), for instance, noted:

> A definite usage of the term stuttering to designate repetition of consonants (K-K-K-Katie), and stammering a spasm which temporarily inhibits speech altogether. ... The difference between the two disabilities, though easily recognized, has never been studied, and the two are generally considered as different forms of the one defect (p. 33).

It is also relevant that laypersons, too, understand these phenomena as reflecting the same disorder. As Stein (1942) put it: "It is interesting to note that, in spite of the multiformity of its character, even the layman, with few exceptions, is able to comprehend the various types of this disorder under one concept" (p. 109).

These salient features of stuttering, the clonic and tonic symptoms, are directly observable events that provide the first level of descriptive characterization of the disorder. They are phenomena that reflect anomaly in the flow of connected speech. As such, it is most appropriate to consider them to be intrinsic "markers" of the disorder they characterize.

The second level of descriptive characterization is to identify the dimension that these markers have in common. This common dimension is well represented in the word "block," another widely used term, which means a (variable and temporary) inability to move forward in the speech sequence.

The designation block (or blocking) is a particularly appropriate word. To begin with, it captures the impression gained from direct observation of stuttering, not only because of the suggestion of difficulty inherent in the elemental repetitions and prolongations themselves, but also because this suggestion of difficulty is frequently confirmed by other signs of effort that occur either during the course of the elemental repetition or prolongation, or in the speech activity immediately sequential to their occurrence. The stutterer appears to be blocked in his evident intention to proceed.

The term block is also consistent with the testimony of stutterers themselves. In fact, stutterers frequently use the word block to describe their experience of a stutter event, or say of the experience that they know what they want to say but cannot say it. Bloodstein (1958) attests to the ubiquity of blocking in his description of

> the one attribute of this disorder which typifies it above all: the person who exhibits it knows precisely what word he wants to say:[16] he is simply unable for the moment to say it (p. 3).

Moreover, blocking describes the essence of both elemental repetitions and prolongations, as noted some time ago by Travis (1933b):

> The repetition consists of alternate blocks and releases. It is clonic activity. In this sense there is no fundamental difference between repeating (clonic activity) and blocking (tonic activity), the latter being merely a marked prolongation of the block phase of the former. Generally speaking, every stutterer presents both types of difficulty (p. 652).

Identifying stuttering in its peripheral aspect as an inability to move forward in the speech sequence has been expressed in terms of a difficulty in transition. Most recently Wingate (Wingate, 1969b; 1976, p. 253ff.) has discussed stuttering as a phonetic transition defect in which the failure of transition is related to linguistic stress. The essential idea of transition difficulty has appeared a number of times in the past, although with different emphases regarding the nature of the obstacle to transition. Aristotle (Forrester, 1947) seems to have expressed the crux of the idea rather clearly in his description of stuttering as "due to an inability to join one syllable to another sufficiently quickly." In 1870 Hunt (1967) explained that

> the stutterer ... has no difficulty of articulating the consonants individually, for we hear him repeat them in rapid succession, b, b, b, b, t, t, t, and so on. What is it then that distresses the stutterer, surely not the initial explosives? Why it is the enunciation of the *following* sound, be it a vowel or a consonant, which is his difficulty; he cannot join them, and it is this which makes him repeat the explosive until the conjunction is effected. It is, therefore, during the transition from one mechanism to another that the impediment chiefly takes place (p. 21).

Froeschels too (1913–1914) said that "the speech of stutterers fails not at the single sound but only at the connection between sounds." Kussmaul (1877) also held that the individual sounds are made correctly but that the trouble lies in connecting consonants and vowels. Bluemel (1913) emphasized that the difficulty is not with the consonant, as might appear, but with the following vowel. Van Riper (1954, p. 440) noted that "most stutterers fail to realize that in stuttering it is not the sounds that are faulty but the transitions between sounds." I will return to such analyses in Chapters 6 and 9.

The idea that the classic features of stuttering are, in essence, surface markers of the actual stutter event (the inability to move forward) is consistent with the long-term identification of these two "symptoms" as reflecting the same disorder. It is also consonant with the rational integration, or reduction, of the two features as stated by Travis (1933b). Moreover, identifying them as the characteristic markers of stutter events, rather than actually being the stutters, allows one to incorporate the fact that occasionally elemental repetitions and prolongations, particularly the former, may occur as benign events. In addition, the concept of markers provides a focus for reconciling the fact that occasionally normal nonfluencies (such as word or phrase repetitions, certain filled or unfilled pauses, revisions, and so forth; see Chapter 2) may accompany a stutter event.

Most likely there is more than one reason why a normal nonfluency may occur in proximity to a stutter. A nonfluency at such loci might represent the stutterer's effort (whether within or outside of awareness) to pass through or circumvent a block that suddenly occurs. Similarly, a normal nonfluency might be an attempt to effect some kind of adjustment to an impending difficulty, for which he happens to have some level of prescience on that particular occasion. At other times both the nonfluency and the stutter may have something of a common origin, reflecting different levels of disturbances in the process of oral language production.

The external appearance of these concurrences, of normal nonfluency and stutter, varies. There are times when the nonfluency obscures a mild stutter event, at least sufficiently that it is difficult to detect. At other times a momentary ability to move forward is not masked but the image of the marker may be faint and transient.[17] Often, of course. both the normal nonfluency and the marker of the stutter event are obvious. It is important to note that when a normal nonfluency occurs at the site of a stutter event the normal nonfluency occurs *prior to* the characteristic clonic or tonic marker.

Table 1.1 presents 10 samples of ways in which a normal nonfluency may occur at the site of a stutter event. In most cases a characteristic marker is evident; however, items 5, 6, and 10 are ones in which the marker is faint or obscured, assuming that there are no attendant accessory features of the motor type.

The foregoing analysis illustrates how normal nonfluencies may appear as one of the "other" (accessory) acts that sometimes occur at the site of a stutter event, yet still retain their own identity separable from the cardinal features of stuttering. Giving special attention to normal nonfluencies in this role seems indicated at this time not only to identify how they fit into the concept of markers of stuttering but also to reduce the considerable, and unnecessary, confusion that has been generated by the claim of an essential similarity between stuttering and normal speech (with its normal nonfluencies).

As emphasized before, the study of stuttering has always proceeded in fundamental, ultimate reference to certain distinctive speech features. The data bases and subject matter to be introduced and discussed throughout this book represent evidence accumulated in specific reference to these distinctive speech characteristics, which are the classic features of stutter-

TABLE 1.1. Example utterances containing various disfluencies associated with a stutter event

	Locus of the stutter event ↓
1.	ai sɔ ɪt ɪn ðə deilɪ p-p-p-peipə̹
2.	ai sɔ ɪt ɪn ðə deilɪ pə pə pəeipə̹
3.	ai sɔ ɪt ɪn ðə deilɪ p-----eipə̹
4.	ai sɔ ɪt ɪn ðə deilɪ pəəəəeipə̹
5.	ai sɔ ɪt ɪn ðə deilɪ deilɪ peipə̹
6.	ai sɔ ɪt ɪn ðə deilɪ ɪn ðə deilɪ peipə̹
7.	ai sɔ ɪt ɪn ðə deilɪ--ɪn ðə deilɪ---əpeipə̹
8.	ai sɔ ɪt ɪn ðə deilɪ--deilɪ-p-eipə̹
9.	ai sɔ ɪt ɪn ðə deilɪ--ə---ə--peipə̹
10.	ai sɔ ɪt ɪn ðə deilɪ--əpeipə̹

ing identified in this chapter—the elemental repetitions and prolongations, the clonic and tonic features.

The material, relative to stuttering, to be presented for review and analysis in Parts I and II of this book represents data obtained from subjects who had been selected for study because their speech evidenced (at least) these essential characteristics. Although these specific speech criteria might not have been stated explicitly in some of the reports to be considered, we can be confident that the speech of those individuals who were identified as stutterers did evidence these classic features. Similarly, the basis for selecting the "experimental" subjects of Part III was that their speech was characterized by these markers of stutter events.

In contrast to the implications of the various "definitions" of stuttering reviewed earlier, and the prevailing orientation they reflect, this book pursues the study of stuttering with the assumption, based on direct observation, that stuttering is a bona fide disorder of speech in which the distinctive events, by which stuttering has always been identified, are anomalies that reflect some kind of error in certain processes involved in speech production. Moreover, "speech" is understood here in the broad sense of the term, namely, as equivalent to "oral language expression" rather than in the narrower sense of motor performance. The objective, then, is to explore and analyze various language dimensions of stuttering in reference to findings that have been reported previously (Part II) and to data that will be presented in this book for the first time (Part III).

A Suspicion of Language Disorder

For a long time there have been good reasons to suspect language involvement in stuttering. Almost 60 years ago, Orton (1927, 1929) noted that certain common observations about stuttering suggested a language base for the disorder instead of the (ever popular) explanation in terms of emotion. Orton said:

> The emotional element has received much attention in stuttering and has long been popular as an explanation of its occurrence. It is, of course, true that stuttering is not only more frequent but more severe in embarrassing situations and that it rarely occurs in singing or in repetition of material learned by rote. This immediately suggests for us that the difference here is related to the plane of the speech effort rather than to the emotional content of the speech. This brings into relief the propositional element of speech and with one exception this seems to be the plane at which stuttering is most severe and most frequent, and it is often of course in embarrassing and strange situations that the propositional effort is most stressed (1929, p. 1047).

Orton's statement is almost certainly the first to carry the suggestion that stuttering might be a disorder of "propositional" speech. Orton, a neurologist, was undoubtedly familiar with the writings of Hughlings Jackson, an eminent neurologist of the late 19th century, who, from his insightful studies of aphasia, described the limited and seemingly bizarre utterances of aphasic patients as "automatic speech" which contrasted dramatically with the "propositional speech" of ordinary normal discourse. Orton's reference to "the propositional element" in stuttering implied that the disorder represents an intrinsic anomally in language function (in contrast to the belief that stuttering is a disruption, occasioned by external circumstances, of an otherwise normal language function).

Research evidence of language involvement in stuttering has appeared intermittently since Orton's time. Certain dimensions of support have turned up in the evidence of delays in articulation and language development that emerged from research having rather broad objectives in the study of stutterers; for example, work by Andrews and Harris (1964), Berry (1938), Darley (1955), and Milisen and Johnson (1936). Suggestive evidence has also appeared in the results of work that has made use of either formal tests or informal measures to assess certain aspects of language abilities: for example, studies by Blood and Seider (1981), Murray and Reed (1977), Perozzi and Kunze (1969), Wall (1980), and Westby (1979). There is, in addition, one line of research that has centered around the study of a set of "language factors" in stuttering. This line of research has yielded a considerable fund of data relative to language aspects of stuttering, and it will serve as the focal reference for the psycholinguistic analysis of stuttering developed in this book.

A review and analysis of the language factors research is presented in Chapters 3 and 4. Before proceeding to that material it is necessary to consider, first, certain basic problems existing within the field of stuttering that persistently obstruct progress toward understanding the essential nature of the disorder. As indicated in this chapter, these problėms involve, most importantly, the very core of the topic, namely the identification of stuttering. They include the closely related matter of the presumptive explanations of the nature of the disorder.

The important negative effect of these problems is well reflected in their influence on the evidence, mentioned before, of language aspects of stuttering. All of the indices of language involvement in stuttering, to be considered in ensuing chapters, have been submerged in one way or another by the orientations that explain stuttering as a psychological (emotional or learned) problem. In particular, much of the valuable information in this area has been compromised by the way in which it has been treated via the position that stuttering is not different from normal speech. The typical treatment of this information has been incomplete and provincial: incomplete because certain obvious, or clearly suggested, leads for further investigation were not pursued; provincial because the analyses made and the interpretations offered were consistently done within the circumscribed focus of a specialized and artificially stabilized view of the nature of stuttering.

These faults in dealing with relevant, valuable information are also reflected in the extent to which pertinent findings regarding normal speech and language function, from sources independent of stuttering research, have typically been ignored or considered only obliquely. Such limitations are exemplified in the contrasts that can be drawn relative to investigation of (normal) nonfluency, which is the principal topic of Chapter 2, and to other aspects of language function that will be considered later, particularly in Chapters 3, 4, and 5.

Footnotes

[1]Earlier writers, properly, accepted a definition that was essentially desciptive. For example, Potter (1882, p. 74): "Definition—an intermittent functional disorder of speech, characterized by irregularly spasmodic action of the muscles concerned in articulation, more rarely of the muscles of phonation and respiration." Similarly, from Hunt (1870/1967, p. 13): "Stuttering . . . is a viscious utterance, manifested by *frequent repetitions* of initial or *elementary* sounds, and always more or less *attended with muscular contortions.*"

At the same time, the most careful and thorough definition of this kind is the one written by West (West, Kennedy, & Carr, 1937, p. 53) that appeared in the brief era of the 20th century just before psychological explanations of stuttering inundated the field. West's statement has received little recognition.

[2]See also Fletcher (1928).

[3]See also Sheehan (1958, 1975).

[4]See also Brutten (1975).

[5]The Johnson position is presented in many sources authored by him and associates; for example, Johnson (1942; 1961b), Johnson and Knott (1955), Johnson and Associates (1959).

[6]Quoted by Beveridge (1957, p. 15).

[7]May 8 and 9, 1981.

[8]Italics mine. Johnson made the same claim in many other places (e.g., Johnson, 1942, p. 255; 1944b, p. 333; 1946, p. 445; 1955, p. 67; 1963, p. 241).

[9]The three other sources consulted were: *Funk and Wagnall's Standard Dictionary of the English Language,* 1963; *Random House Dictionary of the English Language,* 1973; and *Webster's Third New International Dictionary of the English Language,* 1981.

[10]In his initial works in this line Johnson (1961a; Johnson and Associates, 1959) used the term "nonfluency."

[11]This issue of "overlap" has been extended out of all proportion to the miniscule findings on which it is based. It is more a rhetorical device than a bona fide issue. The reader should consider that there are many valid distinctions that we make routinely in which one can find much more overlap than one finds between stuttered and normal speech. For instance: cars versus trucks, boys versus girls, house cats versus panthers, horses versus cows, and so forth.

[12] It is pertinent to recall West's remark that "everyone but the expert knows what stuttering is . . . " (West, Ansberry, & Carr, 1957, p. 15).

[13]See Wingate (1976, chap. 4) for elaboration of these lines of evidence.

[14]Once again, Wendell Johnson was responsible for the change. During the 6 years he was editor of the *Journal of Speech and Hearing Disorders* (1943–1948) he made it

editorial policy to actively discourage use of the word "spasm." See Johnson and Knott, 1955 (footnote, p. 28).

[15]It is significant that the Sheehan article, actually prepared in 1946, was just as pertinent when eventually published in 1974.

[16]We shall find later that there is reason to question whether the stutterer really does "know precisely what word he wants to say."

[17]It seems very likely that circumstances such as this underlie "borderline" instances that present difficulties for discrimination, and thereby contribute to whatever "unreliability" judgments of stuttering may have.

2
The Study of Nonfluency

As discussed in Chapter 1, stuttering is manifested as a unique disturbance in the forward movement, or continuity, of speech—a disturbance in fluency.

Fluency—The Essential Reference

For purposes of the analysis to be undertaken in this chapter, I will use *fluency* in its behavioral or superficial sense, the principle sense in which it is generally understood. Studies of various kinds of nonfluency have proceeded in reference to the descriptive, or surface, meaning of fluency, which happens to be the sense in which the term is standardly employed in both lay and professional usage. In this common usage of fluency the reference is to final output, the continuity perceived in speech utterance; essentially, the sequential concatentaion of words.

Actually, fluency implies complex psycholinguistic functions that, as Leeson (1979) pointed out, receive little attention in the linguistics literature, even from within the professional discipline most likely to be concerned with fluency, namely, foreign language teaching. Although this is not the appropriate juncture to consider the intricacies of fluency in this sense, it is necessary to introduce here certain general matters regarding fluency that are basic to an appreciation of the use of the term and, in some measure thereby, its broader significance.

First, it is pertinent to note that fluency is used primarily and predominantly, to refer to speech. Many other words, such as "flowing," "fluid," "liquid," etc. are used to describe other events that move, or appear to move, continuously. However, fluency and fluent are reserved, almost exclusively, to describe continuity of speech. Although these terms are used occasionally to characterize certain other functions (e.g., *associative fluency* or *ideational fluency*), such use is always in allegory of the basic reference to speech. The *Oxford English Dictionary*, representative of other similar sources, gives the meaning of "fluency" as: "A smooth and easy flow; readiness, smoothness, especially with regard to speech; readiness of utterance, flow of words" (Vol. IV, p. 357).

Second, fluency is simultaneously concrete and abstract. It is concrete in respect to the events (words in sequence) implied in its standard usage. It is abstract in the sense that, in spite of its focal reference to the audible speech sequence, other aspects of the speaking performance (such as, the speaking circumstances; the content of the discourse; etc.) are considered implicitly. Similarly, fluency is simultaneously objective and subjective. It is objective relative to the events that are clearly in focus. At the same time it is subjective because it always involves a judgment based on unspecified, and usually unverbalized, criteria.

Third, fluency has a broad range of reference. In general usage it refers to the ordinary speech of almost everyone, in spite of the fact that we may sometimes be aware, at some level, of the individual differences in fluency that exist among ordinary speakers of the language. In this general sense, fluency describes the speech one is accustomed to hearing from most people in almost all circumstances. Such a broad-spectrum meaning is exemplified in the standard use of fluent to describe performance in a second language. A person is considered to be fluent in a language if he speaks it in a manner comparable to the generalized, abstracted, "average" native speaker of that language. Here the broad limits are applied in two directions simultaneously—to the actual speaker in question and to the idealized, or normalized, native speaker.

Although fluency has a broad reference it also has identifiable limits. These limits are recognized in everyday observation and sometimes are denoted through descriptive phrases, such as "spoke haltingly" or "was very fluent." But, just as fluency is specific to speech, there are also words that are specific to the identification of the upper and lower limits of fluency. The upper limit of the standard sense of fluency is reflected in the word articulate (the adjectival form) which, in addition to its denotative meaning, carries a value of approbation, if not admiration. Above this level, however, one finds that the speech-specific descriptive terms have a less favorable connotation. For instance, *voluble* refers to speech that is "characterized by a great flow of fluency."* It carries a connotation of excess, and the suggestion of at least potential annoyance. If speech is produced "in a manner too smooth and easy to be convincing"* it is described as *glib*, a word that typically carries a negative implication, usually the sense of insincerity or deception. Although the upper limits of fluency are not clearly defined it seems evident that there are bases for, and vehicles for expressing, judgments of high levels of fluency and, moreover, distinctions between those high levels that are acceptable and those that are excessive.

The lower limits of fluency are also identifiable, even though they, too, are not well defined. Leeson (1979), noted, in discussing the fluency level typical of an individual speaker, "in operational terms, it is impossible to talk about any one single level of fluency below which the speaker can be adjudged to be non-fluent (in a language)" (p. 2). Nonetheless, there are bases for identifying, and means of describing, speech that falls below the lower periphery of the broad limits of ordinary fluency. One can, of course, characterize such speech by descriptive phrases, such as "spoke haltingly" and the like. But, importantly, there are also formal speech-specific terms that are used regularly to refer to speech lacking ordinary fluency. To *hem and haw* means "to pause and hesitate in speaking."* Significantly, these words are essentially denotative or descriptive; their only (minimal) negative connotation might be to suggest, in some cases, possible evasiveness, for instance to imply that the speaker was attempting "to avoid saying something definite."*

It is of considerable interest that the words *hem* and *haw* are onomatopoeic. *Hem* is "a conventionalized expression of the sound made in clearing the throat to attract attention or show doubt."* The word *haw*, meaning specifically "to grope for words, to falter"* is a conventionalized representation of the most common filled pause, the so-called neutral vowel, usually written as "ah" or "uh."

At this point it becomes especially pertinent to recall that the word *stutter* is also onomatopoeic. The language thus has three different conventional referents that identify three separate kinds of events constituting departures from ordinary fluency, all three being departures that fall *below* the range of ordinary fluency. It is significant that all three words derive from the same primordial source of word origin, *onomatopoeia*, in which the character of the referent is reflected concretely in the structure of the word itself. It is equally significant that there are three different words, with three different referents, within this seemingly ill-defined area. This fact constitutes persuasive evidence that events occurring in the course of ordinary speech, events that are the basis for judgments of departures from fluency, are not only readily identifiable but also differentially discriminable.

It seems clear that judgment of departures from fluency is based on events that disturb the impression of continuity in oral expression. As noted previously, fluency, even though it focuses principally on continuity of word sequences, has rather broad limits of reference. As ordinarily used, the term is most appropriately considered to mean "the *apparent* flow of connected speech." The key word here is "*apparent*" for, as will be documented later in this chapter, through evidence of the nonfluent character of ordinary speech, the impression of continuity underlying our common use of the word fluency is largely illusion.

Eventual understanding of the nature of stuttering will be tied closely to an understanding of the nature of fluency, in the full sense of the term, and to the relationship of fluency to processes of speech production. One source of information that can contribute materially to understanding fluency is to be found in the findings of research addressed to "nonfluency," both normal and abnormal.

Investigation of Nonfluency: Origins and Directions

Study of nonfluency has proceeded along two separate lines: one line of investigation addressed to normal speech, the other based in a concern with stuttering. Some information regarding fluency irregularities in normal speech is to be found in the stuttering literature, largely from those studies whose expressed focus was to compare stuttered and normal speech. However, the literature based in stuttering has remained insulated from the fairly extensive research on nonfluency in normal speech that has developed within the field of psycholinguistics, where interest has centered on fluency interruptions of normal speech alone. Research in these two lines of investigation differ in several important ways: orientation and interest, investigative approach, vocabulary, course of development, findings, and interpretation and use of the data. The objective of this chapter is to identify and discuss comparatively certain basic contributions of these two lines of research and their significance for understanding stuttering relative to normal fluency.

Formally derived information bearing on nonfluency first appeared in professional literature sources in the early 1930s as a by-product of research addressed to language development in children. Before then, the study of language growth had been largely biographical and had centered almost exclusively on vocabulary acquisition. In contrast, investigations reported in the 1930s (Adams, 1932; Day, 1932; Fisher, 1932, 1934; Lewis, 1934; McCarthy, 1930) obtained data from rather large numbers of children, pursued a scope of inquiry much broader than assessment of vocabulary and, among other advances, were basically quantitative. The reports of these investigations contained some data on nonfluency but these data were not very extensive nor routinely expressed quantitatively. However, they served as a source of reference and a background for one line of nonfluency research that soon followed.

The earliest developing line of research addressed specifically to nonfluencies emerged as a facet of a primary interest in stuttering. Most of this early work was done at the University of Iowa and represented the views of Wendell Johnson. The bulk of this work was done under his direction, and much of the subsequent investigation in this line has continued to reflect his influence. Because of the prevailing preoccupation with stuttering, this line of research has been predominantly comparative in nature, that is, comparing speech samples of stutterers versus nonstutterers. Although some work in this line has investigated disfluencies of normal speakers only (e.g., Chaney, 1969; Kools & Berryman, 1971; Silverman & Williams, 1967a; Yairi & Jennings, 1974), the orientation to stuttering has remained clear in this research as well.

A straightforward research interest in nonfluencies of normal speech was to develop some 15 years later than the disfluency interest based in stuttering; it began at about the same time that the stuttering-based (comparative) research had become more formalized and had begun to appear in publication. The nonfluencies identified in this line of research came to be called "hesitation phenomena."

Research interest in hesitation phenomena originated in curiosity about what certain nonfluencies might reveal about the psychology of the individual. The early work in this line (and in a persisting branch of this line) was pursued with the objective of learning something about the psychological status of individuals, proceeding from a clinical hunch that irregularities in the continuity of speech are occasioned largely by affective factors. However, subsequent work in this line soon began to reflect a major shift of interest toward what hesitation phenomena might reveal about language processes and cognitive aspects of language.

As might be expected, these two separate lines of investigation, one based in stuttering, the other addressed only to normal speech, have yielded some data that are comparable, but in certain important respects the findings differ, often substantially.

Nonfluency Findings from the Stuttering-Based Research

As noted earlier, the background and initial reference source for this line of analysis was supplied in the nonfluency data that had emerged in the course of some quantitative studies of language development done in the early decades of this century.

During the middle 1930s articles on stuttering by Wendell Johnson began to reflect the extent to which his thinking had become influenced by General Semantics, the font from which his "evaluational theory" of stuttering emanated. One of the major tenets of the evaluational position is that *all* children evidence irregularities in fluency, to which is added the claim that the speech of children who stutter (by Johnson's claim, are only "said to be" stuttering) is, at least originally, no different from the speech of children who are considered to be speaking normally. The nonfluency data contained within the reports of early studies of language development apparently suggested to Johnson[1] what he thought constituted support for this claim, and he soon sought further support for it in research that paid special attention to irregularities in fluency. Some of the early work in this line analyzed the speech of evidently normal children

(Branscom, 1942; Hughes, 1943; Oxtoby, 1943)[2] or predominantly normal children (Davis, 1939, 1940), but these studies were undertaken with a clear interest in stuttering and from the beginning were intermingled with studies that compared the speech of stutterers and nonstutterers (Egland, 1938; Johnson, 1942; Mann, 1937).[3]

As suggested earlier, the actual descriptors that have come to be used in the two separate lines of fluency investigation bear a certain significance in and of themselves, for they identify the kinds of fluency irregularities, present in the speech samples studied, that were evident to the investigators. As we shall see, certain important differences in descriptors emerge in the two different lines of research.

The nonfluency descriptors used in early studies varied considerably from one study to another, and although a number of the descriptors recurred in much of the literature, patterns of difference were evident from the beginning. Interestingly and significantly, the investigations of normally speaking children (Adams, 1932; Fisher, 1932, 1934; McCarthy, 1930) reported only "repetitions," whereas descriptors that appeared in the studies comparing stuttering to normally speaking children (Egland, 1938; Johnson, 1942; Mann, 1937) included three classes of repetition (sound and syllable, word, and phrase) and, in addition, "prolongations" and "breaks." In the latter studies, too, the most commonly recurring descriptors were "repetitions" and/or the three separate subclasses of repetition. A category of "hesitations" does not appear in any of this literature. The designation, "pause," appears only in Mann's (1937) study wherein pauses were described as instances "... in which no sound was uttered and no apparent effort was made to say a word ...." Unlike the other studies, which investigated spontaneous speech, Mann's data were obtained from the reading of a list of words and a passage containing the same words; this qualifies additionally the nature of the "pauses" considered in the Mann study.

The first publication in this area authored by Johnson himself had a much broader scope of inquiry than the study of nonfluencies or their variation (Johnson, 1942). That study was concerned with a number of developmental factors that might help to differentiate stuttering children from normally speaking youngsters. Speech and language development, of course, were among the variables considered. All of the information gathered in that study was obtained indirectly, primarily from parents; therefore, comparison of the fluency irregularities of the two groups was not extensive or well elaborated. However, most of the normally speaking children were reported to evidence "nonfluency" ("repetitions and hesitations")[4] under some conditions similar to those reported to be associated with stuttering in the case of the stuttering children.

In *The Onset of Stuttering*, Johnson's major work comparing child stutterers and normally speaking children (Johnson and Associates, 1959), he reported an extensive fund of information accumulated for 150 stuttering youngsters and a matched group of 150 normally speaking children. Again, much of this information dealt with developmental and medical history variables and, again, a good deal of the information was obtained from indirect sources, primarily parents. However, in this study recorded speech samples were obtained, making possible a direct comparison of speech characteristics of the two groups.

It was in *The Onset of Stuttering* that Johnson first presented the list of (at that time) "nonfluencies" that has been used regularly in subsequent studies of stuttering. However, this list of eight categories was actually developed during "studies of speech fluency of college-age male and female stutterers and nonstutterers" (Johnson and Associates, 1959, p. 201), a study completed some time before publication of the *The Onset of Stuttering*. This research on college-age groups, his other major comparative work, was published 2 years later (Johnson, 1961a) and became the primary reference source for many subsequent publications by investigators in the field of stuttering, most of which have compared the speech irregularities of stutterers and normal speakers, although some have extended such study to the speech of normal speakers only.

The eight descriptor categories of the Johnson list are:

1. Interjections of sounds, syllables, words, or phrases. (Includes "extraneous sounds . . . and words," such as "uh" and "well".)
2. Part-word repetitions. (Repetitions of sounds and syllables.)
3. Word repetitions. (Repetition of whole words, including words of one syllable.)
4. Phrase repetitions.
5. Revisions. (Change in content or grammatical structure of a phrase; change in pronunciation of a word.)
6. Incomplete phrases. (Thought or content not completed.)
7. Broken words. (Words not completely pronounced; words in which smooth flow is interrupted; words not associated with any other category.)
8. Prolonged sounds. ("Sounds judged to be unduly prolonged.")

Johnson described these categories of disfluency as

> the features of speech identified in the evaluation of the samples [which] were . . . thought to represent the various aspects of speech nonfluency, *with the exception of pause time.*[5] This measure was not used because of the practical difficulty of deciding whether or not given pauses were part of meaningful or expressive speech (Johnson and Associates, 1959, p. 201).

It is worth noting that Johnson implicitly identified pausing as a kind of nonfluency, and further, that he considered pauses to contain two types: those that are "part of meaningful or expressive speech" and those that are not. At the same time, he evidently did not consider pausing of sufficient value in the study of nonfluency to merit attempting to resolve "the practical difficulty" to which he referred. The exclusion of pause was a major omission. Further, the "practical difficulty" was not a bona fide problem. The research on normally fluent speech (e.g., Goldman-Eisler, 1968; Mahl, 1981) has shown that a fruitful study of pause is not contingent on a resolution of this "difficulty." One must also question Johnson's claim that, except for a category of pause, his list of nonfluencies is complete. Material to be presented later in this chapter shows that, in addition to pause, there are other kinds of nonfluency also worth noting.

Some years after publication of this list, Williams, Silverman, and Kools (1968) noted that Johnson had completed an unpublished revision of the list shortly before his death in 1965. The revision involves only two categories: "broken words" and "prolongations." For these two categories Johnson substituted the catagories of "disrhythmic phonation" and "tension" (sometimes referred to as "tense pause"). It is of considerable interest that only these two categories of disfluency evidently required some adjustment; a commentary, it would seem, on the uniqueness of these descriptors. The matter of their uniqueness will be addressed further in subsequent pages.

As noted earlier, this list of descriptors has been the reference for, if not actually used in, a considerable amount of research appearing since the late 1950s. Recent publications by Adams (1982), Bloodstein (1981), Daughtry (1982), Hegde (1982), and Prins and Beaudet (1980) exemplify its continuing usage. Not only has it been the reference in studies of the speech performance of stutterers, and (most often) in studies comparing the speech of normal speakers and stutterers, it has also been the standard used in certain studies of normal speakers only that were conducted by investigators interested primarily in stuttering (e.g., Kools & Berryman, 1971; Silverman, 1973; Silverman, 1970; Silverman & Williams, 1967a; Yairi & Jennings, 1974).

It is important to recognize that this set of descriptors was developed in reference to stuttering, and that it is not only incomplete but biased as well.[6] These faults, particularly the latter one, make the Johnson list unsuitable for at least general use in the study of nonfluency; the extent to which it is unsuitable should become evident later in this chapter, in discussion of the "hesitation phenomena" research on nonfluency in normal speech. For the present, it is pertinent to point out that the correct methodology for developing and implementing a behavioral measurement device calls for the study of samples that can be considered representative of the normal population. In particular, considerable care should be taken to ensure that the reference samples represent the normal population in respect to special features, if any, that are focal to the area of investigation. In contrast, the Johnson list is based on the study of population samples in which half of all the individuals studied are known to represent abnormality, and specifically on the focal dimensions of study.

Data generated from such methodology quickly creates problems. Throughout the line of investigation comparing "disfluencies" (originally "nonfluencies") of stutterers and normal speakers one finds the interpretation of an essential similarity in the disfluencies evidenced by the two groups (the guiding premise of this line of study, as described in Chapter 1.) This interpretation has been buttressed by minimizing the demonstrable differences in disfluency types between stutterers and normal speakers and, instead, emphasizing the "overlap" between them. Inherent in such analyses, and attendant interpretations, is the assumption that stutters and other irregularities of fluency are simply variants of the same phenomenon; that is, that they are all varying degress or expressions of "disfluency." However, this assumption is rarely stated as an assumption; in fact, it is often well obscured by appearing as the conclusion of a study.

Silverman and Williams (1967b) give a representative summary statement of this position, and note some of the effect it has had. They refer to "a series of investigations which demonstrated that stutterings could not be reliably differentiated from other types of disfluencies in speech" (p. 1085). Such contention ignores the very substantial contradicting evidence from many research sources, representing different orientations (e.g., Lanyon & Duprez, 1970; MacDonald & Martin, 1973; Runyan & Adams, 1979; Sheehan, 1974; Williams, Wark, & Minifie, 1963; Wingate, 1977a). Moreover, it overlooks the fact that high levels of inter- and intra-judge agreement have been required, and found, as a routine part of the methodology in many studies of stuttering having various foci of interest. It also ignores the fact that in the study that yielded the Johnson list of disfluencies (Johnson, 1961a), inter- and intra-judge reliabilities for the various disfluency categories were reported to range between .91 and 1.00.

Silverman and Williams go on to say that "as a result, some of the more recent investigations of lawfulness in stuttering have been based upon what have been termed disfluencies (Johnson, 1961a) rather than upon judgments of the occurrence of stutterings" (p. 1085). Note that although the investigations mentioned in the quotation are investigations of *stuttering*, "disfluencies" is offered as the preferred term to use in such investigations. At the same time, it is significant that Silverman and Williams do acknowledge in a footnote that "disfluencies include all types of disruptions in the rhythm of speech whereas judgments of stuttering do not necessarily" (p. 1085). This statement acknowledges that there is a distinction to be made between what is likely to be judged as stuttering and what is not; and also that "disfluencies" and "stutterings" are not equivalent or interchangeable terms. Nonetheless, as Silverman and Williams stated, many studies have used "disfluency" or "disfluent speech" as an all-encompassing term in which stutters are evidently mixed in with other disfluency types in the speech samples being analyzed (e.g., Horovitz, Johnson, Pearlman, Schaffer, & Hedin, 1978; F.H. Silverman, 1974; Williams et al., 1968). Such use of terms is not conducive to the clarity of reference standardly valued in scientific circles. I have discussed elsewhere (Wingate (1984a) the dimensions of this problem as found in the literature on stuttering.

Lay sources echo the confusion created by this improper use of "disfluency." An article on stuttering in *Changing Times* ("Spotting and Stopping Stuttering," 1983) states that "the technical term for it is disfluency . . . " (p. 64). The muddle surrounding such unclear usage is evident at the practical level as well. Clinicians in many places in the United States (at least) are encouraged to think of working with "the disfluent child" (e.g., Cooper, 1977; Zwitman, 1978). Now, it is widely accepted that all children evidence disfluencies, a fairly safe claim when using a word that has such a broad reference. But clinicians do not give professional attention to the disfluencies of all children. They also do not work with all children who evidence disfluencies. "The disfluent child" who is referred to, and accepted for treatment by, the speech clinician is one whose speech is characterized by the kinds of disfluencies traditionally called "stuttering."

The foregoing problems reflect some of the serious limitations inherent in, and associated with, the descriptors of disfluency emanating from the line of research based in a concern with stuttering.

Some years ago Sanford (1942), discussing evidence then current regarding the relation of speech and personality, commented briefly on the likely contribution from the literature on speech disorders. He said:

> Just as insanity attracts more attention than sanity, disorders of speech have been studied more intensively than normal linguistic phenomena. While it is impractical here even to scan the literature dealing with disorders of speech, it is worthwhile to point out that researchers are almost unaminous in insisting that linguistic disorders, especially stuttering, are closely related with broad aspects of personal adjustment. There is no unanimity, however, as to what the relation is.

He went on to say that

> the whole literature pertaining to this disorder [stuttering] is contradictory and difficult. One is given to wonder if some of the verve that has gone into the investigation of stuttering might not have been better spent upon the less dramatic, but potentially significant, "roughnesses" that occur in normal speech (pp. 838–839).

His comment is as relevant today as it was when written. The following section is addressed to pertinent research of such "roughnesses" in speech, which are identified in the literature on normal nonfluency as *hesitation phenomena.*

Nonfluency in Normal Speech

The hesitation phenomena research, concerned solely with the description and analysis of nonfluency in normal speakers, developed over approximately the same period of time as the comparative research that emanated from a focus on stuttering. Although the findings of the early stuttering-based studies appeared in a compilation prepared by Johnson and Leutenegger in 1955, this line of disfluency analysis did not appear in print as an area of research until the 1959 and 1961 publications by Johnson. A sizable body of literature has accumulated in both areas since that time, but there is scarce indication that writers in either area have taken notice of the literature in the other. In the 15-year period from 1965 to 1980 the *Journal of Speech and Hearing Research* published 25 articles that focused on the topic of disfluencies. The only reference to the normal nonfluency research in any of these articles appeared in Silverman and Williams (1967a) and consisted simply of the notation that two (hesitation phenomena) sources had reported finding that "instances of disfluency tend to be associated with lexical rather than function words" (p. 790).

A comparable situation exists in the nonresearch literature of stuttering, where reference to the hesitation phenomena research is rare and typically cursory. Van Riper (1971, p. 186) covers the area in two sentences; Bloodstein (1981, p. 312) simply cites several references in a footnote—after indicating in the text that the findings from this research are essentially the same as that found in stuttering research. Dalton and Hardcastle (1977, chap. 3) give more consideration to work in this line, but their discussion is limited to (silent) pause.[7]

The psycholinguistic research on normal nonfluency contains no reference to the disfluency research based in stuttering.

The lack of cross reference between the stuttering-based and the normal nonfluency lines of research is more detrimental to an understanding of stuttering than vice versa. As indicated previously, broadly based and objective investigation of normal speech should be the basic reference for the study of nonfluency of all kinds.[8]

In contrast to the stuttering-based studies, the hesitation phenomena research has been undertaken independently of an established orientation having a well-developed set of assumptions. Moreover, it has proceeded from a broad base, with different investigators making independent approaches to the recording and analysis of data, rather than all of the research reflecting essentially the same orientation and focus. Important among other advantages, it has yielded a comprehensive set of nonfluency categories appropriate for describing normal speech. As might be expected, the expanding literature in the hesitation phenomena line of research has revealed a considerably different picture of fluency and nonfluency than that typically presented in publications emanating from an orientation to stuttering.

The beginnings of the normal nonfluency research are marked by the early work of two investigators, Goldman-Eisler (1952, 1954a, 1955, 1956) and Mahl (1956a, 1956b, 1956c, 1958, 1959a, 1959b, 1960), who pursued their investigations independently, and evidently unaware, of the other. This early work was psychological in orientation; the interest in nonfluencies was based on a hypothesis that these aspects of speech might have value in personality assessment. In fact, some of the normal speech protocols were obtained from interviews with persons being seen for psychological counseling. The fact that some of the data base in these early studies was obtained from persons being seen in counseling interviews does not in any way qualify the relevance of these data. Whatever the nature of the problems these individuals may have had, they were not speech problems. Briefly stated, the nonfluencies noted were not ones that attracted attention; to the contrary, they were noticed only after being discovered in the course of research designed for other purposes. This "low profile" is a significant characteristic of normal nonfluencies; they are unobtrusive.

From the clinical orientation in which these analyses were approached nonfluencies were conceived originally to be *disturbances* in speech, as "extralinguistic events" that disrupted the normal flow of speech. The "disruptions" were typically conceived to have a motivational origin, that is, to reflect affective factors that interfered with the ongoing process of speech generation and expression.

Mahl was interested in using speech disturbances as a measure of anxiety in patients, and he believed that different kinds of disruptors might signal different psychological influences. Similar suggestions appeared in the early work of Goldman-Eisler although originally her essential interest was to study the technique of interviewing in order to improve interviewer skills. However, the direction of her interest soon took a different turn; her work became the principal source of a newly developing interest in normal nonfluencies for their potential contribution to understanding speech and language processes.

By the late 1950s research on disfluencies in normal speech was being pursued for its contribution to linguistics, psycholinguistics, and cognitive theory. A frequently cited contribution from this period is a paper by Maclay and Osgood (1959), which pointed to the linguistic and psycholinguistic nature of a variety of fluency irregularities. However, the major influence in this development was the program of research that Goldman-Eisler extended from her work in interview analysis. This work (Goldman-Eisler, 1954b, 1957, 1958a, 1958b, 1958c, 1961a, 1961b, 1964), and the work of others which followed, have provided evidence that many kinds of fluency irregularities, especially certain ones, are not appropriately considered as intrusions or disturbances in speech, as originally thought. Instead, this line of research has shown that many forms of interruption in the flow of speech are intrinsic to the speech production process.

The studies of nonfluency in normal speech have characteristically used the generic term *hesitation phenomena* as a general referent for the fluency irregularities studied. There have been some differences in the range of hesitation phenomena under scrutiny in the various studies, with some studies having a different focus or a more limited scope than others. Also, all studies have not used the same labels for the various kinds of hesitation phenomena. It is significant, however, that although labels sometimes differ among the various studies, the descriptors used are comparable from one study to another. The similarity of descriptor categories across studies is evident even among some of the later studies that have not built directly on preceding work in the hesitation phenomena line of research. Some of the descriptors used in these "independent" studies have been developed from other sources, largely in the linguistics literature, that have made some sort of reference to one or another kind of fluency irregularity during the course of studying other aspects of normal speech.

Table 2.1 presents a list of descriptor categories utilized in five publications that can be considered to represent basic references for work in this area. These publications are considered representative because they contain the earliest classifications, on which most subsequent work has been based, and also include sources having a broad range of interest. For instance, the works of Mahl and Goldman-Eisler, and also the analysis presented by Maclay and Osgood, are early sources. The Goldman-Eisler (1968) reference is to a book that summarizes her work in this area to that date, including her initial studies. The work of Blankenship and Kay (1964) had a somewhat different orientation and is also of particular interest because it, uniquely, is the only work in this line that mentions some sources in the stuttering literature.[9] The work of Levin and Silverman (1965) was based on a variety of sources in the linguistics literature that were not directly related to nonfluency interests. Moreover, their investigation was addressed to hesitation phenomena in the speech of children.

Table 2.1 is arranged so as to identify the similarity in descriptor categories across the five publications. Although category names differ almost as often as they are identical, the referents of the descriptors in any one category are clearly the same.

There are several important points to be drawn from the information presented in Table 2.1. The first point has already been identified, namely, the essential similarities in categories from one study to another, regardless of the labels used to denote the categories, and in spite of the fact that all lists do not contain all categories found in all other lists.

A second point concerns category five. As indicated in the footnote, Mahl's transcription example for this category indicated that the reference is to *sound and syllable repetition* for which he used the simpler designation "stutter." Similarly, Blankenship and Kay indicate that their use of the word "stutter" refers to "sound and syllable repetition *as a type of nonfluency in 'normal' speech*" (p. 361).[10] The point here is that "stutter" is used in both publications to refer to a unique kind of repetition—"elemental" repetitions. Further, in both instances the types of repetitions called stutter were considered to be benign. The use of stutter is descriptive, as it should be; it simply refers to a discriminable type of fluency irregularity for which this word is a well known and appropriate term. The term is appropriate on several dimensions, which include: the structure of the word, its semantic derivation, and its metaphorical use (see Chapter 1, pp. 9). The fact that the term is used most often in reference to events that are not benign is another matter.

It is germane to note that Blankenship and Kay referred to "two possible types of hesitation," which they did not record. One of these types was "unfilled pauses," which they chose not to deal with; the other kind was "nonphonemic lengthening of phonemes," which they did not include because there was no recognizable instance of such hesitation in their data. Blankenship and Kay considered these types of hesitation phenomena as "delaying devices," and also that they are types of nonfluency "very closely related to individual speech style" (op cit, p. 361). Some writers in the field of stuttering might wish to claim that nonphonemic lengthening of phonemes could be equivalent to "prolongations." Note, however, that Blankenship and Kay were the only authors who registered an awareness of the stuttering literature and therefore could be expected to know the term prolongations. Instead, these authors made some effort (a 10-syllable phrase) to describe this type of (normal) nonfluency appropriately. Although they gave no examples of nonphonemic lengthening of phonemes, this description, plus their identification of this nonfluency type as a kind of "delaying device," would suggest examples such as "We::l now" and "Ye::s but . . . ," and the like, with which we are all familiar as maneuvers occasionally made by many speakers.

Comparison and Integration of the Two Lines of Research

The nonfluency categories of the five studies presented in Table 2.1 can be collapsed readily into one composite list of hesitation phenomena that appropriately represents the types of nonfluency revealed in the research on normal speech. Mahl's categories will be used as a base for the collapsed

TABLE 2.1. Descriptors for various categories of "hesitation phenomena" appearing in five example sources reporting study of such phenomena in normal speech*

	Mahl (1956a)	Maclay & Osgood (1959)	Goldman-Eisler (1968)	Blankenship & Kay (1964)	Levin & Silverman (1965)
A. Audible					
	"Ah"	Filled pauses		Nonlexical intrusive sounds	Vocal segregates
	Sentence correction	Retraced false start	(Reconsideration)[a]	Sentence correction	Sentence correction
	Sentence incompletion	Nonretraced false start	(False starts)[a]	Sentence incompletion	Sentence incompletion
	Repetition (of one or more words)	Repeats		Repeat (of one or more lexical items)	Repetitions of a word or phrase
	Stutter[b]	(Repeats)[c]		Stutter[d]	(Repetition of less than a word)[c]
	Intruding incoherent sound				
	Tongue slips				Slips of the tongue
				Word change	
			(Parenthetical references)[a]		Parenthetical remarks
				(Nonphonemic lengthening of phonemes)[a]	Drawls

TABLE 2.1. (*Continued*)

	Mahl (1956a)	Maclay & Osgood (1959)	Goldman-Eisler (1968)	Blankenship & Kay (1964)	Levin & Silverman (1965)
B. Silent					
	Omission (of words or parts of words)[e]			Omission of part of a word	Omission of words or parts of words
	Silent pauses	Unfilled pauses	Hesitation/pause 1. (Grammatical) 2. Nongrammatical	(Unfilled pauses)[a]	Zero segregates

*Goldman-Eisler explored primarily nongrammatical silent pauses. Certain other authors (Boomer, 1965) have focused on filled and unfilled pauses, or (Boomer & Dittman, 1962) on two kinds of silent pauses: "juncture" pauses and "hesitation" pauses. The latter correspond to Goldman-Eisler's "grammatical" and "nongrammatical" categories. Grammatical or juncture pauses are not treated as actual hesitation phenomena.

[a]Mentioned as a category but not studied.

[b]Transcription example indicates reference is to sound and syllable repetition.

[c]Not treated by these authors as a separate category; included as part of category 4.

[d]Specifies "sound and syllable repetition as a type of nonfluency in 'normal' speech."

[e]Mahl stated that "most omissions are of final syllables of words."

combination of these nonfluencies because his list was the first in this line of research and is also as comprehensive as any other list.

Table 2.2 presents a comparison of the combined "Hesitation Phenomena" categories with the categories of the Johnson list, denoted here as "Disfluencies" because this term has been favored by persons in the stuttering line of research.

Two of the categories, three and five, have a direct equivalence in the two lists. Several other categories seem comparable, though there is a superficial difference across lists because the category in one list is more specific than the other. The "Hesitation Phenomena" list includes two kinds of *revision* and three kinds of *interjection*, each of which is a single category in the "Disfluency" list. The latter list specifies *whole-word repetition* and *phrase repetition* separately, whereas the normal speech list combines them into one category. Until research indicates that such categories can be combined without loss it seems prudent to keep them separate. For instance, although *word change* and *sentence correction* are appropriately identified as revisions, the two events might be found to reflect different processes (or errors therein). Similarly, there is conceivably some substantive or relevant difference between the repetition of a word and the repetition of a phrase.[11] One should keep in mind that findings from the normal

TABLE 2.2. Comparison of descriptors for categories of "hesitation phenomena" emerging from studies of normal speech and of "disfluencies" developed in studies comparing stuttering with normal speech

"Hesitation phenomena" (normal speech)	"Disfluencies" (stuttering versus normal speech)	
A. Audible:		
"Ah"	Interjections	
Sentence correction	Revisions	
Sentence incompletion	Incomplete phrases	
Repetition (of one or more words)	Phrase repetitions	
	Word repetitions	
Stutter	Part-word repetitions	
Intruding incoherent sound	Interjections	
Tongue slip	—	
Word change	Revisions	
Parenthetical references	Interjections	
Drawls	—	
—	Broken words	Tension
—	Prolonged sounds	Dysrhythmic phonation
B. Silent:		
Omission (of words or parts of words)	—	
Silent pauses	—	

nonfluency research indicate that the two kinds of pause (filled and unfilled) may serve different functions (Goldman-Eisler, 1961a; Maclay & Osgood, 1959). Similarly, four different functions of interjections can be identified (Wingate, 1976, p. 46). The latter category, in particular, deserves special mention. There is no doubt that the category of interjections in the "Disfluency" list is a confounding gloss. The three equivalent categories in the "Hesitation Phenomena" list clearly represent different kinds of nonfluency—and other pertinent refinements are appropriate, as described in Wingate (1976). Moreover, the interjections category obscures two other differences that are of substantial proportions. First, it makes no provision for the potentially important dimension of length; the number of units in an interjection. Second, it ignores another dimension, iteration, essentially of "uh" (or equivalent), whose importance has already become evident. Even in the data from which the "Disfluency" list originated (Johnson, 1961a), the difference between single and repetitive occurrences of "uh" emerged as a dimension on which stuttered and nonstuttered speech samples could be separated. Johnson found only 12 iterative interjections in the speech samples from the 100 normal speakers; the stutterers had 66.

Although the two lists contain certain evidently comparable items, there are also real differences between them. In a very basic sense the categories developed from these two different lines of research reflect differences in the subject matter being analyzed. The normal speech list contains four categories that do not appear in the Johnson list: tongue slip, drawls, omissions, and silent pauses. The latter category was intentionally omitted by Johnson; instances of the other three categories evidently were either not observed in Johnson's work or were disregarded. The categories of tongue slip, omissions, and silent pauses seem self-explanatory. However, "drawls" merits special comment.

Again, some writers in the field of stuttering might contend that drawls could be comparable to prolongations. However, drawl seems more equivalent to nonphonemic lengthening of phonemes, discussed earlier. Although it might be said that, in drawling, one extends (i.e., prolongs) a sound, any similarity to prolongation ends there. Drawl, a common word, is used exclusively to refer to speech, and with the clear connotation of normal occurrence. Moreover, the word has a specific reference to vowels, only, that are often dipthongized as well as lengthened. In contrast, prolongations is not a common word and its use in regard to speech is secondary and esoteric. Except for certain arcane uses, it refers to an abnormal event. A prolongation may involve a vowel, but it also often involves an abortive vocal gesture, a voiced or an unvoiced consonant. These differences are reflected, significantly, in the fact that the two words occur differentially in their respective literatures. The fundamental distinction between the two can be stated in terms of syllable locus. A drawl is a syllable-completion phenomenon; a prolongation is an event of syllable initiation.

For practical purposes, however, the issue regarding drawls is of little consequence here; in the only study noting drawls (Levin & Silverman, 1965), they occured so rarely as to be excluded from the analysis. (Note that Blankenship and Kay also omitted nonphonemic lengthening of phonemes because of their rarity.)

Of related interest regarding rarity of occurrence of certain nonfluency types in the normal speech research, Levin and Silverman (1965, p. 75) reported that "*corrections* and *repetitions* presented some problems. Any single one of the four subcategories of correction or of the three subcategories of repetition was too rare to be useful." Special attention should be paid to the fact that subcategories of repetition were rare in these normal speech samples. Tongue slips and omissions were also infrequent.

Two categories in the "Disfluency" list (Table 2.2) do not have a comparison category in the "Hesitation Phenomena" list: the categories of "broken words" and "prolonged sounds," or the categories later substituted for them, "tension" and "disrhythmic phonation." Either of these pairs of descriptors can be incorporated into a single category of prolongations (Wingate, 1964, 1976, pp. 44–46). The fact that disfluencies of this type appear only in the list based on work concerned with stuttering indicates that they are characteristic of stuttering. This finding clearly corroborates evidence consistently revealed in the results of the comparative stuttering research itself (see Wingate, 1962, 1976, pp. 55–58), including Johnson's own data (see Johnson and Associates, 1959, tables 38 and 39, pp. 134–135, and tables 69 and 70, pp. 206–207; also Johnson, 1961a, table 6). In fact, it seems very likely that the (actually miniscule) amounts of this category reported for those samples of normal speech studied in the stuttering-based research (e.g., Johnson, 1961a; Johnson and Associates, 1959; Yairi & Jennings, 1974) reflect the constraint imposed by the limiting categories of the Johnson list.

Comparison of the nonfluency categories from the stuttering-based and the hesitation phenomena research contradicts an assumption in the stuttering-based research noted earlier, namely, that all kinds of disfluency are common to all speakers. Instead, the nonfluency categories developed in the study of normal speech provide a basic reference for pointing up the kinds of disfluencies characteristic of stuttering. Prolongations (or their equivalents) do not show up in assessments of normal speech. Another category of disfluency, sound and syllable (part-word) repetition, also does not appear routinely in the studies of normal speech. When it is included in one of the lists based on normal speech, it attracts use of the term "stutter," but with the qualification that, in this instance, the immediate referent lies within normal speech. It is entirely admissible to employ the term "stutter" in such qualified descriptive usage; this term has been widely used for a long time to refer to the kind of repetitions identified here, and in its essential descriptive reference nothing more need be intended.

Interpretations of much of the stuttering-based research have made a point of the "overlap" between stuttered and normal speech samples in the disfluencies contained in the Johnson list (e.g., Johnson, 1961a; Silverman, 1974; Silverman & Williams, 1967b). But the predominant overlap is to be found in precisely those nonfluency categories reported regularly in the extensive research on normal speech, summarized in Tables 2.1 and 2.2, and only negligible amounts in those categories typically identified as stutters.

There is no logical reason to expect that the speech of stutterers should differ from the speech of normal speakers in regard to the types of nonfluency found regularly in normal speech.[12] These nonfluencies constitute a "given"—they are common, regular components of speech. Comparison of stuttered and normal speech in respect to these (normal) nonfluency categories may have some value for purposes as yet undetermined, but in respect to the issue at hand comparison is, at best, superfluous. Actually it is misleading. To claim similarity, or continuity, between stuttering and normal speech on the basis of the nonfluencies found in everyone's speech is an oblique interpretation that diverts attention from the central issue.

In contrast to the many kinds of fluency interruptions that do occur commonly in the speech of stutterers and normal speakers alike, two types occur differentially in the two groups and characterize stuttered speech. These categories show up as differential even in the data to be found in the stuttering-based research, as well as by their absence (or special qualification) in the research on normal nonfluency. Moreover, they have been considered distinctive of stuttering for a very long time. The case in point is that these two categories were known by the terms "clonic" and "tonic" for considerably more than 100 years, and well into this century. The terms were well accepted and widely used, evidently because of their succinct and appropriate descriptiveness. However, as noted in Chapter 1, these terms, evidently by virtue of their frequent use with the word "spasm," were expunged from the professional literature over the past 30 years through the influence of a prevailing ideology that could not tolerate the suggestion of neurologic involvement that the terms implied (see Chapter 1, footnote 14). Nonetheless, by whatever names, these two categories continue to be revealed as the essential discriminanda of stuttering, identified in Chapter 1 as the characteristic markers of stuttering.

Differences between stuttered and normal speech are also to be found in comparisons of simply the amount of disfluency present in each of them. This level of comparison has generally been ignored, although it has important implications for understanding the nature of stuttering.

The dimension of amount of disfluency is considered in the following section, within which the differences in type of disfluencies is also clearly revealed.

Amounts of Disfluencies: Comparative Data

The research to be reviewed in this section was mounted from an orientation to stuttering. Therefore, the term *disfluency* is used as the general referent for fluency irregularities because it is the term that has been favored by authors writing from the field of stuttering.

In his efforts to demonstrate "overlap" between the disfluencies of stutterers and those of normal speakers Johnson often[13] made the point that some persons "regarded as" normal speakers are more disfluent than some individuals "classified as" stutterers. Such comparison turns out to be another example of the contradiction and illogic in the Johnson position. Although the intent of the comparison was to illustrate how stuttering and normal speech are alike, it actually gives clear indication of their difference and, as well, the nature of the difference. Persons identified as stutterers are not "so-called" because of the number of their disfluencies. Stuttering is not distinguished from normal speech in terms of the amount of disfluency, but in terms of the kinds of disfluency.

Additional testimony that frequency of disfluency is not the determining criterion is contained in studies such as those of Muma (1971), Westby (1979), and Yairi (1972). The 26 normally speaking, 4-year-old children studied by Muma had been assigned individually to one of two groups: one being "low-disfluent" and the other "high-disfluent." Each child in both groups was classified independently by their teacher and the author, neither of whom questioned whether children in the high-disfluent group should be considered to stutter. Yairi was able to divide both his stutterer and normal speaker groups into two subgroups, one of each being low-disfluent, the other high-disfluent. Westby was readily able to establish three separate groups of 10 kindergarten/first-grade children classified in terms of being either stutterers, or "highly disfluent," or "typical of kindergarten/first-grade disfluency." The classification was based on the concurrence in assessments of teacher, parent, and school clinician. Actually, a third level of normal speech was implied, in view of the fact that the selection process excluded "children who are not noticeably disfluent" or are "highly fluent" children (Westby, 1979, p. 140).

The claim that some normal speakers are more disfluent than some stutterers leads to another contradiction of the Johnson position. The normal speakers that are more disfluent than stutterers are few in number. As a general rule, stutterers are much more disfluent than are normal speakers. Actually, this difference qualifies as a basic fact about stuttering, and one that is hardly ever recognized. This fact has not been given the consideration it merits for its potential contribution to understanding the nature of stuttering.

Evidence for the fact that, in general, stuttered speech contains many more disfluencies than does normal speech is to be found in the data of many studies, undertaken with a variety of different objectives and involving stutterers of all ages from preschool to adulthood.

Mann (1937) compared oral reading samples of 29 stuttering children between the ages of 7 to 14 years with those of a matched group of children with normal speech. All subjects read a list of 490 words and a 950-word passage. The average percent of disfluencies for the stuttering children was 11.8% in reading the word list and 12.3% when reading the essay. In contrast, the respective values for the children with normal speech were only 3.7% and 3.3% disfluencies.

Egland (1938) compared spontaneous speech samples of three preschool age stutterers to those from a normative group of 26 youngsters of comparable age. His data revealed a 13.8% disfluency in the stuttered samples but only 5% in the speech of the normally speaking children.

Minifie and Cooker (1964), attempting to develop a "disfluency index," compared the disfluency scores of 37 college-age stutterers and 22 normal speakers. Although the extent of disfluency evidenced by several stutterers was within the range found in the samples from the normal speakers, "in general, the stutterers received much larger disfluency scores" (p. 191).

Knabe, Nelson, and Williams (1966) recorded the frequency with which 10 dimensions of "linguistic output" occurred in the speech of 16 college-age stutterers, and a matched group of normal speakers, in their replies to 10 questions. The only dimension on which the two groups differed significantly was the extent of disfluency: the stutterers had a mean score of 3.1 compared to a value of 1.1 for the normal speakers.

A study by Cooper, Cady, and Robbins (1970) was designed to compare the efficacy of three different words presumed to act as "contingent punishment" of disfluencies in the speech of both stutterers and normal speakers. Their subjects were 14 adolescent-to-young adult stutterers and 14 matched normal speakers who read aloud in 3 separate 7-minute segments in each of 3 different conditions. Since the reported data were fairly extensive and were presented separately for each segment, they are summarized here in Table 2.3. In each segment the stutterers evidenced many more disfluencies than the normal speakers; from two-and-a-half to four times an many.

Floyd and Perkins (1974) compared the "disfluent syllables" in the free play of four preschool stutterers with that found in comparable speech samples from 20 normally speaking children of the same age. The stut-

TABLE 2.3. Average overall disfluency for 14 stutterers and 14 normal speakers in each segment of three contingency conditions*

	Condition 1			Condition 2			Condition 3		
Subjects	1	2	3	1	2	3	1	2	3
Stutterers	78.5	51.5	70.4	88.1	69.6	75.6	87.5	66.7	79.6
Normals	25.4	19.6	24.1	22.3	20.4	27.9	24.7	18.6	20.4

*Data from Cooper, Cady, and Robbins (1970).

terer speech samples contained an average of 9.9 disfluencies whereas an average rate of only 1.2 disfluencies characterized the speech of the normal children (respective ranges were 7.3 to 14.3 versus 0.1 to 2.6).

The foregoing studies have reported findings only in terms of overall disfluency. Other studies have made more detailed comparative analyses, recording the frequency of various kinds of disfluency. The latter research thus has yielded separate results for disfluency types as well as overall disfluency comparisons. In some of this work disfluencies were tallied separately for males and females. Because male-female differences were rarely notable within the main categories of stutterer and normal speaker, I have combined the data for the sexes in reporting the findings of these studies. Also, instead of presenting the separate data for each kind of disfluency, I have combined certain disfluency categories into composite types. The rationale for the combinations is based on the analysis presented earlier in this chapter regarding: (1) the distinction between stutters and normal nonfluencies, and (2) the problems posed by the two disfluency categories of word repetitions and interjections.

As discussed earlier, although any disfluency type may be involved in the occurrence of a stutter event, the characteristic and most frequent markers of a stutter are the elemental repetitions and prolongations. Therefore, I have combined as *Type S* (for stutter) the data for the following kinds of disfluency: part-word (sound and syllable) repetitions, broken words, and prolonged sounds.[14] The data for revisions, phrase repetitions, and incomplete phrases have been combined as *Type N* (for normal). I will list word repetitions and interjections under a general heading of *indeterminate*, for several reasons. First, they have been the greatest source of confusion and equivocation in the identification of stuttering. Both classes lack specificity: "words" includes polysyllabic and monosyllabic items; "interjections" includes syllables, words, and phrases as well as filled pauses, and also gives no indication of possible iteration. Second, even when each class is represented by its most frequently occurring item—the repetition of a single-syllable word or the occurrence of a filled pause, respectively—it may or may not actually mark a stutter event. Although these two kinds of disfluency share the Indeterminant status, I continue to list them separately largely to call attention to the frequency with which word repetition occurs in this research.

It is appropriate that the first two sources of these data should be the studies reported by Johnson (Johnson, 1961a; Johnson and Associates, 1959) that have been so determinate in the study of disfluency from an orientation based in stuttering.

Of the 150 stuttering youngsters who served as the essential reference group in *The Onset of Stuttering* (Johnson and Associates, 1959), actual recorded speech samples were available for 89 children, 67 males and 21 females, between 2½ and 8½ years of age (an average age of 5 years). Comparable speech samples were obtained from their matched, normally speaking control subjects.[15] All samples were of spontaneous speech, elicited by use of cards from the Children's Apperception Test; the average sample size was approximately 500 words.

The results obtained for these 178 children are summarized in Table 2.4. The data are presented in decile format, as they were in the source cited. Clearly, the figures corroborate the findings of the research previously reviewed in regard to overall disfluency, namely, that stutterers evidence considerably more disfluencies than do normal speakers. Moreover, the separate tabulation of the different kinds of disfluency reveals the major dimensions of the overall difference. In contrast to the normal samples

TABLE 2.4. Types of disfluencies per hundred words in spontaneous speech samples[a] of 89 stuttering and 89 normally speaking children, ages 2.5 to 8.5 years[b]

Disfluency type	Deciles								
	1	2	3	4	5	6	7	8	9
Type N									
Stutterers	0.3	1.4	2.2	2.7	3.7	4.7	6.6	8.4	10.9
Normals	0.7	1.2	1.9	2.9	3.3	4.3	5.6	7.2	9.7
Type S									
Stutterers	0.9	1.6	3.2	5.2	6.6	9.5	13.1	17.4	29.4
Normals	0.2	0.3	0.5	0.7	1.1	1.2	1.9	2.8	4.5
Indeterminate									
Word repetitions									
Stutterers	1.2	2.5	4.5	5.4	6.3	7.6	10.4	12.1	15.7
Normals	0.5	0.6	1.0	1.2	1.7	2.4	2.8	3.4	4.6
Interjections									
Stutterers	1.4	2.9	4.2	5.4	6.3	7.6	10.4	11.9	15.7
Normals	0.6	1.2	2.2	3.2	3.7	6.0	8.0	10.8	16.9

[a]Responses to the Children's Apperception Test.
[b]Data from Johnson and co-workers (1959, Tables 69 and 70).

the stuttered speech samples contain huge quantities of Type S disfluencies, and considerably more word repetitions. The samples are comparable in regard to Type N disfluencies and interjections. It does not seem unreasonable to suggest, at least on a statistical basis, that the disfluencies making up the Indeterminate categories are divided between stutter events and normal disfluencies in a proportion that mirrors the relative differences between the Type S and the Type N categories.

The data base for Johnson's other major publication (Johnson, 1961a), on disfluencies in adult speech, was also extensive. Speech samples were obtained from 100 college-age stutterers, 50 males and 50 females, and 100 normally speaking matched control subjects. Each subject performed three tasks: (1) talking "for three minutes or so" about a future job or vacation; (2) telling a story based on card number 10 of the Thematic Apperception Test; and (3) reading a 300-word passage. The normal speakers produced larger spontaneous speech samples than did the stutterers but, on the average, the stutterer samples were adequate (means of 264 and 336 words in Tasks 1 and 2 respectively).

As in the publication from which the data were taken, they are presented here in separate tables for each of the three tasks (Tables 2.5, 2.6, and 2.7) and are given in the format of decile values. These data also constitute evidence that stuttered speech contains many more disfluencies than does normal speech and, further, that Type S disfluencies clearly characterize stuttered speech. Again, stuttered speech is shown to contain higher frequencies of the Indeterminate types of disfluency. Again the

TABLE 2.5. Types of disfluencies per hundred words in spontaneous speech samples[a] of 100 young adult stutterers and 100 normal speakers[b]

Disfluency type	Deciles								
	1	2	3	4	5	6	7	8	9
Type N									
Stutterers	0.0	0.5	1.3	1.7	2.7	4.0	5.3	7.3	11.2
Normals	0.5	0.8	1.2	1.4	1.7	2.7	3.5	4.5	5.9
Type S									
Stutterers	1.5	2.2	3.9	6.3	9.5	15.7	22.8	36.1	80.1
Normals	0.0	0.0	0.0	0.0	0.2	0.4	0.6	0.9	2.3
Indeterminate									
Word repetitions									
Stutterers	0.7	1.4	2.8	3.9	5.1	6.5	8.3	10.0	15.0
Normals	0.0	0.0	0.5	0.8	1.1	1.4	1.8	2.2	3.1
Interjections									
Stutterers	4.6	6.6	9.3	10.8	14.8	19.6	23.2	31.3	46.4
Normals	1.9	3.9	5.0	6.0	7.2	8.7	10.3	12.7	14.9

[a]Telling about job or vacation plans.
[b]Data from Johnson (1961a, Table 4).

TABLE 2.6. Types of disfluencies in the spontaneous speech samples[a] of 100 young adult stutterers and 100 normal speakers[b]

Disfluency type	Deciles								
	1	2	3	4	5	6	7	8	9
Type N									
Stutterers	0.3	1.0	1.7	2.5	3.5	4.8	6.2	8.7	11.8
Normals	0.8	1.1	1.4	2.0	2.6	3.1	4.1	5.7	7.2
Type S									
Stutterers	1.4	2.4	3.5	7.8	11.4	15.5	27.1	37.2	85.7
Normals	0.0	0.0	0.0	0.1	0.4	0.5	0.7	1.2	2.0
Indeterminate									
Word repetitions									
Stutterers	1.1	2.3	3.0	3.7	6.0	7.5	9.6	12.6	18.5
Normals	0.0	0.4	0.7	0.9	1.0	1.2	1.7	2.3	3.4
Interjections									
Stutterers	2.6	8.1	9.8	13.3	16.0	19.7	25.4	34.8	52.5
Normals	1.1	1.7	2.7	3.6	4.6	6.8	10.7	12.1	16.9

[a]Telling a story to card No. 10 of the Thematic Apperception Test.
[b]Data from Johnson (1961a, Table 5).

TABLE 2.7. Types of disfluencies in samples of oral reading from 100 young adult stutterers and 100 normal speakers[a]

Disfluency type	Deciles								
	1	2	3	4	5	6	7	8	9
Type N									
Stutterers	0.0	0.0	0.0	0.5	0.6	1.0	1.2	1.9	2.7
Normals	0.0	0.0	0.3	0.3	0.5	0.5	0.7	1.0	1.3
Type S									
Stutterers	0.7	1.0	1.3	2.5	4.0	6.7	12.1	20.9	33.6
Normals	0.0	0.0	0.0	0.1	0.1	0.3	0.5	0.7	1.0
Indeterminate									
Word repetitions									
Stutterers	0.0	0.0	0.0	0.3	0.3	0.9	1.2	2.0	2.7
Normals	0.0	0.0	0.0	0.0	0.0	0.0	0.1	0.3	0.5
Interjections									
Stutterers	0.0	0.0	0.0	0.3	0.5	1.0	1.5	2.4	11.3
Normals	0.0	0.0	0.0	0.0	0.0	0.0	0.0	0.0	0.1

[a]Data from Johnson (1961a, Table 6).

suggestion arises that in stuttered speech a sizable proportion of the latter kinds of disfluency are involved in an abnormal event.

A report by Silverman and Williams (1971) contains pertinent data obtained in the course of three studies addressed to the adaptation effect. In each study the principle objective was to compare, for stutterers and normal speakers, the extent to which six[16] kinds of disfluency evidenced the adaptation effect. In two studies the subjects were English speaking but of different age levels; in the third study all subjects spoke Japanese. One of the two English-subject studies dealt with elementary school (second to sixth grade) children and included 67 stutterers and their matched controls. The second English-subject study was conducted with 24 junior high school (seventh to ninth grade) stutterers and matched normal speakers. Subjects in the Japanese language study were 30 fourth to sixth grade stutterers and matched normal speakers.

The data from the three studies are presented in Table 2.8. The tabled values represent the occurrence, per 100 words, of the total disfluencies occuring during the course of a 3-trial adaptation sequence.

As with the evidence from the foregoing research, the data from each of these studies reveals that stuttered speech has considerably more disfluency than normal speech and, again, that the substantial difference is occasioned particularly by Type S disfluencies. Of additional significance is the evidence that these same comparisons hold true for a language other than English.

Silverman (1974) recorded the frequency with which each of the dis-

TABLE 2.8. Average disfluencies per hundred words in the oral reading of three groups of stuttering and normally speaking school children during a 3-trial adaptation sequence[a]

	Disfluency type			
			Indeterminate	
Subject group	Type N	Type S	Word repetitions	Interjections
American, 2nd–6th grade				
67 Stutterers	1.7	5.6	1.9	0.4
67 Normals	2.3	1.4	0.6	0.2
American, 7th–9th grade				
24 Stutterers	1.1	8.4	1.2	2.3
24 Normals	1.0	1.0	0.2	0.0
Japanese, 4th–6th grade				
30 Stutterers	1.2	8.8	0.5	1.1
30 Normals	1.0	0.8	0.1	0.0

[a]Data from Silverman and Williams (1971, Tables 1–3).

fluency types in the Johnson list occurred in the oral reading and elicited spontaneous speech of 56 stuttering boys in grades two through six and their matched normal speaking controls. The data for the spontaneous speech samples are presented, in the quartile format of the reference source, in Table 2.9. The data for the oral reading samples, not presented here, were comparable to those for spontaneous speech. These findings concur with those of the other research reviewed, in terms of both overall extent of disfluency and the relative proportions of the different types.

Yairi and Lewis (1984) obtained spontaneous speech samples, of approximately 500 syllables each, from 10 very young stutterers, age 2 and 3 years, in whom stuttering onset had occurred within 2 months prior to the time they were seen. The disfluencies, using the Johnson list, in these speech samples were compared with those occurring in similar speech samples obtained from normal youngsters matched individually for age and sex with each stutterer. It is pertinent to mention that, in six cases in which either of two normally speaking children would have been an appropriate "match" for a stuttering child, the authors chose the more disfluent of the two in order to reduce the possible bias of the findings resulting from having unusually fluent children in the control group.

The findings are presented in Table 2.10. The difference in total disfluencies between the two groups is significant, a difference due essentially to the categories of part-word repetitions and dysrhythmic phonation.

The evidence is consistent, and clear, throughout all of these studies

TABLE 2.9. Types of disfluencies per hundred words in spontaneous speech samples[a] of 56 stuttering and 56 normally speaking elementary school boys[b]

Disfluency type	Lowest index	Quartiles Q_1	Q_2	Q_3	Highest index
Type N					
Stutterers	0.3	1.7	2.4	4.0	11.0
Normals	0.5	1.7	3.1	5.1	12.1
Type S					
Stutterers	0.0	1.4	3.6	9.8	64.2
Normals	0.0	0.3	0.9	1.5	6.2
Indeterminate					
Word repetitions					
Stutterers	0.0	1.3	2.5	4.4	3.6
Normals	0.0	0.4	0.8	1.3	3.3
Interjections					
Stutterers	0.0	0.2	0.8	1.9	10.7
Normals	0.0	0.3	0.5	1.5	8.5

[a]Responses to the Children's Apperception Test.
[b]Data from Silverman (1974).

TABLE 2.10. Average disfluencies per hundred words in spontaneous speech samples of 10 stuttering and 10 normally speaking children, age two and three years[a]

	Disfluencies			
			Indeterminate	
Subject group	Type N	Type S	Word repetitions	Inter-jections
Stutterers	2.6	12.8	3.6	2.5
Normals	1.7	2.1	0.9	1.4

[a]Data from Yairi and Lewis (1984).

that stuttered speech contains many more disfluencies than does normal speech. In fact, in all of this research the frequency of disfluencies in stuttered speech is at least twice as much as that found in normal speech (and often the ratio is substantially greater than 2:1). As mentioned at the beginning of this section, this evidence deserves recognition as an important fact about stuttering. The significance of this fact will be developed in later parts of the book.

For the moment the pertinence of the findings from this comparative research centers mainly in the consistent evidence that stuttered speech is characterized by certain observable types of disfluency. This is not to say that stuttering is to be identified, or differentiated from normal nonfluency, solely in terms of observable disfluency types. One must recognize that stutter events are occasionally accompanied by Type N disfluences, as well as by a certain number of those types listed here as Indeterminate. Also, what at least appears to be a Type S disfluency evidently occurs, infreqently, in normal speech. Endeavoring to differentiate stuttering from normal nonfluency solely on the basis of the classes of observable disfluencies is a confounding and hopeless undertaking. Ever since Johnson created this diverting issue, primarily through his singular emphasis on the "overlap" between groups, it has constituted a major, persisting obstacle to progress in understanding the nature of stuttering.

The essential points regarding the fact that Type S disfluencies characterize stuttering are: (1) these types are not themselves the stutters but are the distinctive markers of a stutter event; and (2) the nature of these distinctive markers provides us with our best clues as to the essence of stuttering, in at least its phenomenal aspect. As I will develop later in the book, these clues articulate well with other lines of evidence that, together, point to the basic nature of the disorder.

The differences between the disfluencies of stuttered speech and those of normal speech continue to be revealed in recent studies of the speech of very young normally speaking children (Bjerkan, 1980; Silverman, 1972; Wexler & Mysak, 1982; Yairi & Clifton, 1972). Also, the study by Yairi and Lewis (1984), which is particularly pertinent to the contentions of the Johnson position, presents evidence that the markers that characterize stuttered speech are present from the time of onset of the disorder.

The Nonfluent Character of Ordinary Speech

The hesitation phenomena research, addressed specifically to the study of normal nonfluency, has identified several kinds of nonfluency that are found regularly in normal speech and that contribute to a description of the fluency dimension of ordinary speech. A more comprehensive characterization of normal fluency is realized through the addition of pertinent information derived from three other sources: (1) corroborative evidence regarding nonfluencies that has surfaced during the course of research on normal speech that was undertaken for other purposes; (2) data regarding the extent of nonfluency in ordinary speech; and (3) the degree to which listeners, and the speakers themselves, are unaware of normal nonfluency.

Evidence from Elsewhere

A Linguist's Description of Spontaneous Speech

Abercrombie (1963),[17] writing from the standpoint of a linguist's concern about the proper subject matter for study, complained that linguistic study actually had not been addressed to what linguists presumably investigated. He noted that linguists regularly contended that "the main business of linguistics is the investigation of spoken language," which implies a study of the ordinary speech of everyday life. He pointed out, however, that linguistics had concerned itself almost exclusively with what he called "spoken prose"—the discourse of stage, screen, and radio, and the speech of monologues and prepared lectures. He emphasized that these forms of speech are regularized, highly specialized abstractions from conversation that account for only a small part of spoken language.

Speaking of the substantial differences between ordinary speech and "spoken prose," Abercrombie quoted T.S. Eliot's characterization of ordinary talking as being replete with "fumbling for words, its constant recourse to approximation, its disorder and unfinished sentences." Characteristics such as these, Abercrombie emphasized, are not to be found in spoken prose. He then went on to describe how ordinary speech differs from spoken prose in kind, not simply in degree, and he listed several ways in which such differences are manifested. Some of the items he mentioned are among the features identified, independently, in the research on nonfluency in normal speech.

Abercrombie also drew attention to the frequency with which nonfluencies appear in ordinary speech, remarking that "it comes as quite a surprise" to discover how often they occur. At the same time he noted that, in spite of the extent of its occurrence, "What has been called 'normal nonfluency' attracts no attention" (op cit, p. 15).

Research Confirmation

Abercrombie's observations are well supported by a wide range of evidence, a substantial proportion of which is supplied by the hesitation phenomena research. As noted earlier in this chapter, discovery of the variety and extent of nonfluency in ordinary normal speech constituted a real revelation, which initiated a whole new area of research.

Other aspects of the hesitation phenomena research, also pertinent to the characterization of ordinary speech, will be reviewed presently. However, I would like to first present additional documentation of Abercrombie's description of ordinary speech that has emerged from research undertaken for purposes unrelated to the study of nonfluency.

French, Carter, and Koenig (1930) reported a landmark study of spontaneous speech undertaken from the standpoint of telecommunications interests. These authors were interested in certain structural aspects of conversational speech, primarily word and sound frequencies. They analyzed speech samples obtained from 1,950 different telephone conversations, mostly business calls, that yielded an eventual corpus of almost 80,000 words. Our present interest in this research is the fact that 20% of the original material consisted of half-completed words and sentences, and nonwords like "uh," "ah," "yeah," and "er" (French et al., p. 291).

Another line of evidence comes from research in the field of elementary education. Research reported by Strickland (1962) was actually addressed to the study of reading skills. For purposes of reference and comparison she analyzed spontaneous speech samples obtained from 575 children in the first six grades. She excluded from the analysis certain features of the speech samples, called "mazes," that were "not pertinent to the structure or meaning of what they are saying." She identified mazes as consisting of the following categories:

> *Noises* were unintelligible sounds such as "ah," "er," and the like. *Holders*, such as "well," "you see," and "now uh," were used to hold attention. *Repeats* were repetitions of words such as "you—you." "I think—I think." *Edits* were words used by the speaker which indicated a correction or change of direction in what he was saying (op cit, p. 24).

Strickland's category terms differ somewhat from the normal nonfluency descriptors found in the hesitation phenomena research, yet reference to the appropriate list in Table 2.1 will reveal clear correspondences to each of these items. Strickland did not compute the relative frequency with which mazes occurred in her samples, but the relevant data suggest that they amounted to approximately 15% of the total corpus of about 180,000 words.

Strickland indicated in a footnote (op cit, p. 24) that the designation mazes was borrowed from research by W.D. Loban, but she did not cite a publication. However, it is almost certain that the work to which she referred was the research reported the preceding year (Loban, 1961). That research, eventually published in summary form (Loban, 1976) was an extensive longitudinal study of language use in over 200 elementary school children[18] who had been chosen to constitute a representative sample of the population, stratified according to socioeconomic status, sex, racial background, and range of intellectual ability. The research was "concerned with [children's] use and control of language, their effectiveness in communication, and with the relations among their oral, written, listening and reading uses of language," (Loban, 1976, p. 1).

Appropriate language measures, including recorded samples of spontaneous speech, were obtained at regular intervals for each of the children from their kindergarten year through the sixth grade. Fluency, in a broad sense, was one of four major dimensions of the appraisal and was itself based on four measures: (1) amount of language used, (2) manner of speaking (readiness of response), (3) extent of vocabulary, and (4) freedom from mazes. Loban used the term mazes because "the linguistic troubles of the subjects resemble very much the physical behavior of a person looking for a way out of an actual spatial maze . . . [as characterized by] many hesitations, false starts, and meaningless repetitions" (op cit, p. 8). Mazes tended to be rather long, averaging 2.6 words per maze at the kindergarten level and gradually decreasing to 2.1 words, on the average, by the time the children were in sixth grade.

More recently Fagan (1982), studying specially elicited speech samples of fifth graders, noted yet another type of maze, a kind of unintended redundancy. Fagan's analyses led him to suggest that a maze is "not a stumbling block or a tangle in oral language but an aid to achieve fluency" (op cit, p. 94).

Similar findings are contained in research reported by Carterette and Jones (1974). These authors, noting the extent to which existing statistical studies of language were based on written sources, undertook to collect data that would represent informal spoken language. The objective of their research was to obtain a sizable corpus of the ordinary everyday speech of normal speakers (any individual with "even minor" speech defect was excluded) who represented a fairly wide age range. To this end they obtained extensive conversational speech samples, averaging 21,000 words each, from four separate groups: three children from each of the first, third, and fifth grades, and one group of young adults. Carterette and Jones reported that "it became immediately obvious upon listening to the tapes that the language was quite different from linguistically ideal or written language" (p. 18). Their efforts at accurate linguistic transcription of each corpus led to a designation of units that they called "phonemic words." Such units, determined by pause boundaries, included some true words and word combinations that occurred as "routinized insertions," but also contained many nonwords like those noted in the French, Carter, and Koenig findings. It is impossible to tell, from their data, the relative frequency of nonfluency types listed in Table 2.1 but, altogether, phonemic words made up 26 to 28% of the lexical corpus of the individual group samples. The authors commented that "to normalize such data is to edit out what is most characteristic of speech" (op cit, p. 27).

It bears emphasis that the nonfluencies identified in all of the research reviewed in this section have been of the order of Type N disfluencies, and that none of this research has included mention of Type S.

The Extent of Normal Nonfluency

In addition to yielding detailed information about types of nonfluencies typical of normal spontaneous speech, the hesitation-phenomena research has concurrently documented how frequently these features occur.

Goldman-Eisler's work, which was addressed to silent pause alone, clearly revealed the discontinuity in speech. Her findings led her to describe ordinary speech as "fragmented," a description suggested, for example, by her evidence that "50 percent of speech is broken up into phrases of less than three words, 75 percent into phrases of less than five words" (Goldman-Eisler, 1968, p. 17).

The fragmentation of ordinary speech is occasioned not only by silent intervals but by other kinds of nonfluency as well. Mahl (1956c, 1959a, 1959b, 1960, 1981) also pointed to the very frequent occurrence of "speech disturbances." "Speech," he said (1959b, p. 251) "may be literally peppered with various disturbances," a comment supported by his finding that one or another of the nonfluency categories he identified occurred approximately once every 10 words.

Other studies of nonfluency in normal speech corroborate the reports made by Goldman-Eisler and Mahl. Wyrick (1949), studying nonfluency in the conversations of normal young adults, found that some form of nonfluency occurred in one out of every eight words. Voelker (1944), in a study of normally speaking adolescents, also found that some kind of nonfluency occurred, on the average, once every eight words. Kowal, O'Connell, and Sabin (1975), reporting on only four kinds of nonfluency (false starts, filled pauses, repeats, parenthetical remarks) in the speech of children and adults, found average nonfluencies to range from 1 per 9.4

words for children to 1 per 14.6 words for adults. These figures would undoubtedly have been higher if all kinds of nonfluencies had been recorded.

Awareness of Nonfluencies

Listener Awareness of Nonfluencies

As noted earlier, Abercrombie (1963) pointed out that normal nonfluency attracts no attention. Evidently the vast majority of normal nonfluencies go unnoticed because both speaker and listener are intent on the message being expressed. It is axiomatic within disciplines concerned with the study of language that both speaker and listener are intent on the meaning embedded in utterances. The speaker's energies and attention are focused on transforming thought(s) into communicable form; the listener is intent on comprehending the message being generated.

McNeill and Lindig (1973), discussing the issue of the "unit" of language perception, note: "in normal language use the focus of attention . . . is the meaning of an utterance. Subordinate levels become the focus of attention only under special circumstances" (p. 430). The "special circumstances" mentioned here refer to whatever conditions might occur that would draw attention to aspects of speech other than the embedded meaning; in a word, they are distractions from meaning. Clearly, such circumstances must cross a certain level of perceptual threshold, a threshold that is undoubtedly conditioned by the listener's focus on the embedded message.

There is evidence that listeners not only "do not notice" normal nonfluencies but (subconsciously) intentionally ignore them. For example, Martin and Strange (1968) found that requiring subjects to attend to hesitations (nongrammatical pauses) in speech samples interfered with their comprehension of the message. As the authors pointed out, attending to these two dimensions of the signal constitutes a set of competing tasks. From a somewhat different angle, Cole (1973) found that listeners did not detect contrived errors of pronunciation contained in connected speech but readily discerned the same errors is isolated syllables. Failure to detect the errors was clearly dependent on their being embedded in a larger word-level context. Conversely, many actual errors of listening are evidently occasioned by contextual influences; that is, errors in the perception of segments and of words are induced as a function of the meaning apprehended by the listener (Garnes & Bond, 1975).

The hesitation phenomena research, in addition to yielding evidence of the type and extent of nonfluencies in normal speech, has concurrently documented how regularly these nonfluencies escape notice, thereby leaving a (false) impression of fluency. Goldman-Eisler (1968) described very clearly the contrast between perception and reality in regard to the perceived fluency of ordinary spontaneous speech. She wrote:

> Somehow the phenomenon of speech has become associated with images which suggest continuity of speech production. We speak of the even flow, of fluency of speech, of a flood of language, and many words relating to speech derive from descriptions of water in motion, such as "gush, spout, stream, torrent of speech, floodgates of speech, etc." The facts, however, show these images to be illusory; if we measure vocal continuity by the numbers of words uttered between two pauses and call "phrase" the sequence uttered without a break, we obtain a picture of fragmentation rather than of continuity (p. 15).

Mahl, too, observed that, in spite of the frequency with which nonfluencies occur, the vast majority of them escape the awareness of both listeners and speakers. He noted (1959b) that listeners are more likely to perceive the nonfluencies of normal speech only when they are "bunched," that is, when they occur with unusual frequency within a certain span of time.

Most likely there are other circumstances that can bring at least certain nonfluencies of normal speech into listeners' awareness; for example, the overuse of the same interjection such as "y'know" or excessive use of "uh." Ordinarily, however, listeners take little note of such nonfluency. Some nonfluencies may not be perceptible to the listener, yet many are well above threshold but ignored. Others are undoubtedly registered subliminally but disregarded. For instance, Boomer and Dittman (1962) demonstrated, in an experimental condition, that listeners could differentiate juncture pauses from hesitation pauses even when the two pause types were of comparable length. Under the conditions of ordinary conversation, listeners are likely to be completely unaware of their capacity to make such distinctions, even though probably registering them subconsciously. Such functioning is akin to the phenomenon called "linguistic transparency" (Polyani, 1964), meaning that a listener is ordinarily not aware of normal phonological and grammatical structures even though they must have been perceived in some sense.

Thus, normal speech, although containing many departures from literal fluency, is regularly *misperceived as fluent.* In contrast, stuttered speech is not misperceived as fluent. Unlike the nonfluencies of ordinary speech, stutters come into perceptual prominence very quickly, by virtue of the "special conditions" they embody.

A widely accepted principal criterion of defective speech is that it calls attention to itself (see Van Riper, 1963, p. 16). This criterion is of particular relevance to the present discussion. Normal speech, in contrast to defective speech, does not call attention to itself in spite of the fact that it contains many irregularities. It is pertinent to recall here the earlier discussion regarding the fact that the difference between normal and stuttered speech is not drawn in terms of the *amount* of nonfluency but in respect to *kind.*

Speaker Awareness of Nonfluencies

Normal nonfluencies ordinarily escape the awareness of speakers as well as listeners. In fact, the speaker is usually even less aware of his nonfluencies than are his listeners. Consider, for instance, the examples cited in the previous section; frequent interjection of "y'know" or the like, or excessive use of "uh." Listeners may become keenly aware of, even annoyed by, such recurrent nonfluencies. Actually, such excesses are widely regarded as (nonconscious) "bad habits" that the speaker would undoubtedly remedy if aware of their occurrence. But compelling irregularities of this kind are not common in ordinary speech; most speech contains a much less dramatic set of nonfluencies, although a wider array of them. Speakers are routinely unaware of these nonfluencies as they are unaware of other ways in which their speech departs from idealized form.

Again, Abercrombie (1963) observed:

> When you look at the written text of a genuine spontaneous conversation, it is pretty horrifying—particularly when it is a conversation in which you yourself have taken part. It is sometimes unintelligible, and it is always illogical, disorganized, repetitious, and ungrammatical. I have several times heard people remark, on seeing the text of a recorded conversation, that it is illiterate. But of course it *should* be illiterate—literally. It should be different from written language (p. 14).

Some of Mahl's work provides documentation of this analysis, in specific regard to nonfluency. He reported (1959a, 1960, 1981) that, when confronted with transcripts of their own speech, speakers were invariably surprised at the extent of nonfluency recorded. Most of them were interested in this new information about their speech, but some were defensively disbelieving or registered dismay, shame, or anger. As Mahl noted, all of these reactions reflect the extent to which the vast majority of normal nonfluencies go unnoticed, and particularly by the speaker himself.

It is of considerable interest that, even in the case of stuttering, the listener is more likely to be aware of stutters than is the speaker. Research findings in studies by Hahn (1940), Porter (1939), and Razdol'skii (1965) provide persuasive evidence that stutterers are unaware of many of their stutters (see Wingate, 1976, pp. 25–26). The research evidence on this point corroborates clinical experience. I have found regularly that stutterers do not notice some (sometimes many) of their stutters, particularly the less dramatic instances. Other clinicians concur in this observation. From his lengthy clinical experience Van Riper (1973, chap. 10) considers that the basic procedure in therapy is to train the stutterer to identify his stutters. The task is to identify not only the acts that are part of his more obvious stutters ("he rarely recognizes what he does . . ." p. 246) but also the stutters of which he remains unaware. In Van Riper's words, "next we ask him to identify those short, easy stutterings which serve as our temporary primary target and *which already exist unrecognized in his speech"* (p. 249).[19]

Commentary

From its inception the research on nonfluencies in normal speech has been guided by an interest in the significance of nonfluencies and of the different forms of nonfluency. This interest progressed from the original expectations—that nonfluencies might have clinical value—to a gradually broadening scope of inquiry into the linguistic, cognitive, and psycholinguistic implications of nonfluencies. This line of research has moved continuously toward a fuller understanding of the nature, role, and import of nonfluencies.

In contrast, over the same span of time the stuttering-based research addressed to the characterization of disfluency has consistently reflected an interest in simply recording occurrences of the disfluencies on the Johnson list, summing up their frequencies of occurrence, and computing their relative proportions for purposes of making comparisons. This line of research has remained static. We know very little more now about the nature of stutters, or normal nonfluencies, or the relationship between the two, from this line of research than we did when it began.[20]

It seems clear that progress in understanding stuttering and its relationship to fluency will require expanding the scope of research that relates stuttering to normal nonfluency. The existing research on nonfluency in normal speech has very substantial import for stuttering, not simply for its corroboration of what is meant by "stuttering" but also for what needs to be learned about the nature of fluency. Broadly based data on the speech of normal speakers, obtained and analyzed independently of some special bias, should be the basis for any range of interest in fluency and nonfluency. The study of fluency disorders should be undertaken in full cognizance of, and relevance to, research on normal fluency—and the nonfluency intrinsic to it.

Much could be learned simply by applying the approach and methods for the normal nonfluency research to stuttered speech samples. Further, a whole new area of direct comparative research suggests itself. Presumably such research would proceed in reference to an extended list of nonfluency categories as suggested in the discussion developed here. Investigation of pause would seem to merit early attention, inasmuch as the study of pause has figured substantially in the analyses of normal nonfluency, but has been neglected in the mainstream of the stuttering-based research. Some comparative work, done several years ago (Love & Jeffress, 1971; Zerbin, 1973) and a more recent study (Wingate, 1984b) suggest the promise in this area of investigation. I will return to this matter in Chapter 8.

There is one remaining contrast that deserves special mention in the context of the comparisons presented in this chapter because it epitomizes the differentiation made. In the literature of stuttering one frequently encounters consideration of the consonant–vowel distinction, in reference to evidence that consonants are "more difficult" than vowels. In contrast, concern with the consonant–vowel distinction is not to be found in the literature dealing with "hesitation phenomena." The reason is not hard to find: normal nonfluencies involve units larger than the syllable; stutters are characterized by syllables broken into their constituents.

I turn now to a consideration of research findings that bear on the issue of language involvement in stuttering. The contents of Chapters 3 and 4 present a review and analysis of the fairly extensive research addressed specifically to language factors in stuttering. Chapters 5 and 6 focus on relevant information about the structure of English that has derived from broadly based research on the language in ordinary, normal usage. The background created by this information serves to highlight certain salient linguistic features of stuttering.

Footnotes

*These quotations are taken from *Webster's New World Dictionary of the American Language, College Edition,* 1964. However, similar entries will be found in any regular dictionary source, for example: *The Concise Oxford Dictionary of Current English,* Clarendon Press, 1982; or, *Webster's New World Dictionary, Second Concise Edition,* Simon and Schuster, 1982, or similar references.

[1]This inference is based on the fact that the studies by Branscom (1942), Davis (1939, 1940), Hughes (1943), and Oxtoby (1943), all directed by Johnson, cite pertinent findings of the relevant early language studies.

[2]The studies by Branscom, Hughes, and Oxtoby were eventually published in a combined version, as chapter 5, "Studies of Nonfluency in Preschool Children," in W. Johnson, and R. Leutenegger (Eds.), *Stuttering in Children and Adults,* 1955. Modifications of the reports by Mann, Egland, and Johnson also appear in the same source as, respectively, chapters 7, 6, and 3.

[3]*Ibid.*

[4]The nonfluency of the normally speaking children was eventually described, as "repetitions and hesitations," when this study was reported "in full" as chapter 3 (same title) in *Stuttering in Children and Adults* (Johnson & Leutenegger, 1955, p. 67).

[5]Italics mine.

[6]The list might also be criticized for having been developed on adults. Periodically in the literature of stuttering one finds complaint, however valid it may be, that the speech of children should not be assessed in reference to adult level speech.

[7]I should probably include, as part of the nonresearch literature, my own reference to this research (Wingate, 1976, chap. 4). This reference, though brief, stresses the relevance of the normal fluency research to the identification of stuttering.

[8]It is of some interest that definitions and illustrations of Mahl's categories of "speech disturbances" appeared in a 1963 article in the *Journal of Speech and Hearing Disorders* (Zimbardo, Mahl, & Barnard, 1963). Mahl is one of the earliest and

continuing contributors to the study of normal nonfluency (see later in this chapter). Evidently his contribution aroused little interest among persons interested in stuttering, even though this article appeared in a principle publication source for stuttering literature only 2 years after the Johnson publication (Johnson, 1961a) that provided the "disfluency" categories used thereafter in the stuttering-based research. Also, 3 years later Jakobovits (1966), writing in the same journal, called attention to the normal nonfluency research and suggested that research in stuttering should make use of this fund of information. Clearly, the suggestion has been ignored.

[9]Their citations are limited to references dealing with the loci of stutter events.

[10]Italics mine.

[11]The category of "word repetitions" is confounded. Words differ in length, a dimension that is evidently pertinent to the issues considered here. The matter is discussed in Wingate (1976, pp. 42–44).

[12]Actually, the only reason to expect a difference should be posed by the very theoretical position that presses the issue of similarity: to wit, if stuttering develops as a fear of nonfluency (and/or whatever it is associated with) and if stuttering represents the effort to avoid nonfluency (and/or whatever it is associated with) then one should expect the speech of stutterers to contain only stutterings and not the disfluencies of ordinary speech.

At the same time, it may eventually be found that certain types of normal nonfluency are associated with different processes in stuttered as compared to normal speech.

[13]See, for example, Johnson (1961b, p. 211, 1963, p. 241) and Johnson and Associates (1959, p. 216).

[14]Or the descriptors later substituted for the latter two, namely "dysrhythmic phonation" and "tense pause."

[15]These data were taken from a masters thesis by Kools (1956).

[16]Evidently there were no instances of "incomplete phrases" or "tense pauses."

[17]The article by Abercrombie was originally presented in 1959 as one of four public lectures on Spoken Language. It was later reprinted (1965) in *Studies in Phonetics and Linguistics,* Oxford University Press.

[18]At the kindergarten level the sample contained 338 children. This number dropped to 260 in the first grade; further attrition decreased the number to 236 at the sixth-grade level.

[19]Italics mine.

[20]Within the spectrum of research interests in stuttering some of the work concerned with loci of stutters and disfluencies can be considered to have made an initial contribution in this direction. However, other areas of research interest in stuttering are affected in one way or another by the limitations discussed in this chapter.

Part II: Language Factors: Accumulated Research and a New Analysis

The four chapters of Part II focus on sources of evidence pertinent to considering stuttering in terms of oral language variables ("speech" in the broad sense). Chapters 3 and 4 consist of the review, critical analysis, and integration of the research, addressed specifically to language factors in stuttering, that has been published in the 50 years since this topic was broached. Chapter 5 contains a review of relevant findings from research into structural aspects of normal speech, followed by discussion of the significance of these findings for understanding the evidence obtained from the research in stuttering. Chapter 6 develops a characterization of stuttering that encapsulates the focal aspects of the analyses developed up to that point in the book.

3
Language Factors: Early Findings

Formal inquiry into langauge factors in stuttering can be said to have begun with a series of articles that appeared between 1935 and 1945 largely in the *Journal of Speech Disorders.* These publications, authored principally by S.F. Brown (Brown, 1937b, 1938a, 1938b, 1938c, 1943, 1945; Brown & Moren, 1942; Johnson & Brown, 1935, 1939), reported the results of research he had undertaken originally for his master's thesis (Brown, 1935) and continued for his doctoral dissertation (Brown, 1937a). Although the findings of this early work were of immediate (and lasting) significance, they evidently did not generate much interest in the era during which they were published. The major aspects of the Brown investigations were quickly replicated by Hahn (1942a, 1942b) but, with the exception of a different form of language study (Eisenson & Horowitz, 1945), there was otherwise no evidence of interest in this topic.

Inquiry into language factors in stuttering subsided in the middle 1940s and was not pursued again for almost 20 years. A revival of investigation in this area that began during the early 1960s has been somewhat more broadly based, and longer lasting. Still, interest in language factors in stuttering has generally been limited, and often peripheral to other directions of interest in stuttering.[1]

Brown's work had a heavy—in fact, determining—influence on subsequent investigation of language function in stuttering. The influence of his writings was expressed not only in respect to the dimensions of inquiry and the foci of analysis but, probably even more important, in terms of the assumptions, guiding hypotheses, and interpretative orientation of his work. For these reasons it is appropriate to first review the series of Brown's publications in sufficient detail to provide a frame of reference for the discussion of subsequent contributions, which will be considered in Chapter 4.

The Object of Study

Although certain structural aspects of (the English) language are the immediate foci in the "language factors" research, stuttering is the ultimate referent, the actual object of study.

In overall perspective the study of language factors in stuttering has been unnecessarily complicated by the kinds of problems discussed in Chapter 2—the identification of stuttering and its differentiation from normal nonfluency. Actually, the problem did not arise until after the revival of interest in language factors that appeared in the 1960s. However, because the research reported since that time is generally assumed to be continuous with, and consistent with, the Brown series (and certain work in the 1950s that utilized Brown's findings), the whole scope of the study of language aspects of stuttering is affected in some measure by these problems.

The fact that the Brown series was free of this complication is both significant and curious. It is significant because, as I will document shortly, the referent for "stuttering" in the Brown series squares very well with the descriptive identification of stuttering that emerges from a careful and objective analysis of the relevant data contained in many different sources of observation and inquiry. The fact is curious because, first, Wendell Johnson was directly involved in the work that eventuated in the Brown series (see next section), and the influence of his psychological orientation is clearly evident throughout the series. Second, as discussed in Chapter 2, Johnson was primarily responsible for clouding the differentiation between stuttering and other kinds of nonfluency through his "evaluation" conjecture, which embodies the contention that stuttering and normal nonfluency are simply degrees of the same thing. The Brown series, however, was not constrained by this complication because that work was undertaken, and completed, in a period prior to the time that Johnson's evaluation conjecture had come to preoccupy his thinking. In those days the effect of the "evaluation" notion was largely one of biasing the interpretation of research findings. It had not yet been pushed to the point of distorting the identification of stuttering. In fact, the identification of stuttering stated by Johnson and Brown (1935), in the first article of the Brown series, was straightforward and realistic:

> A stuttering spasm was taken to be any interruption of the normal rhythm of reading. It might take the form of a complete block, undue prolongation of a sound, a repetition of the initial sound of a word or syllable, saying "uh-uh-uh," repetition of the previous word or words, or a complete cessation of all attempts to speak for a moment. It was necessary to interpret these various interruptions of rhythm carefully for each case, in the light of what was known about the type of stuttering characteristic of each stutterer. For example, saying "uh-uh-uh" before beginning a word was a definite indication of a spasm in some cases, while other stutterers

never hesitated in this way before words in relation to which they had spasms. In these latter cases the "uh-uh-uh" was either a mannerism or an indication that the stutterer had momentarily lost his place, while in the former cases it was marked as a spasm in relation to the word before which the "uh-uh-uh" came (p. 484).

Here the identification of stuttering is not glossed, as it would be later, but is done carefully. Note the effort to distinguish between variants of "uh-uh-uh." Later, Johnson would encompass all such variants, along with certain other kinds of disfluency, in an undifferentiating category of "Interjections." This careful statement of stutter identification has particular relevance to the concept of "markers" of stutter events, presented in Chapter 1. Note especially that when word repetitions signal a stutter, the actual locus of the stutter event is revealed by the "repetition of *the previous* word or words," and that when an uh-uh-uh reflects a stutter, the stutter event is "in relation to the word *before which* the uh-uh-uh came." These descriptions clearly express the marker concept, in direct reference to two potentially troublesome categories of disfluency.

The Brown Series

As an overview statement, it is relevant to note that Brown's more important findings regarding language factors in stuttering were bona fide, although largely serendipitous, discoveries. These discoveries derived from sequential analyses of a substantial language corpus, in which each analysis in the sequence led to the next one.

The Phonetic Factor

The research began with Brown's M.A. thesis (Brown, 1935), which was published in the same year as the first article in the series (Johnson & Brown, 1935). The study had a rather limited scope, the simple objective being "to ascertain whether stutterers experience more stuttering in relation to one speech sound than in relation to another" (Johnson & Brown, 1935, p. 481). The major impetus for this inquiry derived from the not uncommon testimony of some stutterers that they find certain sounds "difficult"—testimony that ranges from claims of trouble with general categories of sounds (e.g., "gutturals") to specification of particular phones. The notion that stutterers have more difficulty with certain sounds than with others has a lengthy history, and still persists. This notion overlaps extensively with the claim of "feared" sounds, a description that appears in many different accounts of stuttering where it carries varying explanatory loads. It has long been closely associated with the purely psychological explanations of stuttering; one will find references to "difficult sounds" and "feared sounds" intermingled within the series of articles to be discussed in this chapter and Chapter 4.

As noted in Chapter 1, analytic observation of stutter events made by several authorities of the 19th and early 20th centuries provided grounds for seriously questioning that the problem in stuttering lies with certain sounds per se. Apparently Johnson and Brown had some awareness of the views expressed by certain of these writers but considered them to be essentially subjective opinions not supported by research. The intent of the initial study, as Brown (1945) later described it, was to "investigate objectively the introspective reports of stutterers as to their phonetic difficulties and the many widely variant statements found in the literature as to sound difficulties for stutterers" (p. 190). However, the objectivity of this initial study, and of the several that were to follow, was compromised by the orientation from which the work was approached. Johnson and Brown, both stutterers, evidently were persuaded that stuttering is a psychological problem. Johnson, whose influence on the Brown series is clear, had already (Johnson, 1934) given evidence of developing his extreme position that "what is called" stuttering is due entirely to external environmental factors.[2] There is no evidence that this psychological bias influenced the collection or compilation of data in any of the work reported by Brown, but its influence was unmistakable in the analysis and interpretation of the results obtained. Equally important, this bias materially affected the analyses and interpretations of much of the subsequent work that was addressed to the study of language factors in stuttering.

The psychological orientation dominating this research was expressed clearly in the brief introduction of the initial publication (Johnson & Brown, 1935):

> The point of the present investigation may be seen in the probability that if stuttering were due entirely to physical factors—were in no sense due to psychological factors—stuttering would occur with approximately the same relative frequency in relation to all sounds, or if significant differences were found they would be consistent in terms of the relative phonetic or physical complexity of each sound in question. The degree to which data accruing from this investigation cannot be accounted for reasonably on phonetic or physiological grounds should indicate within due limits the degree to which the occurrence—or rather the occurrences—of stuttering are to be accounted for on psychological grounds (p. 482).

The first study was addressed to the initial sounds of words during the course of oral reading, rather than from samples of spontaneous speech. Use of reading material, rather than samples of spontaneous speech, was intentional because of the various controls made possible. Accordingly, the authors prepared the "Iowa Oral Reading Test for Stutterers" which consists of 5 sections of 1,000 words, each made up of excerpts from various publication sources. Such material, properly described as "written prose," presents certain limitations in the study of oral language. Written prose is rather different from "spoken prose" which, in turn, is considerably different from ordinary speech (see the discussion in Chapter 2, p. 47 ff, and Chapter 5, p. 133 ff).

Nonetheless, a great deal of valuable information about language factors in stuttering has derived from work making use of written prose (and, as well, from other material even less like ordinary speech). In many important ways a reading of this fairly extended connected material could be considered analogous to ordinary speaking, at least in comparison to reading a series of unrelated sentences or words. At the same time, as I will discuss later in a more appropriate context, this particular set of passages has two features that make it unrepresentative of even written prose, and have contributed to certain inaccurate interpretations relative to stuttering.

The passages were constructed to include as many different word-initial sounds as possible, each of them being employed "a sufficient number of times" to permit statistical analysis. The material was kept simple in vocabulary and syntax, and as free as possible from emotional coloring. Note that a guiding principle in preparation of the material was to incorporate an adequate sample of the phones of the language in word-initial position. This consideration reflects an important point that is often lost sight of, namely, that the "difficult sounds" reported by, and of, stutterers are word-initial sounds (more properly, syllable-initial sounds; see later). This characteristic feature of the locus of stutter occurrences is so ubiquitous, and perhaps therefore so taken for granted, that much of its deserved significance is, thereby, frequently ignored. The fact that the great preponderance of stuttering occurs in word-initial position turns out to be one of the most central elements in the phenomena of stuttering. I will have much more to say about this fact in later analyses and discussions.

Data in the Johnson and Brown (1935) study were obtained from 32 young adult stutterers (26 males, 6 females; average age, 22 years), each of whom read the five passages twice. The resulting corpus thus consisted of 311,903 words spoken. A total of 30,131 stutters were recorded, amounting to 9.7% of the corpus (this value would later serve as a critical reference point).[3] From the data on stutter occurrences the authors were able to establish a rank order of difficulty of sounds, reproduced in Table 3.1. As shown in the table, most of the consonants rank much higher in stuttering occurrence than all of the vowels and diphthongs. This finding established one of the major conclusions of this study, and of the series, namely that "in general more stuttering is associated with consonants than with vowels" (Johnson & Brown, 1935, p. 494). Note that the word "initial" is omitted before the words "consonants" and "vowels." Almost certainly "initial" was implicit in the sentence, but its omission illustrates the point made earlier regarding the regularity with which this most im-

TABLE 3.1. Rank order of difficulty of sounds according to mean percent of stuttering[a]

C	%	V	C	%	V
d	21.7		t	9.1	
z	20.9		hw	8.7	
g	19.8		w	7.6	
tʃ	19.1			6.7	ɜ
dʒ	18.9			6.0	ɛ
v	17.4			5.0	ɪ
k	16.3			4.8	ɔɪ
θ	15.8			4.7	i
l	15.6			3.8	ou
r	14.6		ð	3.7	ʌ
m	13.6			3.5	eɪ
p	13.0			3.5	aɪ
s	12.4			3.2	ɔ
b	12.3			2.7	ɒ
ʃ	12.1		h	2.4	
n	12.0			1.8	ɑ
f	11.6			1.6	au
j	11.3			1.3	æ
				.8	ə

[a]In this arrangement of the data the "easy" sounds appear in the right hand columns. (Data from Johnson & Brown, 1935, Table IV.)

portant aspect of stutter events is, in effect, minimized. In this particular study, 92% of the stutters occurred in word-initial position; later analysis of the data in terms of syllable-initial position would bring this figure close to 100%.

Johnson and Brown noted in their introductory statement the possibility that stuttering might be found to occur with approximately the same frequency on all sounds, which they believed would suggest that stuttering could be due to physical factors. On the other hand, if evident differences in stuttering among phones were found, these differences might be rationalized on phonetic grounds; that is, stuttering might be found to be related to certain classes of phones, their manner or place of production, or some similar variable.

Their findings showed clearly that all sounds were not stuttered comparably, let alone equally. In their view, this finding eliminated an explanation in terms of physical factors. At the same time, there was also no discernible phonetic principle evident within the rank order of "difficulty" that emerged. Also, the general ranking did not apply directly and consistently to all individuals. Rank order of stuttered phones varied somewhat from one individual to another; in fact, the stutters observed in the individual speech samples even posed varying degrees of exception to the "general rule" that more stuttering occurred on (initial) consonants than on (initial) vowels.

The results of this first study thus turned out to be somewhat equivocal. Although the finding of individual variation among stutterers lent a certain support to the authors' preference for a psychological explanation of the results, individual stutterers were not sufficiently consistent in regard to sounds they stuttered to support adequately the original assumption that stutter occurrences are caused by fears of certain sounds. Nonetheless, the authors continued to believe that a phonetic variable, especially the consonant-vowel distinction, was an important source of stutter occurrences. Although the "general phonetic factor" suggested by the ranking was apparently not a strong factor (because all individuals did not conform closely to it) it also clearly could "not be accounted for by chance." To the authors (Johnson & Brown, 1935) it thus seemed "probable that this general factor is really a number of factors which combine to influence the stutterer's difficulties in relation to various sounds (p. 494).

This conviction regarding the focal role of "difficult" sounds was maintained consistently throughout the Brown series of publications, even though in the later studies other dimensions of language-relevant factors came into principal focus at the time. In fact, in the final article of the series (Brown, 1945) a phonetic factor was identified as one of the four dimensions by which words most likely to be stuttered could be characterized. This "phonetic factor" consisted of all consonants other than the five "easiest" ones, determined in reference to the general rank order yielded in this initial study (Table 3.1). As noted earlier, stutters occurred on 9.7% of the total words making up the data base; therefore, sounds having an overall mean percentage of stuttering greater than 9.7% were included in the phonetic factor. Reference to Table 3.1 will show that this 9.7% criterion excluded all vowels and diphthongs and, as well, the five consonants /h/, /ð/, /w/, /hw/, and /t/, in that order. These five phones were thereafter referred to as the "easy" consonants. It is pertinent to note that the rank levels of the five easy consonants clearly aligns them with the vowels and diphthongs; in particular, the rank values of /h/ and /ð/ are lower than that for half of the vowels. Of special significance is the fact that the lowest rank of all is occupied by the /ə/, the reduced or so-called neutral vowel.

The Phonetic Factor and Context

Apparently the authors, in reviewing the data obtained in this initial study, considered that factors other than phonetic ones—factors related to context—might also be related to stuttering occurrence, possibly confounding or masking the expression of difficult sounds. Therefore, a second study was undertaken to extend the analysis of "difficult sounds."

This second study (Brown, 1938a)[4] was designed to eliminate possible contextual effects and thereby permit isolated expression of sound difficulty. In this study the same 32 subjects were asked to read a list of 700 words consisting of 70 groups of words, each group made up of 10 words beginning with one of the following: 23 different consonants, 29 different consonant blends, and 18 vowels. Care was taken to separate, within the list, words beginning with the same or similar sounds and, as well, to prevent word orders that, spoken in sequence, might suggest or resemble a contextual sequence.

The results obtained through use of this word list made it clear immediately that context did have an effect on the occurrence of stutters. In fact, the effect was pronounced: only 14 of the 32 subjects[5] stuttered enough to make collection of data worthwhile; further, the majority of the remaining 18 subjects stuttered fewer than three times on the entire 700-word list.

This finding of a dramatically higher incidence of stuttering when speaking contextual material was one of the most compelling features discovered in this first series of studies investigating language factors in stuttering. Clearly, its importance was not appreciated adequately in this first series, and subsequent work has yet to develop its full significance. Brown accounted for the effect of context largely in terms of the grammatical classes of words, an analysis that will be reviewed presently.

Brown (1938a) reported a high correlation (.91) between the overall rank of sound difficulty revealed in the reading of the 700-word list and the rank order that had emerged from the same subjects' reading of the contextual material used in the initial study (Johnson & Brown, 1935). Of particular interest (especially for purposes of our analysis in later chapters), this correlation between the two rankings of sound difficulty for the group of 14 subjects was considerably higher than any similar correlations for any individual in the group.[6] At the same time, the rank difficulty of sounds derived from the results of the 14 subjects reading the list of words correlated .73 with the rank difficulty of sounds for all 32 subjects reading the contextual material.

The several findings showing concurrence among group-based rankings of stuttered sounds suggested to Brown (1938a, p. 395) "that the phonetic factor is important and that its influence is fairly constant in various situations." However, the essence or the nature of the phonetic factor was not evident. Except for the apparent consonant-vowel difference, itself not complete, the rank position of the various phones, particularly the consonants, still could not be rationalized. A satisfactory explanation could not be mounted in terms of either phonetic principles, or the underlying physiological actions that might be attributed to them, nor in terms of a psychological reality they might have for stutterers. In neither study did individual stutterers show notable consistency in respect to sounds stuttered. Moreover, analysis of stuttering on consonant blends, done for the data of the second study, added to the evidence that, by and large, individual stutterers did not stutter repeatedly on a certain individually specific set of phones. In fact, 10 of the 14 subjects showed significant differences (in all, 63 significant differences) between the percent of stuttering on single phones and the percent of stuttering on consonant blends containing those same sounds as the initial component of blends. Brown (1938a, p. 396) endeavored to account for these "quite unpredictable and eccentric" differences as probably due to "the effects of emotional associations." However, this explanation was entirely conjecture; he made no reference to any evidence or indication from the data that might have supported this guess.

Clearly, the considerable amount of pertinent evidence that had been revealed in these analyses did not support the notion of "difficult" or "feared" sounds as either the source, or precipitant, of stutter events specific to individual stutterers. However, Brown, and many others to follow, could not abandon the notion of "difficult sounds." For Brown, at least, this conviction may have found support from the finding that the group-based rankings of stutter occurrence on the various sounds did show considerable stability across the two different circumstances (contextual versus noncontextual).

Again it seems appropriate to mention that, in contrast to all the variability, inconsistency, and differences found among individual stutterers, one finding did remain constant across, and within, all individuals: for all subjects the stutter occurrences involved, almost entirely, word-initial phones.

Grammatical Class

The focus of the third study in the series (Brown, 1937b) developed directly from the evidence of contextual factors that had been revealed so dramatically in the preceding study. It occurred to Brown (1937b, p. 207) that "one of the most obvious of these other [contextual] factors is the grammatical one." He therefore made a grammatical analysis of the reading selections used in the first study. Initially he used a refined system of word classification that yielded 23 "parts of speech" categories, of which 18 occurred with sufficient frequency in his reading material to permit statistical treatment. A rank difficulty of these parts of speech was established according to the record of stuttering occurrences obtained in the first study; this ranking is reproduced in Table 3.2. Statistical analysis yielded no significant differences between subcategories of the same general grammatical class, so Brown collapsed the data into the "conventional eight parts of speech." The ranking for these combined categories is reproduced in Table 3.3.

TABLE 3.2. Rank of difficulty of parts of speech based on the median percent of stuttering for 32 cases[a]

Participial adjectives	14.1
Proper noun	9.6
Gerunds	8.05
Adjectives	8.0
Adverbs	6.95
Nouns	6.6
Root verbs (in verb phrase)	5.25
Simple verbs	4.7
Subordinating conjunctions	3.8
Relative pronouns	3.15
Personal pronouns	2.55
Infinitives	2.1
Coordinating conjunctions	2.0
Prepositions	1.9
Auxiliary verbs	1.6
Possessive pronouns	1.2
Articles	0.6
Prepositions linked to verbs	0.0

[a]Data from Brown (1937b).

Grammatical class turned out to be a much more substantial and consistent factor than the phonetic variable. Some amount of individual variation was found, but individually based rankings generally corresponded well to the group ranking, namely a median rank correlation of .85. Also, individual consistencies were considerably better for grammatical class than they had been for phones: only four subjects showed consistency measures below .63. Further, in contrast to the phonetic data, the grammatical data did not evidence extreme variations for either the

TABLE 3.3. Rank of difficulty with parts of speech grouped into conventional eight classifications (median percent of stuttering for 32 cases)[a]

Adjectives	8.2
Nouns	7.65
Adverbs	6.5
Verbs	3.75
Pronouns	2.45
Conjunctions	2.0
Prepositions	1.75
Articles	0.6

[a]Data from Brown (1937b).

individual-group correspondences or differences for any particular individual. Brown observed that a relationship existed between the grammatical and the phonetic variables, noting that "a considerable proportion of the words included among the easier parts of speech begin with sounds toward the lower end of the phonetic rank of difficulty, whereas the more difficult sounds are found more frequently in the initial position of adjectives and nouns" (p. 212). This correspondence led him to question whether an actual grammatical factor existed or, instead, "if all the differences found can be accounted for on a phonetic basis." Here again, it seems, one finds expression of the persisting influence of the original beliefs regarding "feared" or "difficult" sounds; Brown was inclined to translate the clear grammatical variable into a phonetic one.

Brown undertook to resolve this question, of a grammatical versus a phonetic factor in stuttering, by making a comparison of stuttering frequency in two word classes, each representing an opposite end of the grammatical class ranking. He selected proper nouns as representing high stuttering frequency and articles as representing low incidence of stuttering (see Table 3.2). He then compared the frequency of stuttering on words of each of these classes to the frequency of stuttering on all other words that had the same initial sounds. He found that most subjects stuttered less on articles than on other words beginning with the same sound as the articles but, in contrast, more stuttering on proper nouns than on other words having the same initial phones. These comparisons indicated that the grammatical class of words was related to stuttering independent of a phonetic factor and, additionally, that grammatical class is more significantly related to stuttering occurrence than are particular phones. These comparisons thus augmented the principle findings of this particular study in the series, namely, that the relationship of stuttering and grammatical class was consistent from one stutterer to another and, as well, for individual stutterers from one time to another. Obviously, grammatical class had an important connection with stutter occurrences. Consistent with his orientation that stuttering is a psychological problem, Brown interpreted the findings regarding grammatical class by assuming that they reflected the stutterer's concern about conveying meaning. The point of departure for this interpretation was the clear evidence that so much stuttering was associated with nouns, verbs, adjectives, and adverbs, and so little stuttering occurred in relation to pronouns, conjunctions, prepositions, and articles, the word types often identified as "function words."[7] Brown (1937b) described the latter word types, or form classes, as "the parts of speech . . . which contribute least to the meaning which the speaker wishes to convey" (p. 213). In support of this claim he offered, as "empirical demonstration," the observation that in a telegram or a newspaper headline such words could be omitted with "the least sacrifice in meaning." In contrast, nouns, verbs, adjectives, and adverbs, often called "content words," were *pari passu* assumed to be word types critical to the meaning of an utterance.

Evidently Brown was satisfied that the clearly evident effect of context was adequately explained as an influence expressed in the grammatical classes of words. He did not pursue further, either here or in later publications, the matter of context and its broader implications which, of course, extend beyond the dimension of the grammatical class of words.

The final step in the rationale Brown developed, at this point in his series of publications, was to introduce an assumption with which to relate his appraisal of the meaningfulness of word classes to their different levels of association with stuttering. This rationale is best expressed in his own words:

> Certainly the stutterer is more unwilling to stutter on words which are crucial for the meaning of what he is saying than on words that are relatively unimportant to this meaning... the increased unwillingness to stutter on words crucial for sentence meaning should make stuttering more likely to occur on those words (Brown, 1937b, p. 214).

Stress and Position

The fourth article in the series (Brown, 1938b) dealt with stuttering occurrence relative to word stress (in his usage, word accent) and to words in early sentence positions. Brown explained that the reason for studying stuttering occurrence on words found in early positions (of what might be called expressive units: sentences, paragraphs, sections of the reading material utilized) was based on the frequent testimony of stutterers that they have trouble "getting started" but then have less difficulty in later parts of an utterance. He gave no reason for studying stuttering occurrence relative to word stress, nor why investigation of word stress was pursued jointly with the study of word position influences. Since, of the two variables, word position turned out to be the less impressive in its relation to stuttering, I will discuss it first.

Brown focused his investigation of word position on the first three words of sentences and paragraphs, evidently in consideration of stutterers' complaints, as mentioned earlier, but perhaps also from an awareness of findings obtained somewhat earlier in an unpublished study by Milisen (1937). Again, Brown's analysis was based on the same corpus utilized in the preceding studies. He compared the relative frequency of stuttering on words occupying each of the first three positions in a sentence to the proportional incidence of stuttering on all words in sentence positions other than the first three. This analysis revealed that stuttering did indeed occur considerably more often on the first three words than on words in other positions. Eighty percent of the subjects stuttered first words approximately 80% more often than succeeding words. Stuttering on the second and third words occurred less frequently, but still notably more than on words succeeding them (approximately 60 to 70% more for second words; 40 to 50% more for third words).

Brown recognized that these findings might accommodate a physiological, or motor, explanation of stutter occurrence in that, with the beginning of a new unit of expression a change is made, rapidly, from a condition of comparative relaxation to one of more or less tension. However, consistent with his preference for explaining his findings in terms of the psychology of the individual, he accounted for these findings in terms of "prominence," an explanatory vehicle he would later use in a more comprehensive matter. In this instance he claimed that words in early utterance positions are more prominent (than later words) in the speech sequence "because they introduce a new statement or idea," and that therefore a stutterer will make more of an effort to speak these words fluently (such extra effort presumably resulting in the word being stuttered).

Brown's analysis regarding word stress revealed a very high correspondence between this variable and stutter occurrences. Actually, this particular concurrence was the most impressive finding newly revealed in Brown's work. Even more than for grammatical class, stuttering was consistently associated with word stress. All 32 subjects stuttered much more on stressed than on unstressed syllables in the 3,276 polysyllabic words contained in the material he used. In fact, for 28 subjects these differences were statistically significant. The concurrence of stuttering and stress was even more impressive when word stress occurred on the first syllable of the polysyllabic words: all subjects had significantly more stuttering on stressed first syllables than on any unstressed following syllables. The variable of word stress even showed some salience over word-initial position. Stuttering was much more likely to occur on stressed first syllables than on unstressed first syllables; also, for words in which stress occurred on a syllable other than the first, stuttering was more likely to occur on the stressed syllable than on the first syllable.

Brown mentioned more than one possible explanation for these findings, including consideration of data from sources that were pertinent to a physiological account of the results. However, consistent with his psychological orientation, he accounted for the evident influence of both sentence position and word stress in terms of their "prominence" in the speech sequence—a prominence that presumably excites the stutterer's effort to avoid stuttering at those points. Such effort or "struggle," it was presumed, is manifested as stuttering.

In spite of his results that revealed the marked concurrence of stuttering and word stress, the original supposition regarding "feared" or "difficult" sounds continued to have a determining effect on his analyses. In this particular instance, Brown noted a possible physiological explanation of the effect of stress, and he cited evidence from relevant research by Tiffin and Steer (1937),[8] conducted with normal speakers, which showed that stressed syllables are characterized by longer duration, greater intensity, and higher pitch than are unstressed syllables.

Brown acknowledged that such differences between stressed and unstressed syllables "may be in part responsible" for the substantial incidence of stuttering on stressed syllables, but he discounted this possibility because, in his conception, these differences were not focal to the stutter event. He pointed out that the increased duration, intensity and pitch reported for stressed syllables involved the vowels of the syllables. Vowels, he pointed out, were usually not the initial sounds of syllables, and also not often stuttered. To the contrary, he emphasized, those sounds most often stuttered, and also most often syllable-initial, were predominantly consonants. Thus, stress could not be directly responsible for stutter occurrences, he maintained, because stuttering occurred on consonants.[9] His only adjustment to the possible involvement of the stressed vowels was his suggestion that perhaps *anticipation*[10] of the greater demands posed by these stressed vowels, rather than the demands themselves, elicited the increased stuttering on the consonants of the stressed syllable. This suggestion was consistent with his notion of "prominence," and preserved the role of consonants as the difficult sounds. The essence of his view of the matter is summed up succinctly in his statement (Brown, 1938b) that "the majority of syllables, however, whether accented or not, begin with consonants" (p. 117).

An Interim Review

In the next two papers (Brown, 1938c; 1943[11]) Brown reviewed the results he had reported to that time, namely, the evident relationship of stutter occurrence to the variables of phonetic type, grammatical class, sentence position of words, and syllable stress of words. The reviews included a restatement of his analyses and a consolidation of the general psychologically based interpretation that focused on "prominence" or "conspicuousness" of words, presumably expressed through the agency of the four variables noted previously. In both of these papers he attempted to interweave prominence with meaningfulness, but could do so only for the variables of grammatical class and phoneme type. He related meaning to grammatical class as he had before, namely that content words (those stuttered most) are more important to the meaning of an utterance. The phonetic factor, in the form of the consonant-vowel distinction, was now rationalized as representing meaningfulness through the claim that consonants have "greater relative importance for clarity and distinctness, and hence meaning" (Brown, 1938c, p. 227; 1943, p. 197). Brown acknowledged (1943, p. 198) that sentence position does not contribute to meaning, but early sentence position seemed to be easily explained as another form of prominence. Word stress was also included under the rubric of prominence, although Brown did not explain his reasons for placing it under that heading.

Word Length

Brown's next analysis, addressed to the variable of word length (Brown & Moren, 1942), was precipitated by the study by Milisen (1937) in which it was found that frequency of stuttering varied directly with word length. The Milisen data were derived from a study addressed to anticipation of stuttering in which the procedure employed a format using single words. Brown believed that the effect of word length should be assessed relative to connected utterance which, of course, his corpus could provide.

Rather than analyze the lengths of all the words stuttered in his extensive data, Brown limited the analysis to two grammatical classes: adjectives, the word class having the highest incidence of stuttering, and prepositions, the class having next to the lowest incidence. Use of these two representative classes also provided a control for the grammatical factor. He used two measures of length: number of syllables and number of letters; he did not explain why he used letters instead of phones. The "phonetic difficulty" of each length level was then recorded in order to assess the extent to which this variable might contribute to, or qualify, the variable of word length.

Results of the analysis revealed that word length was directly related to stuttering occurrence. A steady increase in percent stuttering accompanied a progressive increase in number of syllables; a similar, although somewhat irregular, relationship was found using number of letters as the measure of word length. The phonetic variable had some positive relationship to word length, more so for prepositions (rho = .68) than for adjectives (rho = .48), but overall this concurrence was not sufficient to raise question about the evident influence of word length itself.

As one could have expected, Brown's explanation for the relationship of stuttering to word length was that longer words "are more prominent in the speech sequence because of their greater duration in time" and that therefore stutterers would try harder to avoid stuttering on such words. According to the avoidance conjecture, such effort to avoid stuttering constitutes stuttering.

The Final Review

The last publication of this series (Brown, 1945) was a kind of recapitulation combined with a reanalysis of what were, to Brown, the most important findings of the several studies in the series. He identified phonetic type, grammatical class, sentence position, and word length as the four variables that his previous work had shown to be clearly associated with stutter occurrences and he presented, as the objective of the final study, the intention to address "the question ... whether these rather obvious characteristics are the only important determinants of the loci of stutterings, or whether there are other, possibly more subtle, attributes of words which serve as stimuli which may elicit stuttering" (p. 181).[12] Using a sample amounting to 20% of the words constituting the original corpus on which the preceding studies had been based, he assigned to each word a "plus value" for each of these variables that occurred as an attribute of a word. A word was given a plus value: (1) for "difficult sound" if the word's initial phone were any consonant other than /ð/, /t/, /h/, /w/, and /hw/; (2) for "grammatical class" if the word were an adjective, noun, adverb, or verb; (3) for "sentence position" if the word occupied either the first, second, or third position in a sentence; and (4) for "word length" if the word contained five or more letters.[13]

Figure 3.1, taken from Brown (1945) shows dramatically the relationship between stutter occurrence and the extent to which stuttered words were characterized by the four variables named (note also the relationship of this influence to stuttering severity, a matter that generally has received very little extended comment). Brown reported (p. 186) that the rank-order correlation between number of stutters and the average plus-value of the words stuttered was $.99 \pm .003$, and he referred to this "almost perfect correlation" as "strong evidence that the four factors considered [here] are adequate to account for the loci of stuttering" (p. 189). In fact, he reported that the analysis undertaken in this final study yielded "no indication of any important additional factor" (p. 189).

Commentary

Throughout this review of the Brown series I have reported his work with a minimum of comment, critical appraisal, or reinterpretation, endeavoring to present it succinctly yet comprehensively, with its original form and substance. As noted earlier in the chapter, the findings Brown reported in this series and, as well, his interpretation of these findings, had a profound influence on the investigations of language factors in stuttering that were to follow. It is particularly pertinent to note that the subsequent work proceeded primarily in reference to the substance of Brown's final publication, just reviewed (Brown, 1945). Evidently that article was accepted as the comprehensive integrative summary and denouement of the entire series, as reflected in frequent subsequent references to "Brown's factors" or "the factors discussed by Brown," meaning the four variables that he included in his final analysis (see Blankenship, 1964; Chaney, 1969;

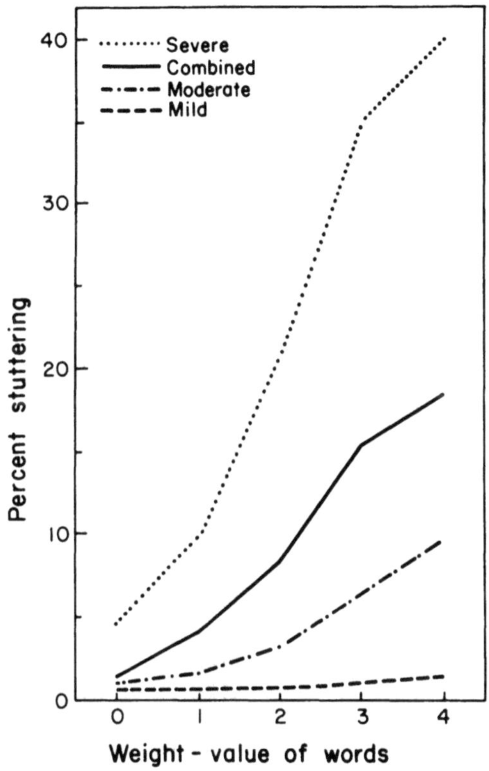

FIGURE 3.1. Stuttering as a function of the number of "Brown's factors" occurring as word attributes (from Brown, 1945).

Meissner, 1946; Oxtoby, 1946; Silverman & Williams, 1967a, 1967b; Williams, Silverman, & Kools, 1969a). Subsequent attention to the variables of phonetic type, grammatical class, sentence position, and word length was due not only to the fact that these were the four variables considered in Brown's final article but also because of his conclusion that these four variables were "adequate to account for the loci of stuttering" and that there was "no indication of any important additional factor."

Actually, this initial series in the study of language factors in stuttering identified *six* variables associated with the occurrence of stutters, not just four. The remaining two variables were: (1) word-initial position and (2) word stress. Brown did not acknowledge either of these variables in his final paper. In fact, he did not even mention them in his introductory statement of review that identified the sources of the other four variables. He gave no reason for excluding the variables of word-initial position and word stress; he simply omitted recognition of them. However, their exclusion was almost certainly not oversight.

Brown might have omitted the word-initial variable because he took this finding for granted, since even at that time the concurrence between stutters and word-initial position was widely recognized. Still, prior to the series of studies by Brown, awareness of this concurrence had been essentially clinically based, contained in the personal testimony of stutterers and noted by professional persons who had varying amounts of opportunity to observe stutterers. However, it had not been documented in any systematic fashion. Brown's evidence regarding word-initial position was therefore a bona fide result of his investigation, as much so as any of the other variables he reported (although perhaps not as much a "finding" in the sense of discovery). On that ground alone this result merited attention.

While word-initial position might have been ignored because it was taken for granted, there is no comparable plausible explananation for Brown's omission of the word stress factor in his final summary. The concurrence of stutters and stressed syllables was a real finding, a clear and impressive discovery revealed through exploratory analysis and disclosed for the first time in this series. On that ground alone it merited attention in the final summation. Moreover there are even more compelling reasons why both of these variables merited not only attention but special consideration.

It seems clear that Brown's concentration on the variables of phonetic type, grammatical class, sentence position, and word length was the result of the psychological orientation, directly representing Johnson's "evaluational" conjecture, that had given rise to this line of investigation and that surfaced persistently in the interpretations of results throughout the series. The four variables that Brown claimed were "adequate to account for the loci of stuttering" were variables that fit well into the notion of "prominence," with its encapsulated features of "importance" and "meaning." Prominence could then be used to explain stutter occurrence through the assumption that stutterers evaluate those words having some form of prominence as being words that require special effort—the special effort, amounting to "struggle," then being expressed as stuttering.

At one point in the series Brown (1943) acknowledged, briefly, that the prominence notion did not have very substantial logical support. However, he then immediately proceeded to contend that prominence, and evaluation were actually revealed by results of his studies. He said (Brown, 1943):

> It is hardly necessary to state that the "normal" speaker rarely "thinks" of the words he is uttering in terms of their grammatical function, the sounds they begin with, their accented syllables, or their position in the sentence, and though the "stutterer" may differ from the "normal" speaker in various other respects, it is highly improbable that he differs in this one.

However, he then continued:

Yet the statistical data clearly indicate that he [the stutterer] is differentiating certain words from the rest. Without being clearly conscious of it, the stutterer is locating an overwhelming proportion of his stutterings on words with certain characteristics of prominence and importance to communication, and this behavior seems to be most adequately described in terms of evaluation (p. 198).

In other words, although it is unlikely that anyone, when speaking, is thinking of the words they are speaking in terms of their prominence, stutterers must be doing so, subconsciously, because the data indicate concurrence of stuttering and certain attributes of words. Now, these attributes were ones that Brown had already decided reflected prominence because they were characteristic of words that were stuttered. The circularity of reasoning, and the non sequitur, contained in the previous quotation reflect the strength of the bias inherent in the orientation underlying these analyses.

By the time the final article appeared the notion of prominence and its presumed potency were well crystallized and firmly installed as a well-known, documented fact, as reflected in the following statement (Brown, 1945):

The findings of this study, and of the previous studies cited herein, demonstrate conclusively that the loci of stutterings in the speech sequence are not determined by chance. They depend on the stutterer's evaluation of words as being prominent and his desperate desire to avoid stuttering at those points at which for any reason stuttering would be especially conspicuous. The evaluation of certain words as being more prominent than others cannot be altered. It occurs in nonstutterers, [sic.] and it is impossible to imagine how speech can occur without some sort of awareness on the part of the speaker as to the relative importance of the words he is speaking . . . [14] It seems reasonable, then, to say that both stutterers and nonstutterers [sic.] evaluate the prominence of the words they speak in terms of the four factors of phonetic value, grammatical function, position, and length (p. 191).

Although he acknowledged that prominence might possibly be occasioned by "other as yet undetermined attributes," he made no mention of word-initial position or word stress, attributes whose concurrence with stuttering had already been revealed clearly and consistently. Actually, either of the latter variables could have been shown to have as much association with stuttering as the combined value of all four of the variables he chose to consider. Word-initial position alone could provide as comprehensive, and considerably more parsimonious, a basis to account for stutter occurrences. If one were to make the slight adjustment from "word initial" to "syllable initial" then in Brown's (1938c) own words: "Less than one half of one percent of all spasms studied did not occur on the initial sound of a syllable, either at the beginning of a word or within it" (p. 227). Brown did not make a comparably relevant statement regarding word stress, and his data for this variable are not as readily amenable to succinct recapitulation. However, the remarkable concurrence of word stress and stuttering (presented earlier in this chapter, "Stress and Position") reveal it as a variable superior in value to all of the four variables that Brown preferred.

I will deal more extensively with all six of these variables in the analyses to be developed in Chapter 5.

Footnotes

[1]Research interest within this general area has placed much more emphasis on possible motor factors (in recent years, for example: Cross & Olson, 1987; McClean, Goldsmith & Cerf, 1984; Tornick & Bloodstein, 1976; Zimmerman, 1980a, 1980b, 1980c; and the International Conference on Speech Motor Dynamics in Stuttering held in Nijmegen, The Netherlands, in 1985). A particular focus in recent times has been the recurrence of attention to phonation (see review by Freeman, 1979; later examples include: Conture, Schwartz, & Brewer, 1985; Ingham, Montgomery, & Ulliana, 1983; Reich, Till, & Goldsmith, 1981). This revival of interest in phonation was precipitated by two articles (Wingate, 1969a, 1970b) that were intended to direct attention to prosodic features in stuttering. In using the term "vocalization" in those articles I had not intended "phonation," as was erroneously assumed (see Wingate, 1979c).

[2]The so-called evaluational "theory" mentioned in the first two chapters. In addition to the reference cited, another publication (Johnson & Knott, 1955) reveals the extent to which the evaluational conjecture had been developed by the time the S.F. Brown series began. The Johnson and Knott reference, although not formally into print until 1955, was written in late 1935 or early 1936. Johnson's statements regarding the "cause" of stuttering gained momentum and captured an increasing audience over the period of time covered by the Brown series (1935–1945). However, as noted in the text, procedure and data collection in the Brown series were not affected.

[3]The phonetic factor (see later in this section) would consist of those phonemes (all consonants) stuttered more frequently than this percentage. Additionally, the 9.7% value, rounded off to 10%, would later become a reference value to indicate "average" stuttering.

[4]Although not published until 1938, this study was completed before publication of the "Grammatical factors" paper, and it was a reference in the latter paper. The only rationale given for the noncontextual (word list) study was "to study the sound difficulties of stutterers in another type of situation" (Brown, 1938a, p. 390).

[5]Of whom "a majority . . . would be classed as severe stutterers" (Brown, 1938a, p. 392).

[6]The highest rank correlation for any individual was .81; the median individual rank was only .68.

[7]Also called interstitial, structural, or grammatical words.

[8]The work of Ortleb (1937), Schramm (1937), and Steer and Tiffin (1934).

[9]Note earlier discussion (Chapter 2) to the effect that stuttering does not occur *on* specific sounds.

[10]"Anticipation" is an absolute synonym for "expectancy" in the orientation to stuttering reflected here; the notions of awareness and apprehension are implicit.

[11]This paper, published in 1943, had been presented to the Congress on General Semantics in 1941.

[12]Note the omission of word stress and word-initial position.

[13]Brown's rationale for using number of letters instead of number of syllables as the measure of word length was: (1) that stuttering was as closely related to number of letters as it was to number of syllables, and (2) that number of letters is the best measure of the space occupied on a printed page. (The latter suggests a belief that seeing the size of a word would affect an evaluation of its difficulty.)

[14]This claim seems to be a direct contradiction of his 1943 statement (preceding quotation). It seems that a speaker's most probable, though still unlikely, awareness of the "relative importance of the words he is speaking" would be in respect to what words he stresses, but Brown ignored the dimension of stress.

4
Corroboration, Extension, Complication

This chapter is principally a synopsis of the research into language factors in stuttering that was published subsequent to the S.F. Brown series. A few of these studies were reported within a short time of Brown's last article (Brown, 1945), but the majority did not begin to appear until almost two decades later.

The chapter includes only that research in which certain language variables were studied directly or were manipulated in one way or another. I have excluded from consideration here the sector of research that assessed language aspects of stuttering from a more general base, namely, research that employed some kind of formal or informal measure of language related function. The findings from such research will be introduced in a more appropriate context (see pertinent sections of Chapter 7).

Early Contributions

Replication of Brown's analyses and corroboration of his findings appeared in the literature even before his series of articles was complete. Nonetheless, as the extension of this line of research proceeded, certain complications and equivocation began to surface, which confounded Brown's original analyses. Before considering this later research, it is appropriate to review the pertinent findings of two studies, done early in the same era as Brown's work, whose contributions to the study of language factors in stuttering have remained obscured.

Two Studies from the 1930s

One of these two studies was part of a doctoral dissertation done by Milisen (1937) that was addressed to the relationship between stuttering "expectancy" and the "frequency, type, and point of occurrence" of actual stuttering. This work, cited by Brown (Brown & Moren, 1942), actually yielded the first research evidence that word length and early sentence position of words are positively related to stuttering. The evidence bearing on these two variables was derived from two separate procedures, and thus the findings are not based on the same corpus as were the results obtained in much of the subsequent work. Still, the evidence is highly consistent with findings yielded in later investigations.

Milisen's data on word length were obtained by having subjects read, twice, 100 different words presented individually on cards. The words were taken from the first 3,000 words of the Thorndike-Lorge word list; 37 were one-syllable, 37 were two-syllable, and 26 were words of three-syllables or longer. The distribution of 32 phonetic sounds in word-initial position was held relatively constant over the three dimensions of length. Milisen found that words of two syllables or longer were stuttered significantly more often than words of one syllable. This finding was notable not only for revealing a relationship between stuttering and word length but also because (1) the effect was evident for words spoken in isolation, and (2) the effect was not linear; evidently the important difference was between words of one syllable as compared to words of more than one syllable.

His data on sentence position were obtained from the same subjects reading four-word sentences, presented individually on cards. The sentences were so constructed that 61 different words occurred in each of the four positions. His results indicated a significant progressive decrease in frequency of stuttering from the first to fourth position. Since the same words occurred in each of those positions the effect was evidently due, at least predominantly, to early sentence position.

The second of these two early studies was not directly concerned with language variables; it was actually the original study of stuttering adaptation.[1] This research, conducted by Van Riper and Hull in 1934–1935 was not published until 20 years later (Van Riper & Hull, 1955). It yielded findings that are particularly relevant to the study of language factors in stuttering, although this contribution has gone unrecognized in the pertinent literature.

Van Riper and Hull were interested in measuring the effect of certain situations on the frequency of stuttering. As a reference base against which to compare the effect of the several situations in which they were interested, they measured the extent of their 31 subjects' adaptation to a constant situation. This was achieved by having the subjects read and reread a 133-word passage a number of times in close succession. This procedure revealed "a progressive decrease in the number of spasms from one reading to the next until finally a relatively stable plateau was reached" (p. 200) after about five readings. Then, with a view to determining whether the decrease in stuttering was occasioned by an increasing familiarity with either the syntax or structure of the passage or with the words or content, the authors introduced two modifications of procedure. They had the subjects: (1) read the passage backward, and (2) read a selection made up of the same words rearranged. They found that in both of these circumstances the extent of stuttering was essentially the same as that occuring at the *plateau level* of the adaptation series, that is, when stuttering had dropped to its lowest level in the readings of the regular passage.

These findings, which showed significantly less stuttering in the speaking of noncontextual material, were the first formal evidence that stuttering is related, as Orton (1929) had surmised, to "the plane of the speech effort" (see Chapter 1, p. 14). However, this evidence that stuttering is related to the propositionality of an utterance has not been noted in the literature concerned with language factors in stuttering.

Early Replication

The first research undertaken specifically in reference to S.F. Brown's work was reported in two articles by Hahn that appeared early in the 1940s. One article was addressed to phonetic factors (Hahn, 1942a), the other to grammatical factors (Hahn, 1942b). Hahn had available the protocols from a previous study (Hahn, 1940) in which he had investigated the influence on stuttering of presumed increments in social pressure. In that study 43 subjects had read prepared materials in four situations that ranged from reading in isolation to reading to a small audience of 5 to 10 persons. The reading material consisted of four versions of a 550-word passage, a different version of the passage being read in each of the four situations presumed to represent increasing levels of social pressure. In preparing the reading material Hahn had taken care to include in word-initial positions all consonants and consonant combinations that appear in that position in English. Evidently he made no attempt to adjust the frequency of initially appearing consonants in his material to represent the frequency of their initial occurrence in a large reference corpus. However, he did report the percentages of initial occurrence of individual consonants in his material, and from these data it is possible to establish a rank order of consonant frequency that can be compared to composite frequency-of-occurrence ranking based on extensive language samples (see Chapter 5). A rank order correlation of initially occurring consonants in Hahn's material with the ranking from reference material yields a value of .83. This value indicates that the Hahn material was adequately representative of word-initial occurrence of consonants in general usage. Hahn reported that the frequency with which a sound occurred in initial position had no appreciable relationship to its difficulty rank, that is, to the frequency of stuttering on that sound. In fact, the sounds that occurred most frequently in the reading material were not the sounds on which stuttering occurred most often. Hahn's report was thus the first to register evidence of a generally inverse relationship between stuttering occurrence and frequency of phoneme occurrence. However, Hahn did not consider the possible significance of this finding.

The rank order of consonant difficulty yielded by the Hahn (1942a) analysis agreed well with the rank order found by Johnson and Brown (1935) and S.F. Brown (1938a). Hahn did not report a correlation value for this agreement, but the present author's computation of a rank order correlation between the Hahn and the Johnson and Brown rankings of consonant difficulty yields a value of .84. The actual correspondence is particularly high in respect to the "easy" consonants, notably /h, ð, w, and hw/.

Hahn's findings regarding phonetic aspects of stuttering corroborated those of Brown in other respects as well. Stuttering occurred almost exclusively at word-initial position: he reported that 98.13% of the stutters involved initial sounds; the remaining 1.87% occurred on medial consonants. This pattern was closely associated with word "accent:" that is, stuttering on medial consonants occurred most often on accented medial syllables.

Hahn's subjects also stuttered predominantly on consonants. Although Hahn did not give overall figures for consonant versus vowel stuttering, his data provide the following contrasts. Approximately 1 in 5 initial phones in the reading material were vowels, giving a 20% opportunity for stuttering on vowels relative to consonants (all consonants combined). However, the overall percentage of stuttering on all vowels was less than the percentage of stuttering on *any* individual consonant, with the exception of /h/. As with the Brown findings, the rank order of consonant difficulty could not be resolved in terms of physical properties of sound production. And again, individual variation was evident in spite of the evidence of a group factor of phonetic difficulty. Only 17 of the 43 subjects had significant difficulty with specific sounds; 15 of these subjects were severe stutterers.

Hahn remarked that his findings relative to phonetic elements in stuttering most likely reflected the operation of psychological factors, but he recognized that such factors were not evident from his data.

Hahn's second article was addressed to the analysis of grammatical aspects of stuttering, using the same corpus used in his first study as the source of data. He, too, found that, for all subjects except one, far more stuttering occurred on nouns, verbs, adjectives, and adverbs than on words of the other grammatical categories. His actual rank order of difficulty of the several grammatical classes varied slightly from that of Brown's (see Table 4.1), but clearly "content" words were stuttered much more often than "function" words. Neither Brown nor Hahn reported the relative frequency of these two broad word classes in their material but, assuming that the material used in both studies contained a representative distribution (see Chapter 5, "Structural Features of Ordinary Oral Lang-

TABLE 4.1. Concurrence among six separate studies regarding the purported "grammatical gradient" in stutter occurrence[a]

Grammatical class	Rank expressing the "gradient"						
	Brown, 1937b (English)	Hahn, 1942a (English)	Eisenson & Horowitz, 1945 (English)	Hejna, 1955 (English)	Quarrington et al., 1962 (English)	Jayaram, 1981 (English)	Jayaram, 1981 (Kannada)
Adjective	1	1	1	2	3	2	3
Noun	2	2	2	1	4	1	2
Adverb	3	4	3	( )[b]	1	—	—
Verb	4	3	4	( )[b]	2	3	1

[a]All studies except the one by Hejna used prepared written material, read by the subjects.
[b]Alone among these studies, Hejna's analysis took into account the frequency with which words of each class occurred in the sample. Verbs and adverbs were not stuttered significantly more often than chance expectancy.

uage") of content and function words, the ratio would have been approximately 50-50. Therefore, stuttering occurrence would not have been a function of the relative frequency of occurrence of content and function words.

Hahn's data, like Brown's, also revealed the grammatical factor to be more consistent than the phonetic, with evidence of a strong group tendency that was "far more significant than individual variations." He, too, pointed to a possible relationship between phonetic and grammatical factors in their association with stuttering, noting that there was some relationship between certain of the easier parts of speech and the relative frequency with which the initial phone of these words was an "easy" consonant or a vowel. Although he mentioned that either factor might explain the other, he favored an explanation centered in grammatical class. Hahn was impressed by the greater consistency of stuttering occurrence on "those words which convey meaning in a sentence rather than on words less important in carrying meaning." Thus he concurred with Brown in judging that the single most important language factor in stuttering occurrence is that certain words (content words) are more important to the meaning of an utterance, and therefore present more of a problem for stutterers.

A Separate Contribution

One of the few studies of language factors in stuttering that evidently did not take Brown's work as its source of departure was the investigation reported by Eisenson and Horowitz (1945).[2] Eisenson's primary interest was in aphasia (e.g., Eisenson, 1947, 1954, 1971) and his writings on stuttering have favored a principally organic account of the disorder (see Eisenson, 1958, 1975). The article under review here (Eisenson & Horowitz, 1945) reflected these interests in that it was addressed to assessing propositionality in stuttering, using the term proposition "in the sense in which Hughlings Jackson first employed it in describing aphasic speech" (op cit, p. 193).

Eisenson and Horowitz had 18 stutterers read 3 selections, each of 130 words in length, that differed in level of propositionality. One selection was simply a list of words, the second was a nonsense passage, and the third was a meaningful paragraph. The same 20 adjectives appeared in each selection, and each selection contained the same proportion of other grammatical classes as determined by their relative occurrence in the meaningful paragraph. The findings are reproduced in Table 4.2.

Clearly the frequency of stuttering on the various grammatical classes of words varies according to the propositional level of the reading material. Of particular significance is the evidence that propositional level affects content and function words differently. For function words, individually and as a group, there is essentially no change in frequency of stuttering with variation in propositional level of the material. In contrast, there is evidence of a steady increase in frequency of stuttering on content words as the propositional level of the reading material increases. The finding that values for adverbs depart from this pattern was almost certainly due to the type of adverb appearing in the three selections, an explanation recognized by the authors. The adverbs in the word list "were all

TABLE 4.2. Percentages of parts of speech stuttered in selections representing three levels of propositionality[a]

Grammatical class	Propositional level: Word list	Nonsense passage	Meaningful passage
Noun	6.8	10.0	15.5
Verb	5.7	5.6	9.4
Adjective	6.7	12.7	19.4
Adverb	8.6	1.0	10.4
$\bar{X}$ content words	6.8	8.5	14.6
Pronoun	3.4	4.8	3.0
Preposition	3.8	3.2	4.4
Article	3.9	1.8	1.7
Interjection	7.7	11.5	7.7
Conjunction	3.4	1.9	2.7
$\bar{X}$ function words	3.8	3.8	3.4

[a]Data from Eisenson and Horowitz (1945, table 1).

formed from adjectives, consisting of words like *merrily, jocosely*, etc.," whereas in the nonsense passage the adverbs consisted of "words like *even* and *enough*." The meaningful paragraph contained both types of adverbs. These two adverbs types are clearly different to intuitive appraisal, which probably reflects at least two dimensions on which they differ objectively. One of these differences involves word length, a dimension already reported (Brown & Moren, 1942; Milisen, 1937) to be related directly to stutter occurrences.[3] The other difference between these two adverb types is in respect to their frequency of occurrence in the language. Word frequency is a dimension that later research would show is also related, inversely, to the occurrence of stuttering. Thus the adverbs contained in the word list of the Eisenson and Horowitz study, being on the whole longer and also less common, were the kind of adverbs that are more likely to be stuttered, whereas the adverbs in the nonsense selection were a kind of adverb less likely to be stuttered. This difference would account for the fact that the values for the adverb category in Table 4.2 do not show the same progressive increase in stuttering with level of propositionality as do the other content words.

Eisenson and Horowitz interpreted their findings in terms of increasing levels of meaningfulness. They characterized content words as "conventionalized symbols of propositionality" which, because of their inherent meaningfulness (they believed), were more likely to be stuttered than were function words. Further, they explained, the greater inherent meaningfulness of content words was accentuated when they occurred in a context, that is, as part of a propositional utterance. Thus, like Brown, and Hahn, these authors also believed that word meaning was the crucial element in accounting for instances of stuttering. Eisenson and Horowitz, however, did point out that meaningfulness is a highly complex factor "which interrelates with others, such as strength of stress, to create difficulty in the flow of speech."

Hiatus and Revival

Overview

For a period of almost 20 years following the publications reviewed above, attention to language factors in stuttering was essentially limited to investigations that made use of "Brown's [four] factors" in the course of research having other objectives (e.g., Jamison, 1955; Meissner, 1946; Oxtoby, 1946; Trotter, 1956; Williams, 1955). A revival of interest in the language factors themselves did not appear until 1962; it was signaled by the publication, in the same issue of the *Journal of Speech and Hearing Research*, of two separate studies, one by Soderberg (1962a) and the other by Quarrington, Conway, and Siegel (1962).

Before proceeding to review the findings of research published in the 1960s and later, several matters of general relevance merit brief discussion.

The Hejna Study

This unpublished dissertation (Hejna, 1955), done in the period between the first and second eras of inquiry into language factors in stuttering, deserves special consideration for several reasons. Uniquely in the extensive literature on the subject, Hejna's work was based on lengthy samples of spontaneous speech. His data were derived from recordings of 18 stutterers speaking individually, for extended periods,[4] about topics suggested by "cue" cards, randomly accessible.

Hejna did not limit his analysis to the four factors emphasized by Brown, but included the variable of "accent" as well. His findings revealed significant group effects for all five factors: grammatical class, phonetic (consonant-vowel), syllable stress, sentence position, and word length. However, certain qualifications in these findings deserve particular mention.

In assessing the phonetic factor Hejna took into account the frequency with which the various phones occurred initially in a representative sample of the total corpus,[5] a matter typically overlooked. With frequency of word-initial occurrence thus "controlled" only /ð/ among consonants, and the vowels /æ, ɑ, ʌ, ɚ, ə/ were stuttered less than might be expected. If he had analyzed his data as Johnson and Brown (1935) had, he too would have found /h, w, t/ among the "easy" consonants.

Hejna remarked on a possible relationship between the phonetic and grammatical factors. He noted that /ð/ is the initial phone of "the," and that vowels in initial position occurred predominantly among function words, "the less important grammatical categories."

Relative to the sentence position factor, Hejna found that the significant group effect was not evident until the second word, and that it extended beyond the third word. He suggested that the difference between his findings and the results of studies using reading material might be due to the greater freedom of word choice in spontaneous speech and "personal habits in structuring sentences."

In regard to the influence of "accent," Hejna remarked that, in view of the recurring clear evidence that this factor determines stutter locus in polysyllabic words, it may also have a similar role with monosyllabic words at points of phrasal accent in connected speech.

Hejna also noted that seldom did one of these five factors occur in isolation, and he suggested that perhaps one factor "may have brought other factors into focus on particular words." Evidently he considered the grammatical factor to be the one most likely to express this focus.

In spite of his astute observations regarding certain of the language factors in stuttering, and evident links between them, Hejna's overall interpretation of his findings expressed the prevailing theoretical focus, which cast explanation in terms of "meaningfulness," anxiety, stimuli, reaction, and the like. Subsequent references to Hejna's work have typically been addressed to his general findings and his overall interpretation, and have overlooked the notable special facts that have been identified here.

An Additional Variable

Research in the era of renewed interest in language factors soon added another important variable to those identified in Brown's reports. This new variable was *word frequency*, the extent to which a word is found to occur in large[6] samples of language use. S.F. Brown (1938c, p. 229) had once mentioned that stutter occurrence might reflect an influence of word frequency; he indicated there that investigation of this dimension was in process but thereafter made no other reference to it. Both Soderberg (1962a) and Quarrington and colleagues (1962) recognized a potential confounding effect of word frequency in their research and constructed their materials with a view to controlling for it. However, actual evidence that stutter occurrence is related to word frequency was first presented in a convention paper by Hejna (1963). Soon thereafter studies published by Schlesinger, Forte, Fried, and Melkman (1965) and Soderberg (1966) presented corroborating evidence. Word frequency thus became a fifth variable subjected to investigation in the revival of interest in language factors in stuttering.

The Assumption of Hierarchy

A second feature of general significance that emerged in this era of renewed attention to language variables was the persisting theme of a search for the most important variable among the five that now constituted the field of attention; at least, investigators seemed intent on developing evidence for a rank ordering of the relative importance of the several variables. The presence of such a theme suggested that investigators expected to isolate the major determinant from among these five variables.

Although there were evident differences among investigators in regard to which variable(s) they believed to be the most important, the phonetic variable (essentially, the consonant-vowel distinction) and the grammatical class variable received proportionately more attention than the others. Grammatical class, in particular, was a major focus and seemed to reflect a persisting persuasion, carried over from Brown's work, that word meaningfulness was at the core of the relation between stuttering occurrence and the language variables. However, in this new era the focus on meaningfulness shifted, for a period of several years, to an emphasis on the notion of "information load."

The Information Load Episode

The "information load" construct appeared in a number of studies over the first 10 years of this era (for instance, Quarrington, 1965; Schlesinger et al., 1965; Soderberg, 1967, 1969, 1971; Taylor, 1966a, 1966b). The notion of information load clearly had considerable appeal to investigators of language factors in stuttering, an appeal that evidently was based on a presumption that information load was both a more objective and more expansive reflection of meaningfulness than the interpretation offered by Brown, for whom the notion of meaningfulness centered in the grammatical class of words. However, it is important to recognize that the information load construct did not add anything to our understanding of the concept of meaning, nor did it provide an improved vehicle for relating stutters to meaning. Meaning, in the information load model, is still restricted to the confines of individual words, as it was for Brown.[7] Actually, research would eventually yield evidence that several of the language factors already discovered by Brown were contributing to what was being identified as information load, but this correspondence was not generally recognized or acknowledged at the time.[8]

The notion of information load has been expressed in certain other terms that are presented as essential equivalents: terms such as "uncertainty," "predictability," or "transition probability." The latter two terms are actually the most identifying, because they reflect both the origin of the concept and the means by which it is measured. "Information load" derives from a stochastic model of the speech sequence in which it is assumed that the significance of units (in this case, words) can be described in terms of sequential, or transitional, probabilities. The sequential (transition) probability, or information load, of a word is determined by recording the ease with which it can be guessed, from whatever context precedes it, by persons reading the protocol containing it. A word's information load is thus represented in its predictability as the next word in the sequence, with predictability expressed as the percentage of readers who guess the word correctly.

There are serious limitations to the information load concept, and it is appropriate to identify these limitations now, so that findings in the stuttering research relative to this concept can be viewed in proper perspective. First, the theoretical basis from which "information load" is derived has been shown to be inadequate as a model of language formulation and expression (e.g., Bever, Fodor, & Weksel, 1965; Chomsky, 1965). Substantial evidence, yielded by several dimensions of inquiry, indicates convincingly that language is not organized or produced simply in strings of individual words. In fact, by 1965 models of the type underlying the information load concept had "lost most of the realism and appeal they briefly held" (Wang, 1965, p. 526). But the information load concept is vulnerable to critical analysis at a level of reflection less sophisticated than that of theoretical models. Even a relatively superficial awareness of the clear-cut differences underlying the production, as compared to the perception, of spoken language should lead one to seriously doubt that the meaningfulness of a word, for any particular speaker, is appropriately reflected in the difficulty with which that word can be guessed by a certain proportion of other individuals. Moreover, even if one draws the issue simply in terms of predictability, the performance of readers guessing items in a protocol is hardly an analogue of the processes by which such items are selected by the creator of that protocol.

Furthermore, the term information load is itself loaded with excess meaning. "Predictability" of words has a clear, direct denotative reference; it is also objective in the sense that it can be expressed quantitatively. The same can be said for "transition probability." In contrast, however, information load carries unwarranted connotations, of which the most insidious is the fundamental implication that the term refers to something more profound than simply probabilistic predictability.

The considerable appeal that the information load construct held for investigators of language factors in stuttering evidently was based on a presumption that information load was both a more objective and a more expansive reflection of meaningfulness than the interpretation offered by Brown, for whom the notion of meaningfulness centered in the grammatical class of words. But whatever breadth this construct may have had derived from the fact that it was compounded of variables that Brown's work had already indentified as relevant attributes of words. The scope of this equivalance should become fully evident from the analyses to be presented in the first part of Chapter 5, which identify relationships that exist among the several dimensions of word characteristics as they find expression in ordinary normal language use. For the immediate discussion, however, it is timely to identify and discuss briefly the language factors that have a clear relationship to predictability.

Information Load Substantives

Information load is, first, intimately related to the sentence position of words. This relationship happens to be intrinsic to the procedure for determining information load. It will be recalled that information load values are computed from readers' guesses of sequential individual words contained in a text with which the readers are not familiar. As one might well have anticipated for this procedure, it has been found that early words in sentences of such texts are generally more difficult to guess than later words. Because fewer readers guess them correctly, these words accrue higher uncertainty values, which marks them as being of "low transition probability" which, in turn, is presumed to indicate that they carry higher information loads. This chain of circumstances, having its origin in essentially a procedural artifact, thus yielded the conclusion that more information is contained in words that occur in the early parts of sentences, a conclusion that was accepted quite literally.

It is pertinent to note that the foregoing conclusion, generated through the information load procedure, is directly contradicted by less mechanistic analyses of the relative sentence loci of nodes of meaning. For instance, Boomer (1965) presented evidence that the point of major uncertainty typically occurs toward the ends of phrases. Similarly, descriptions of sentence structure in terms of "Given-New" strategies (Clark & Haviland, 1974; Osgood, 1971), indicate that the informative parts of a sentence are saved until last.

The fact that early words in sentences are generally more difficult for readers to predict may not have been widely known to investigators who applied the information load construct to stuttering. At the same time, there is reason to question how this fact would have been treated by the several investigators, had they known it. Taylor (1966b), who evidently was aware of the fact, provided a good example of the clouded reasoning surrounding the information load construct with her explanation that "stutterers will be disposed to stutter at the beginning of sentences because of their experiential knowledge that early words will be hard to predict" (p. 240). I doubt the existence of any evidence indicating that a speaker has difficulty predicting the early words in his utterances. In fact, research in the area of hesitation phenomena, using normal speakers (e.g., Boomer, 1965; Levin, Silverman, & Ford, 1967), yields evidence that a speaker typically begins talking before knowing all that he is going to say. In other words, he is relatively less aware of what his later words will be. This evidence is consistent with simple introspection; from well over a hundred individuals to whom I have put the relevant question, all have said that they would be more certain of the early words in what they were planning to say. Taylor's statement is based on a misapplication of the information load research; it contends that the words spoken early in a speaker's sentences are just as uncertain for him, the speaker, as they are for most individuals who might later read a transcription of his utterances. The evident presumption here is that word "uncertainty," which in information load usage is simply a statistical expression of readers' guesses, describes a psychological reality for the speaker. This presumption was criticized earlier in this chapter.

Information load is confounded by another fact of ordinary language structure. Research along differing lines of inquiry into normal language function (Aborn, Rubenstein, & Sterling, 1959; Goldman-Eisler, 1958b;

Nicol & Miller, 1959) have all found that content words are less predictable than function words. Once again, this is a fact that could be anticipated on the basis of even relatively minimal awareness of normal language structure.

Information load also has substantial connections with word frequency, as revealed by the following statement in one of the first publications (Schlesinger et al., 1965) that related information load to stuttering: "It may be concluded that there is slightly less tendency to stutter on words of high transition probability than on words of low transition probability *unless* the latter occur frequently in the language" (p. 35).

Within a few years certain research findings (Lanyon, 1968, 1969; Lanyon & Duprez, 1970; see "Language Factors and 'Disfluency'") provided evidence that word length is a fourth language feature with which information load is confounded.

The information load construct thus not only had certain serious intrinsic limitations, it also turned out to be superfluous. It added nothing of value to this area of research; in fact, to the contrary, the preoccupation with information load was distracting and confounding to efforts toward a better understanding of language factors in stuttering.

Language Factors and "Disfluency"

A third major aspect of the literature in this era was the appearance of reports in which attention was addressed to the relationship between Brown's factors and the disfluencies of normal speakers (Bloodstein & Gantwerk, 1967; Chaney, 1969; E.M. Silverman, 1974; F.H. Silverman, 1965, 1974; Silverman & Williams, 1967a; Williams, Silverman, & Kools, 1969b). Much of this work reported that normal disfluencies, too, were associated with many of the language variables that had been repeatedly found to be linked with stutters. These findings for normal nonfluencies were usually construed as evidence that there is no essential difference between stuttered and normal speech. Such conclusion seems to have been predicated on the motivation to present these findings as evidence that stuttering is simply a *degree* of "disfluency." In turn, this presumed evidence was offerred as support for the theoretical bias centered in the contentions of Wendell Johnson's "evaluation" conjecture. Most likely this predisposing bias was the reason that, as I will point out later, a recurring important difference between the stuttered and normal speech samples in this research was regularly overlooked—the difference relative to sentence position.

The Identification Complication

As discussed at length in Chapter 2, complications in the identification of stuttering arose from Wendell Johnson's effort to normalize the disorder by blurring the lines between stutters and normal nonfluencies. As noted in Chapter 3 these complications did not influence the findings of the Brown series because, at the time, Johnson had yet to develop his extreme position. However, much of the literature of stuttering that appeared after Johnson's major publications, in 1959 and 1961, has borne this burden, and its influence is clear in certain of the studies of language function in stuttering reported since the revival of interest in this area.

This complicating influence has found expression in two forms: a general nondiscrimination in which little or no effort has been made to distinguish stutters from other disfluencies (the form exemplified in the use of Johnson's list of disfluencies); and, a specific nondiscrimination in which one or two categories or interruptions in fluency—word repetitions and interjections, particularly word repetitions—have been recorded, analyzed, and interpreted as instances of stutter.

The second form of nondiscrimination turns out to be the most misleading and troublesome, for several reasons. First, basically because it identifies as stutters events that are not stutters. As discussed in Chapter 2, and consistent with the identification of stuttering stated for the Brown series, word repetitions and interjections may mark an instance of stutter, which they immediately precede, but they are not themselves instances of stutter. Moreover, word repetitions and interjections frequently are simply normal forms of interrupted fluency, which are found in the speech of stutterers as well as normal speakers. Simply tallying the frequencies of each type only helps to obscure the object of inquiry.

Second, these disfluencies, word repetitions in particular, are the most frequent type of fluency interruption, especially in the speech of young children. Third, the most frequently occurring word repetitions (again, especially in the speech of young children) are the conjunction "and" and the pronoun "I." Counting these repetitions as stutters seriously distorts several dimensions of data that are relevant to the analysis of language factors in stuttering. Undoubtedly, this procedure distorts at least three of the language factors: the content-word/function-word ratio, the ratio of consonants to vowels, and the factor of word length. Such distortions can only give an erroneous picture of language factors in the stuttering of early childhood.

Table 4.3 presents the kinds of fluency interruptions identified as stuttering among the studies, to be covered in this chapter, for which the information is pertinent. In most instances, stuttering is identified in terms of those disfluency types that have repeatedly been shown to indicate stutter events.

The Later Research

Some of the research done in this era was addressed specifically to certain of the language variables, considered singly or jointly. Other studies had broader purviews which, while having various objectives, contributed

TABLE 4.3. Kinds of disfluencies identified as "stuttering" in pertinent studies reviewed in Chapter 4

Publication		Revision	Phrase	Repetition: Word: ?[a]	Repetition: Word: Mono.	Repetition: Syllable	Repetition: Sound
Bernstein	1981						
Bloodstein & Grossman	1981		x	x		x	x
Hannah & Gardner	1968		x	x			x
Helmreich & Bloodstein	1973		x	x		x	x
Jayaram	1984					x	x
Kaasin & Bjerkan	1982					x	x
Lanyon	1968		x			x	x
Lanyon & Duprez	1970		x	x		x	x
Ronson	1976	x	x	x		x	x
Schlesinger, Forte, et al.	1965						x
Silverman & Williams	1967b	x	x	x		x	x
Soderberg	1967					x	x
Soderberg	1971					x	x
Taylor	1966a		x	x		x	x
Taylor	1966b		x	x		x	x
Tornick & Bloodstein	1976			x		x	x
Wall	1980					x	x
Wall et al.	1981					x	x
Wells	1983				x	x	x
Williams, Silverman, et al.	1969a	x	x	x		x	x

[a]Word length not specified.

data on all of the language variables, although often just on "Brown's [four] factors." With a view to presenting these findings systematically, the review has been organized in sections, each of which features one of the language variables. In each section the relevant data from pertinent studies will be considered regardless of the individual scope or objectives of those studies, as the data relate to the language variable in focus for each section. Often, of course, it will be necessary to include reference to one or more variables other than the one in focus at the time.

As noted earlier in this chapter, the renewed interest in the language factors of stuttering was weighted toward the phonetic and the grammatical variables, a weighting reflected in the first two publications of this era.

Consonants: The Phonetic Factor

The first publication in the new era (Soderberg, 1962a) was addressed to the phonetic variable in stuttering; specifically, to the frequently reported

Prolongation		Pause					Other	
Audible	Silent	Filled	Silent	Inappro.	Interj.	Staller	Hard attack	Audible access.
x		x			x			
x				x			x	x
x	x	x	x					
					x			
x	x							
x	x							
x					x			
x					x			
x	x							
x						x		
x	x				x			
x	x							
x	x							
x	x							
x	x							
x				x	x			
x	x							
x	x							
x								
x	x				x			

differential frequency of stuttering on consonants versus vowels. Soderberg used three lists of five-syllable phrases, each list emphasizing either vowels, voiced consonants, or voiceless consonants in initial positions. The phrases were "of low propositional value," controlled for Brown's four factors and also for word stress and word frequency. Soderberg found no significant differences in mean frequency or mean duration of stuttering between the three lists; however, he did find a slightly greater duration of stuttering on consonant-vowel syllables than on vowel syllables. These findings clearly served to question the claim that consonants are inherently more difficult than vowels.

Word-initial consonants were reported by Taylor (1966a, 1966b) to be the most important of the four factors featured by Brown. Taylor carried the theme of uncertainty into an explanation of stuttering that centered on the consonant-vowel distinction. These two publications, having similar foci, reported rather extensive analyses of the same limited data. These data were questionably appropriate for the purpose used, for the following reasons. First, they were obtained from nine stutterers reading the same

500-word passage three times in succession. The matter of using data obtained from repeated readings is itself a source of reservation. Furthermore, the data analyses were restricted to the first appearance of words that occurred more than once in the passage. A major effect of this restriction would be to bias substantially the content-word/function-word ratio. Taylor's resulting corpus contained 289 words, of which 239 had a consonant in initial position. Although the initial data analysis showed a differential effect of grammatical class (context versus function words) this difference reportedly disappeared when controlled for initial phone.

Taylor concluded that the combined analyses of her data showed that the consonant-vowel difference made the greatest contribution to stuttering, followed by the variable of word position and then word length. In summary she concluded that these three variables all "describe words of more, rather than less, uncertainty" (1966b, p. 241). This interpretation made it possible to incorporate all three variables into the information load concept.

Apparently Taylor was not convinced that the consonant-vowel factor was adequately explained by "uncertainty."[9] She suggested that "an additional factor of articulatory complexity" contributed to the apparent preeminence of the consonant effect on stuttering. However, she rationalized this hypothesized factor of articulatory complexity only in general terms; she could not justify it in respect to consonant type any more than could Johnson and Brown.

The differential effect of consonants versus vowels continued to be assessed in research that, similar to research in the interim period, pursued other objectives in the course of which speech samples were anayzed in reference to Brown's factors (Bloodstein & Grossman, 1981; Griggs & Still, 1979; Jayaram, 1981; Williams, Silverman, & Kools, 1969b). The results obtained in these studies also corroborated Brown's findings regarding the phonetic factor; namely that, in general, more stuttering occurs on consonants (other than the "easy" ones) but, at the same time, that individual differences are clearly evident within this group pattern.

Several studies extended investigation of the evident consonantal contribution to stuttering by analyzing the influence on stuttering of certain distinctive features of consonants. Soderberg (1972) developed a list of pairs of nonsense syllables in which the second item of a pair differed in either one, two, or three distinctive features from the first item of the pair. The three distinctive features manipulated were: place, manner of articulation, and voicing. Twenty young adult male stutterers each read the paired syllables five times consecutively at maximum rate. Significantly more stuttering occurred on the consonant of the first syllable of the pair when the consonant of the second syllable differed by one distinctive feature than when the second consonant was the same as the first one or differed from it by two or three distinctive features. These somewhat equivocal findings did not conform to expectation, but were considered by the author to suggest that phonetic context contributes to the occurrence of stutters.

A few years later a similar study was reported by St. Louis and Martin (1976). These authors constructed a list of 64 bisyllabic nonsense words, each syllable beginning with one of eight consonants that provided differences in the features of voicing and manner and place of articulation. Each consonant was placed in all combinations of syllable-initial position in either the first or second syllable. Eight young adult male stutterers each read the list twice at his normal speech rate; four subjects stressed the first syllable, the other four stressed the second syllable. As found in the Soderberg study, most stutter events occurred on the first syllables. Evidently some of this stuttering was influenced by distinctive feature contrasts contained in the consonant of the second syllable; significantly more stuttering occurred on the same first consonants when they contrasted with the second consonant in manner and place of articulation. However, the authors indicated that distinctive feature differences did not provide as good an explanation of stutter occurrences as did considering individual consonants. Although the findings of this study suggested, as had Soderberg's, that phonetic context makes some contribution to stutter occurrences, they also indicated that stutter events are not effectively identified in terms of distinctive features.

Wells (1983) investigated distinctive feature influences in spontaneous speech samples obtained from 20 adult male stutterers. She identified, for each subject, the total number of stuttered phonemes occurring at the beginning of sentences and an equal number of nonstuttered sentence-initial phonemes, with the two phoneme pools balanced relative to the number of utterances in each transcript. Consistent with the findings of much previous research, she found that consonants were stuttered significantly more often than vowels and, further, that these consonants were more frequently continuants or voiceless. In terms of the Chomsky-Halle system of distinctive feature analysis the feature (− strident) also was significantly more often associated with stuttered than nonstuttered phonemes. Wells did not present a rank order of stuttered phonemes nor identify the phonemes actually involved in stutter events. Evidently the influence of the four distinctive features identified (+ consonantal, + continuant, − voice, and − strident) was not cumulative; the only feature clearly common to all stutter events was that all phones were consonantal. Since the other three features evidently were represented irregularly in stutter events, Well's findings are consistent with previous findings that, although consonantism is apparently associated with stuttering, any crucial dimensions of that consonantism remain indeterminate.

Most of the research on language factors in stuttering has dealt with data obtained from groups of subjects. A study by Griggs and Still (1979) deserves special mention because of its focus on individuals. In view of the frequent reports of individual differences among stutterers, Griggs and Still studied the individual profiles in frequency of stuttering on Brown's factors in speech samples from six stutterers (two adults and four children). The samples consisted of approximately 3,200 words, overall, of oral reading by each subject, obtained in two separate sessions. Five of the six subjects showed the usual higher rate of stuttering on consonants; again, individual differences were evident in regard to particular consonants.

Content/Function: The Grammatical Factor

In presenting the findings bearing on grammatical class those data pertinent to (young) adults and those relevant to children will be treated separately, primarily because Bloodstein (1960, 1974, and elsewhere) has drawn the issue that "a true grammatical factor" is not present in the stuttering of early childhood. This claim will be discussed later in the chapter.

The Grammatical Factor in Adults

The second study reported in this new era, by Quarrington, Conway, and Siegel (1962), was intended "to clarify relations between grammatical form, word position, and initial phone" even though it "examined only a restricted range" of these three variables. Actually, the theme of this study centered in a concern with "meaning" which, typical of the research developed in reference to Brown's work, was structured in terms of the meaningfulness of individual words. Moreover, the study undertaken by Quarrington et al. was limited to words of the "content" classes. Their experimental materials, consisting of a series of 64 six-word sentences, were made up entirely of nouns, verbs, adjectives, and adverbs which the authors attempted to equate in respect to word length, frequency, and initial stress. The subjects were 27 young adult stutterers.

Quarrington et al. expected to find evidence that stuttering is associated with a "grammatical gradient." This term, and the concept it embodied, were introduced by Quarrington et al. although they erroneously attributed the concept to Brown. Actually, grammatical gradient referred to the rank of the four content-word classes (only) in terms of the relative amounts of stuttering occurring on words of each of these classes. However, the term implied the concept of a gradient of *meaningfulness* that presumably spanned the content-word classes.

Apparently Quarrington et al. believed that the evidence they expected to find would duplicate what they assumed Brown's results had shown relative to the presumed gradient. They seemed disappointed that the rank order of the grammatical classes in their results did not correspond to the one reported by Brown (see Table 4.1). Their results, although not the same as Brown's in specific detail, did show a clear effect for grammatical class (content-words versus function-words) and, as well, for early sentence position.[10] They interrelated these two variables by suggesting that the "unequivocal effect of position may be a function of a gradient of meaning."

As noted previously (Chapter 3), Brown explained the effect of word position as due to the fact that early words in a sentence are more prominent simply by virtue of their position. He did not posit a direct or intimate connection between word meaning and early position; rather, he presented them as different forms of his comprehensive interpretive notion of "prominence." However, Quarrington et al. evidently construed Brown's treatment of meaning and prominence as a statement that early words are more meaningful. This construction of Brown's interpretations was clearly revealed in their next publication (Conway & Quarrington, 1963) where they said:

> Brown suggested that differential stuttering frequencies assignable to word position may be due to differences in the conspicuity or "meaningfulness" of individual items within the speech sequence. That is, the difficulty which a stutterer experiences in beginning to speak may be related to the meaning which those earlier words convey (p. 300).[11]

In fact the main hypothesis of this second study (Conway & Quarrington, 1963) was that word position is interdependent with contextual constraint, that is, with the extent to which word sequences approximate standard English. Evidently they reasoned that in sentences having a low order of approximation to English the early words would be proportionately less meaningful and therefore no position effect would be evident in such sentences. However, their results actually revealed that, in the sentences representing each of the three levels of contextual constraint, stuttering consistently occurred more frequently in early positions. At the same time, the results also showed a direct relationship between extent of stuttering and the degree to which the sentences approximated English; in other words, clear evidence that the frequency of stuttering is related to the meaningfulness of an utterance.[12] Although the authors mentioned that this finding, reflecting a contextual influence on stuttering, corroborated certain evidence contained in the report by Eisenson and Horowitz (1945) relevant to propositionality, their interest remained focused on "the meaningfulness of contextual items in a speech sequence," that is, on individual words.

It is relevant to note here that information bearing directly, and negatively, on the presumed grammatical gradient appeared in publication by Danzger and Halpern (1973). They had 16 stutterers read nouns, verbs, and adjectives that were varied systematically on the dimensions of word frequency, length, and level of abstraction. The mean percentages of stuttering associated with the three grammatical classes were very similar and found to be not statistically significant. Although adverbs were not included in the comparisons, the results obtained for three of the grammatical classes presumed to constitute the grammatical gradient were sufficient to question seriously the notion of a gradient, among these word classes, that had some regular influence on stuttering.

Quarrington (1965) noted, in regard to the two preceding studies he had co-authored, that the "earlier failure to demonstrate the operation of information value at the word level might be due to the restricted nature of the speech act studied (i.e., seven-word sequences)" (p. 222). Note that by this time the notion of information load had supplanted the construct of grammatical gradient, with its emphasis on content words.

Because, as he indicated in the prior quotation, the verbal material used in his previous studies might have been inappropriate, Quarrington undertook to assess the relationship to stuttering of word position and information value in "a 95-word passage of banal prose" read by 24 stutterers. He reported that word position, word length, and word predictability (information load) were each related independently to stutter occurrence, but that word position was the more potent factor.

Somewhat later Lanyon (1969), reanalyzing these data with controls for word length and information load separately, obtained somewhat different results. The studies reported by Lanyon were unique in this area of research in that his analyses were based on sizable samples of spontaneous speech, rather than prepared material that subjects read. The samples, obtained from three (Lanyon, 1968) and eight (Lanyon, 1969; Lanyon & Duprez, 1970) young adult stutterers, were analyzed for the relationship of stutters to information load, word length, sentence position, and initial sound.

Lanyon found that stutters were directly related only to word length. He also found that word length was related directly, but separately, to stuttering and to initial sound. Lanyon reanalyzed Quarrington's (1965) data, which had yielded a low but significant correlation (.32) between stuttering and information load. When these data were recomputed with the effect of word length held constant, the remaining partial correlation between stuttering and information load was much lower (.16), and nonsignificant. Quarrington's data had also yielded a significant correlation (.43) between stuttering and word length; Lanyon found that this correlation remained comparable (.36), and significant, even when information load was held constant. Thus the Quarrington data, obtained from stutterers reading a prepared passage, yielded results consistent with Lanyon's findings based on stutterers' spontaneous speech. Lanyon concluded that the relationship that had been claimed to exist between information load and stuttering was probably mediated by word length, the evidently more basic variable. Later Soderberg (1971) also found that word length and information value are interrelated.

As noted in the "Hiatus and Revival" section of this chapter, information load could be shown to be confounded with word position, word frequency, and grammatical class. Lanyon's work added the dimension of word length.

Attention to content and function words, and their relationship to stuttering, was not entirely eclipsed by the preoccupation with casting explanations in terms of information load. Soderberg (1967) determined the frequency of stuttering on content and function words in speech samples obtained from having 10 young adult male stutterers read a 141-word passage. For his analysis of the data Soderberg made use of the Trager and Smith (1962) *phonemic clause* as the encoding unit of the study. He found that the difference in frequency of stuttering associated with content versus function words was significant for words in medial positions of clauses but not for initial words, final words, and total words. Soderberg noted that his comparisons of stuttering frequency on these two word classes might have been biased against finding consistent content/function differences because of a clause-initial position effect that favored stuttering on function words. The distribution of content/function words in clause-medial position was 41% content words and 59% function words.[13] However, function words and pronouns occurred with a frequency of 86% in clause-initial position, whereas content words occurred 92% of the time in clause-final position.

F.H. Silverman and Williams (1967b) recorded the total disfluencies, rather than only the stutters, of 15 young adult male stutterers reading a 1,000-word passage. They found that total disfluencies were positively correlated with Brown's factors, as had been found repeatedly for stutters.

Data from a study by Wingate (1979a) contributed additional evidence that content words are associated with stuttering more frequently than are function words. That study was concerned primarily with the apparent confounding of grammatical class and early sentence position. The major results of the study, to be presented in Chapter 5, indicated that, indeed, grammatical class and sentence position are confounded. At the same time, the results also showed that, overall, stuttering was associated more frequently with content words than with function words.

Griggs and Still (1979), studying individual stutterer profiles of the frequencies of stuttering associated with Brown's factors, found marked individual differences among their six subjects in regard to the frequencies of stuttering associated with the several grammatical classes. Nonetheless, there was still a significant difference in frequency of stuttering on content words as compared to function words. This difference was found in both group and individual data.

Research reported by Jayaram (1981) made a particularly noteworthy contribution to the study of the grammatical class variable in stuttering because it provides pertinent comparative data for a language other than English. Moreover, Jayaram's findings were based on samples of both oral reading and spontaneous speech in two languages: English and Kannada.

Kannada is a Dravidian language, evidently derived from the Ural-Altaic group, that is spoken by approximately 30 to 40 million people in southern India. Its grammatical classes are similar to English although, typical of Dravidian languages, it is characterized by caste classification of nouns, inclusive and exclusive plurals of the first person pronoun, and extensive use of verbal auxiliaries. The verb almost always occurs at the end of the sentence. Kannada lacks formal conjunctions and, being a "left-branching" language, it has postpositions instead of prepositions.[14]

Jayaram's subjects, all young adult males, were 10 monolingual stutterers who spoke only Kannada, and 10 bilingual stutterers who were competent speakers of both Kannada and English. The oral reading material consisted of English and Kannada versions of the same passage, which numbered 122 words in Kannada and 149 words in English. All words in both passages were from among the 1,000 most frequently occurring in their respective languages. The English version of the passage contained 55% content words[15]; the Kannada version contained 71% content words. The spontaneous speech samples were considerably more extensive; they were obtained in two separate sessions, lasting about 25 minutes overall, during which the subjects spoke on topics of general interest that covered as wide a topic range as possible.

Analysis of these protocols revealed significantly higher percentages of stuttering associated with content words, in both the oral reading and the spontaneous speech samples of both languages. Also, consistent with previous studies in English only, the relationship of stuttering with grammatical class was stable; Jayaram found that intersubject variability relative to grammatical class was considerably less than for the phonetic factor. The frequency of stuttering relative to the various grammatical classes was also generally consistent with previous findings, with the notable exception (see Table 4.1) that the frequency of stuttering associated with adverbs was less than for most function words, in both the oral reading and spontaneous speech samples of both the monolingual and bilingual stutterers.[16]

The report by Jayaram is the only English publication of which I am aware that presents these relevant data for a language other than English. However, Kaasin and Bjerkan (1982) cite a study by Preus, Gullikstad, Grotterod, Erlandson, and Halland (1970) in which Brown's four factors also were found to hold true for oral reading in Norwegian. Norwegian has certain basic structural similarities to English, in that both are derived from the Germanic branch of Indo-European languages.

The repeated finding that content words are more frequently stuttered than are function words has continued to carry the assumption, made originally by Brown, that the difference in frequency of stuttering reflects a difference in word meaningfulness. This assumption was finally tested in two studies that employed the Semantic Differential as a means of measuring meaningfulness. The first study (Peterson, Rieck, & Hoff, 1969) was undertaken to test the hypothesis advanced by Jakobovits (1966) that stuttering adaptation might reflect satiation of meaning. Peterson et al. had 14 stutterers read a list of 100 three-and four-syllable words five times in succession, for which they computed measures of adaptation and satiation of meaning. The data gave clear evidence of both stuttering adaptation and satiation of meaning, but the two phenomena were not related. The findings thus clearly failed to show that a reduction in meaningfulness played any notable role in reduction of stuttering; in other words, no support for the assumption that stuttering is some function of word meaningfulness. In the second study Peterson (1969) obtained semantic differential ratings from the same 14 stutterers on "evaluative" and "anxiety" scales for each of the five most stuttered and the five least stuttered words. Subjects' ratings of the 10 words were highly consistent on both scales. However, differences in scale values assigned to the most stuttered and the least stuttered words were not related to frequency of stuttering. Thus the findings of this study also yielded no support for the assumption that stuttering is some function of word meaningfulness.

Grammatical Function in Children

There are possibly several reasons for considering a separate treatment of language factors in childhood stuttering. However, as noted earlier, the issue has been drawn in specific reference to grammatical factors. Bloodstein has contended that the role of grammatical class is different in stuttering of early childhood than it is in later childhood and beyond; in fact, it is his position that, in early stuttering, "there is in reality no grammatical factor as such" (Bloodstein & Gantwerk, 1967, p. 789).

Early data offered in support of this position were collected in a review of clinical case records of young stutterers ranging in age from 2 to 16 years (Bloodstein, 1960). From information contained in these records he concluded that there is "a marked tendency" for stuttering to involve function words, "especially conjunctions, prepositions, and pronouns." Support for this clinically based description was derived a few years later from data obtained in a study of the influence of the grammatical factor in the spontaneous speech of 13 child stutterers aged 2 to 6 years (Bloodstein & Gantwerk, 1967). The speech samples averaged 883 words in length. The authors reported that their findings "were markedly different from those reported for older stutterers." However, the claim of a "marked" difference must be viewed with some reservation; their summary statement of the findings reveals something less:

> The stutterings of these children occurred on all parts of speech, distributing themselves to a large extent as the parts of speech themselves were distributed. To the degree that a grammatical factor appeared to be present, it was chiefly the pronouns and conjunctions which were associated with larger amounts of stuttering, and this excessive stuttering on minor "function" words occurred in part at the expense of nouns, which belong to the category of important "content" words responsible for most of the stuttering of adults (p. 788).

These findings do not reflect an inversion of the content/function association with stuttering, they only suggest some change in the relative proportions of certain grammatical classes. Moreover, the inflated incidence of stuttering on pronouns and conjunctions (and less stuttering on nouns) can be explained simply as an artefact of three common circumstances, namely that: (1) young children, in particular, speak in short utterances; (2) children frequently begin utterances with a conjunction or pronoun; and (3) stuttering frequently occurs in utterance initial position. Although Bloodstein acknowledged that the second and third of these could provide a likely explanation of their findings, he evidently preferred an account cast in terms of grammatical class.

In this work, as in his subsequent reports, the matter of mean length of utterance and number of utterances were not mentioned. Number of utterances is a potentially critical variable, because it could inflate the number of initial positions, and therefore bias the data as a function of the second and third circumstances listed earlier.

Bloodstein (Bloodstein & Gantwerk, 1967) contends that "a true grammatical factor... apparently comes into being... as the categories of words which are crucial for the meaning of speech more easily come to be regarded as important, conspicuous or forbidding" (p. 789).[17] The "categories of words . . . crucial for the meaning" are, of course, content words. Bloodstein explains how content words "come to be regarded" with such concern by assuming that the child only gradually becomes "aware of the constituent words as such" after which he begins "to formulate his anticipations of failure in terms of particular words in the manner of the older stutterer" (p. 788). It is by no means clear why the child's "anticipations of failure" should suddenly (or even gradually) center on content words, when his "failures" have supposedly occurred so disproportionately on function words. Bloodstein's basic orientation is couched in concepts of learning, according to which stuttering is acquired through experiences. Consistency of explanation would lead one to expect that if the child has experienced disproportionately more stuttering on function words in his early years of stuttering, this pattern should at least persist, if not expand, rather than change diametrically.

There are other serious problems with the account Bloodstein offers. The child's use of content words far predates his use of function words. In fact, his earliest, and fairly long term, use of the language is predominantly of content words: at first nouns, then noun-verb combinations, and the gradual addition of modifiers that are also content-type words. Function words are latecomers in the child's language development, and even at kindergarten age function words make up only a small percentage of children's word usage (Horn, 1926). At the same time, it does not seem reasonable to believe that children, at least by four or five years, are much less conversant than are naive or uneducated adults with a gross but realistic functional distinction between content and function type words. Evidence for this statement is contained in the simple fact that the child's use of his language has achieved essentially adult form by the time he is five to six years of age.

Several years later Bloodstein (Helmreich & Bloodstein, 1973) undertook to determine if the speech of preschool nonstutterers would evidence the same pattern, for normal nonfluencies, that had been found for stutters in the previous study (Bloodstein & Gantwerk, 1967). A similar analysis was made of spontaneous speech samples, averaging 801 words in length, obtained from 15 normally speaking preschool youngsters.[18] Results showed that the nonfluencies of these nonstuttering children followed very much the same pattern as had the stutters of the stuttering youngsters, at least in respect to pronouns, conjunctions, and nouns. Actually, the pattern was more pronounced. There were significantly large amounts of nonfluency on pronouns and conjunctions and a lower incidence of nonfluency involving nouns. Two differences from the stutter pattern were that these normal speech samples had less than chance frequencies of nonfluency on both verbs and prepositions.

In his discussion of these results Bloodstein made no mention of the possible role of sentence position but, instead, spoke of these findings as providing evidence that stuttering and the nonfluencies of normal speech are "in the main, different degrees of the same thing." This conclusion is unwarranted; to find that two sets of events occur under similar, or even identical, circumstances does not indicate identity, or even similarity, of the events themselves.

In the following year Bloodstein (1974) published a general statement, summarizing his previous work, that purported to describe how early stuttering differs from "fully developed" stuttering. The essence of the article is contained in his contention that:

> The stuttering of young children tends to differ from that of adults in three rather conspicuous ways: 1) there is more stuttering on pronouns, conjunctions, and possibly other function words; 2) there is more repetition of whole words; and 3) an unusual proportion of stuttering occurs on the first words of sentences (p. 379).

These three items are not separate characteristics; they are interrelated and, moreover, confounded. They are also inaccurate, and misleading, as statements referring to stuttering.

The key element of these inaccuracies is an error discussed earlier in this chapter: the policy of counting word repetitions as instances of stutter. Word repetitions are not justifiably identified as stutters. They may mark a stutter event, but they may also be benign occurrences—in the speech of stutterers as they are in normal speech, where they reflect some other aspect of the language production process.

This key inaccuracy is expressed as the second item of the foregoing list. However, it is essentially isomorphic with the first and third items, because: (1) most of the repetitions will be of pronouns, conjunctions, and other function words that (2) occur as utterance-initial words.

It is pertinent to make the point that the third item in the list provides another special focus for objection. In a subsequent publication Bloodstein carried this claim to the point of excluding sentence position as a factor in later stuttering. He said "it is significant from this point of view that the factors influencing the loci of fully developed stuttering are mainly attributes of words" (Bloodstein & Grossman, 1981, p. 299). He went on to claim that later stuttering, in comparison to the stuttering of early childhood, is related more to grammatical class, the phonetic factor, and word length. However, as we shall soon see in the section of this chapter dealing with Position, early utterance position is significantly related to stuttering occurrence at all age levels.

The formal embodiment of Bloodstein's effort to have utterance position be unique to early stuttering was that he made less issue of word meaningfulness and began, instead, to speak of early stuttering as being some function of "syntactic structures." In fact, this shift was largely responsible for a number of studies, by various authors, inquiring into possible syntactic variables in stuttering. These studies will be considered presently, in a separate section. ("Syntax: Clause and Sentence").

The most recent in this series of Bloodstein's publications (Bloodstein & Grossman, 1981) reported another study of the spontaneous speech of preschool age stutterers. In this case speech samples were selected from recordings obtained from five children, ages 3–10 to 5–7 years, during the course of diagnostic interviews or clinical sessions. The samples averaged 499 words in length, with an average of 62 words stuttered. Counting pronouns among function words, four of the children were found to stutter proportionately more on function words, one child stuttered content and function words equally. Consistent with findings of the earlier study, the majority of "stuttered" words were pronouns and conjunctions.[19] Again, the authors did not report data on mean length of utterances or number of utterances, but did acknowledge that the findings were evidently due to the fact that children often begin utterances with a pronoun or conjunction.

Three relatively recent studies have yielded findings that bear importantly on two issues in the foregoing paragraphs. It was noted earlier that Bloodstein had not reported mean length of utterance in the samples analyzed, and that utterances of short length might inflate the results found in studies of young stutterers. Findings reported by Kline and Starkweather (1979) bear pointedly on this criticism; they found that four- to six-year-old stutterers spoke in utterances of significantly lower mean length of utterance than did matched controls. It was also noted earlier that young children often begin their utterances with a conjunction or pronoun, and that initial position is where stuttering most often occurs. Recalling in particular that Bloodstein's reports have emphasized the extent of child stutters on conjunctions, it is noteworthy to learn that Wall (1980) and Wall, Starkweather, and Cairns (1981) found a much higher use of "the conjunction 'and' at the beginning of both simple and complex sentences."

In the interval between the first and second Bloodstein studies, Williams, Silverman, and Kools (1969b) reported a study comparing speech samples from stutterers and normally speaking children in the primary grades. The subjects were 76 stutterers, ages 5 to 12 years-10 months, attending kindergarten through sixth grade, who were matched for age, sex, and grade level with 76 nonstutterers. The speech samples, obtained by having each subject read, or repeat, material appropriate to grade level, were analyzed for the relative frequency with which stutters, or normal nonfluencies, were associated with Brown's factors.

Speech samples from the majority of the stuttering children showed a clear association of stutters with all four factors, the same as that reported regularly for adult stutterers. Of particular relevance to the focus of the present section, grammatical class (i.e., content words more than function words) was one of three factors whose association with stuttering was statistically significant (the other two were word length and position). Calculation of the frequencies with which the four factors occurred at successive age levels among these young stutterers revealed that only for the variable of sentence position was there any suggestion of a developmental trend. This factor's association with stuttering decreased progressively from the kindergarten to the sixth grade level. However, there was no concurrent increase in the grammatical factor, as Bloodstein's contention would predict.

D.E. Williams et al. also found that the majority of speech samples from the nonstuttering children evidenced an association of normal nonfluencies with words possessing Brown's factors. This association was, in fact, statistically significant for two factors: grammatical class and word length.

In contrast, the Brown factor least associated with normal nonfluencies was the factor of sentence position. Moreover, on this factor the speech samples from the normally speaking youngsters differed significantly from the samples of the stuttering children.

Harvey-Fisher and Brutten (1977), analyzing part-word repetitions in the spontaneous speech of five 4- to 6-year-old stutterers and nonstutterers, found that the stutterer speech samples contained more part-word repetitions which also were "inordinately likely to occur on conjunctions." The authors related the latter finding to the fact that, especially in the speech of children, conjunctions frequently initiate sentences and clauses.

Overall, the research findings bearing on language factors in the speech of young children indicate that the pattern of occurrence of these factors is the same as that found in the speech of adults, except that the expression of the grammatical factor is heavily influenced by the extent to which children typically use certain function words (mainly conjunctions and pronouns) as the initial word in their utterances. This finding enhances the significance of the early position factor, which will be considered in a later section of this chapter, addressed to Early Sentence Position.

Word Length and Word Frequency

Although the variables of word length and word frequency have occasionally been investigated separately, and also have sometimes been reported to be independently associated with stuttering, they will be considered in a combined section for several reasons. First, less attention has been paid to either one separately; more often the two are mentioned together. Second, in terms of the overall findings regarding their association with stuttering, the evidence is less impressive than for other factors. Third, at least certain sources (Schlesinger et al., 1965; Soderberg, 1966) have acknowledged evidence from the study of normal language statistics (Zipf, 1949) that the two variables are clearly related to each other.

Relatively more evidence has been published regarding the association of word length with stuttering, largely because in those studies making use of Brown's factors word length has been one of the variables patently included (Bloodstein & Grossman, 1981; Griggs & Still, 1979; Hejna, 1955; Jayaram, 1981; Oxtoby, 1946; Silverman & Williams, 1967b; Taylor, 1966a; Trotter, 1956; Williams et al., 1969a). As implied in previous references to these investigations, they have regularly found that long words are more frequently associated with stuttering than are short words. Several other studies, also mentioned previously, that focused on the relationship of word length to information value (Lanyon, 1968, 1969; Lanyon & Duprez, 1970; Soderberg, 1971) revealed that word length was actually the important factor.

Word length and word frequency were first considered jointly by

Schlesinger et al. (1965) who, in their effort to explore stutter occurrences as a function of information load, found that the dimension of word frequency substantially qualified their findings relative to an account in terms of transition probability. They suggested, citing Zipf's (1949) data showing the inverse relationship between word frequency and word length, that their findings regarding word frequency might actually reflect the influence of word length. Although they did not report a numerical value they indicated that their data showed length and word frequency to be highly correlated. In a subsequent study Schlesinger, Melkman, and Levy (1966) had 31 stutterers (20 boys and 11 girls, ages 8 to 16 years) read nine five-word lists that differed in terms of three levels of word frequency and three lengths (one, two, and three syllables) but were matched for initial sound. They found significant differences in frequency of stuttering between the extremes (high versus low) for both dimensions, with word length actually showing a considerably greater difference than word frequency.

Soderberg (1966) had 20 young adult stutterers read nine 10-word lists in which the words were systematically varied in terms of three levels of word frequency and three word lengths (one, two, and three-to-five syllables). He attempted to equate the lists for initial sound, grammatical function, and stress of the initial syllable. He found frequency of stuttering to be related to differences in values of both variables, but word length showed the more definitive relationship. All differences among the three word lengths were significant but only the difference between high and low levels of word frequency was significant. The interaction of word length and word frequency was not significant, yet Soderberg pointed out that his data showed that the least amount of stuttering was associated with short, high-frequency words and the greatest amount of stuttering occurred with long, low-frequency words.

In 1967 Wingate (1967b) reported the results of a study designed to assess stuttering occurrence relative to words of identical phonetic structure but of two different lengths. The test materials consisted of two word lists that were balanced for word frequency (and were roughly comparable relative to grammatical class). One list contained 30 pairs of single-syllable words, the second list contained 30 two-syllable words, each of which was phonetically matched to a word pair in the first list. For example, *fan* and *sea*, matched by *fancy*; *row* and *stir*, matched by *roaster*. The lists were presented to 14 young adult male stutterers through an apparatus that exposed the "items" of each list (a word pair or a bisyllabic word) at comparable intervals, and allowed the word pairs to be said in rapid succession but as separate words. Stuttering occurred significantly more often on the bisyllabic words. Word frequency was also associated with stuttering, but only for single-syllable words. Clearly, word length was the more important factor, and word frequency subsidiary; the two variables evidently were not additive.

Evidence from the study by Danzger and Halpern (1973), mentioned earlier in regard to contradicting the grammatical gradient conjecture, showed word length to be the only feature having a statistically significant association with stuttering. Word frequency was found to be substantially associated with stuttering although this concurrence failed to meet the standard criterion for statistical significance.

A study reported by Hejna (1963) focused specifically on the variable of word frequency. He had 14 young adult stutterers read a list of 50 words that consisted of 25 common nouns matched with 25 uncommon nouns on the dimensions of length and initial syllable and, of course, grammatical class. He found a statistically significant higher frequency of stuttering on the longer words.

The foregoing studies of the word frequency variable had explored it in the isolation of word lists. Ronson (1976) investigated the effect of word frequency within the context of meaningful sentences. He had 16 young adult stutterers, ranked according to three levels of stuttering severity, read aloud 36 sentences specially constructed to meet many requirements. An equal number of declarative, passive, and negative versions of 12 basic sentences were constructed of identical parts of speech in which every word began with a consonant. The sentences were also controlled on other dimensions, such as: sentence length, as measured by number of words and number of phonemes; main verb type; case relationship; and type-token ratio. Each sentence type was varied in terms of three levels of word frequency. Ronson found that word-frequency level was significantly associated with stuttering for the declarative and negative sentence types, but not in the passive sentence forms. He noted that this result was "possibly attributable to the performance of the severe stutterers" in that a statistically significant relationship between stuttering and word-frequency level held only for those stutterers rated as severe. He also found that the significant differences between word-frequency levels were essentially limited to the comparisons between the high and low frequency words.

Recently Palen and Peterson (1982) conducted a study with 15 young stutterers, ages 8 to 12 years, that essentially replicated the work by Ronson. Overall, their findings concurred with those reported by Ronson, indicating that among children, too, the association of word frequency and stuttering is influenced by type of sentence and severity of stuttering.

In summary, the research bearing on the relationship to stuttering of word length and word frequency has consistently shown that both variables are related to stutter occurrence. The findings also indicate that although the two variables are related, they also have partially independent associations with stuttering, of which word length is the stronger.

Cycles?

Although individual frequency of stuttering is some expression of stuttering severity, overall, stutters involve only a percentage of the words spoken by a stutterer. In other words, stuttering typically shows some intermittency. Such intermittency has been described as reflecting "cycles"[20] of stutter occurrence, for which one explanation or another has occasionally been advanced.

The topic of cycles in stutter occurrence is included here because it has been introduced into some of the publications on language factors in stuttering. Such cycles, that is, cycles in the context of language factors, will be referred to as "short-term" cycles, in order to clearly distinguish this as an area of discourse separate from the more general topic of cycles in stuttering which, for present purposes will be called "long-term" cycles.

The observation that there seems to be some sort of cyclic variation in the expression of stuttering has been noted casually by many students of the disorder, and the phenomenon has been considered formally by several authors (Bloodstein, 1969, p. 22, 1981, p. 34; Bluemel, 1957; Sheehan, 1969). Those works speak essentially to the recurrence of episodes of stuttering; that is, periods of time during which stuttering is manifest for several weeks or months, alternating with similarly variable periods during which the stutterer is symptom free. These episodes seem to occur relatively more often in children, but some older stutterers also report them.

The topic of long-term cycles in the appearance and disappearance of overt stuttering is not especially pertinent to the theme of the present discussion, nor of the book as a whole, and therefore it will not be considered at any length. However, a point should be made of the fact that in many individuals, particularly young children, stuttering is episodic, and this fact has a certain clear and potent relevance to understanding the disorder. The valuable contribution made by the fact of long-term variation in stuttering is that the periodic disappearance (or even diminution) of stuttering symptoms contradicts those beliefs about stuttering that attempt to explain it as the product of learning, or the development of attitudes, or the acquistion of certain (presumably unrealistic) beliefs about the difficulty of speaking. Proponents of such views would be hard put to give a sensible account of how such presumed learnings unpredictably vanish and then, after some unaccountable length of time, unexpectedly emerge once again in full potency. In contrast, credulity is not strained by assuming that such variation is an expression of maturational or physiological fluctuations, similar to variations found for many organismic functions.

In contrast to the phenomenon of episodic, or long-term, variation in stuttering are those fluctuations in stutter occurrence that might be said to take place within the span of several utterances. These short-term cycles refer to what is regularly observed in stuttered speech, namely, that relatively few words are stuttered and these stuttered words are interspersed among many other words that are not stuttered. Reference to this level of variation in stutter occurrences as cycles has appeared, almost exclusively, in certain articles published since the revival of interest in language factors in stuttering.

Application of the cycles notion in this short-term perspective first appeared in Quarrington's (1965) attempt to interpret what he called "the word-position gradient" as being a direct reflection of Sheehan's (1953, 1958) "approach-avoidance conflict" account of stuttering. Sheehan, in his efforts to explain stuttering as a form of approach-avoidance conflict, contended that the act of stuttering reduces the "speech-avoidance gradient" which, in Sheehan's assumption, builds up during intervals of fluent speech or of silence. Thus fluency and stuttering alternate. Quarrington extended this argument to claim that stutter events reflect "a cycle of avoidance reduction in the typical act of sentence production" wherein "the likelihood of stuttering on any particular word is some function of the amount of stuttering present on the preceding word or words." (Quarrington, 1965, p. 223). Quarrington presented this account as an explanation for his finding of a highly significant correlation between stuttering and word position, although he did not not present evidence of cycles from his own data. He did, however, mention that Hejna (1955), in his study of the spontaneous speech of stutterers, had found "a second phase" of stuttering "beginning around words occupying the 15th and subsequent positions" (p. 223). Quarrington's citation was evidently a misreading of Hejna's data. The significance values reported by Hejna for the word positions in question all indicate significantly less than the expected amount of stuttering (Hejna, 1955, table 22); that is, the data indicate exactly the opposite of Quarrington's citation. Actually, Hejna's data indicated continuing decrease in the frequency of stuttering over utterance lengths of 30 words.

Taylor's (1966b) data had shown some alternation in frequency of stuttering over a nine-word sequence, with evident increases at certain word positions. However, the overall trend was clearly a progressive decrease. Taylor and Taylor (1967) tested the "conflict" explanation offered by Quarrington, using data from four of the subjects participating in the earlier Taylor research. Sequential probabilites of stuttering computed for these data revealed no evidence of any dependence between successive stutter events for either group or individual data. This analysis indicated that the "conflict" account was "incompatible with the actual statistics of stuttering" (p. 433).

Soderberg (1967) called attention to his finding, based on group data from 10 subjects, that over a 10-word span stuttering occurred "in vollies or cycles of decreasing frequencies" with high points at the first, third, and seventh words. Soderberg suggested that these occurrences were related to increases and decreases in word information. However, this suggestion evidently was based purely on the appearance of two curves on a graphic plot (Soderberg, 1967, fig. 1, p. 805). The relationship of the two curves reflects, at best, only a very rough correspondence.

It is surprising that these expressions of interest in short-term cycles, although appearing in the context of attention to language factors in stuttering, completely ignored the actually very considerable probability that the apparent cycles might be due to some combination of the language factors already identified as being related to stutter occurrences. However, the final two publications concerned with short-term cycles did attempt to incorporate such variables.

Still and Sherrard (1976) and Still and Griggs (1979) attempted to develop mathematically based support for their view of stuttering as a feedback problem. The Still and Sherrard report was based on only a single subject, which is always a questionnable procedure in studying a disorder like stuttering that has so much known individual variation. The study by Still and Griggs analyzed a corpus obtained from four children and two adults reading 200 words in each of two sessions. For their data the authors attempted to conduct a test that would differentiate between three "theories" of stuttering occurrence: the anxiety, the feedback, and the conflict interpretations. In their analysis they attempted to take into account the probable confounding of "sequential dependencies," that is, the relationships between words in sequence. Through rather sophisticated mathematical manipulation they incorporated consideration of Brown's factors and, as well, familiarity of the passages and whether first or second session. The authors interpreted their data as suggesting two probable trends in stuttering probabilities; however, this suggestion was based primarily on the results from two subjects. Although the authors seemed to believe that they could discern, in the findings, support for the particular viewpoint they favored, it is to their credit that they acknowledged that their conclusions were speculative. It is indeed difficult to appreciate the usefulness of their findings to an understanding of stuttering. It seems to me that their overall value rests largely in first providing additional testimony of the individual variation to be found among stutterers, and second, showing that mathematical applications to the sequential probabilities of stutters is no more meaningful than was their application to the sequential probabilities of language features (see previous discussion in the section on "The Information Load Episode").

It is pertinent to mention here a study addressed to short-term cycles in stuttering that was done long before publication of the reports reviewed earlier, but not, however, cited by any of them. This study, by Pittenger (1940), was reported in the same era as the early publications of the Brown series, some time before the study of language factors in stuttering had aroused any interest. The object of Pittenger's research was to determine if stutters recurred in some kind of cyclic pattern, particularly whether stutters were separated by some systematic distribution of fluent intervals. Evidently the research was undertaken in reference to a reasonable supposition that discovery of a cyclic pattern in stutter occurrences would constitute evidence of a physiological substrate to the disorder.

Data were obtained from the oral reading of 20 adolescent and young adult stutterers individually reading a 1,000-word passage. Oscillographic records were made of the intervals between successive stutters, as agreed by two observers, and these values were plotted separately for each subject. Pittenger used four other sets of data to serve as reference criteria for identifying whether the obtained stutter data truly evidenced a cyclic pattern. The four sets of reference data were: a "chance rhythm" obtained by throwing four dice 200 times; relevant data on the respiratory cycle; a normal electrocardiogram chosen at random; and mean values for electroencephalographic tracings from 10 normal individuals. As a direct measure of cyclic recurrence she computed individual correlations between the mean duration of intervals between stutters and the variability in duration of these intervals.

Pittenger's results showed that the length of intervals between successive moments of stuttering varied markedly for any given individual, being more pronounced in some cases than in others. It was also clear that these intervals did not show any consistent cyclic pattern, except that for some individuals the intervals grew progressively longer. In general the curves representing the length of intervals in the stutter data tended to resemble the curve plotted from successive throws of the dice. Generally, however, the variation in the stutter data was considerably larger than those for any of the four comparative criteria.

These findings led Pittenger to conclude that either stuttering is "functional" in origin or it arises from some organic condition that does not produce regularly occurring phenomena. An explanation of stuttering along the lines of the latter alternative is more plausible today than it could have been in Pittenger's time. Certain dimensions of expanded knowledge about stuttering, particularly regarding language factors in stuttering, provide a substantial contribution to understanding how the expression of a basically organic condition might be partially shaped by presumably functional elements. This matter will be considered in Chapters 6 and 9.

Syntax: Clause and Sentence

In relatively recent times some work in the area of language factors research has explored grammatical dimensions beyond the level of the word. Research having this orientation has sought to identify possible relationships between stuttering and sentence organization through the association of stuttering with units of constituent structure, namely, surface clauses and variations in sentence length and complexity.

An article by Hannah and Gardner (1968) was the first to report investigation of a possible relationship between syntactic dimensions and stuttering. These authors had eight moderately severe adult stutterers individually paraphrase a briefy story that had just been read to each of them. The resulting corpus for each subject (length not specified) was then segmented linguistically. From this segmentation the authors chose for analysis those clauses containing "no more than the three major syntactic units characteristic of the simplex sentence."[21] These three units—noun phrase, verb, and "verb phrase" (a noun phrase or adverbial type structure)—usually occurred in the order given here. Hannah and Gardner reported that stuttering was relatively more often associated with syntactic position than with syntactic function; that is, stuttering occurred more often in the postverbal clause than in clauses occupying the other two positions. The authors indicated that this "greater amount of nonfluency may occur coincidentally with greater expansion or complexity of the postverbal unit, particularly when the speaker must structure another complete syntactic unit and embed it within the initial base utterance in order to complete the thought" (p. 858).

It is difficult to know what to make of Hannah and Gardner's findings in respect to their significance for stuttering. Although the corpus was obtained from stutterers, the range of speech irregularities recorded and analyzed was evidently more comprehensive than simply stuttering, as the title of the article indicates. Indeed, they used "nonfluency" and "stuttering" interchangeably and, more specifically, stated that the "moments of stuttering" they recorded "included the sound, word and phrase repetitions, any prolongations, blocks and other filled pauses unrelated to the normal juncture phenomena" (p. 854). Even if this list is all-inclusive it contains more than stutter disfluencies. Other reservations about this study are that first, one has no idea of the extent of the material analyzed (all data were expressed only in percentages), and second, the material actually analyzed consisted of selections, from this corpus, that met certain structural requirements (identified earlier).[22]

With the foregoing reservations in mind it is pertinent to note that only 16% of the nonfluencies observed in the postverbal units occurred at a point where linguistic analysis would establish a functional syntactic unit. The authors noted that this finding suggests that encoding is a complex process and the phenomena related to it "do not routinely conform to syntactic relationships."

It is appropriate to include here a study by Soderberg (1967) which, although designed for other purposes, yielded important information relative to stutter occurrences in early positions. Soderberg analyzed stutter events relative to the *phonemic clause* (Trager & Smith, 1962), identified as "a phonologically marked macrosegment which contains only one primary stress and ends in one of the three terminal junctures." Although the reading material was the same for all 10 subjects, the number (and therefore length) of phonemic clauses varied substantially among subjects as a function of expression style. Significantly, stutters occurred most frequently in early positions, regardless of length of clause.

A study reported by Ronson (1976), reviewed in the previous section, was oriented primarily to the variable of word frequency, yet certain of his findings bear on the relationship to stuttering of syntactic complexity. As noted earlier, he found a significant relation between stuttering and word-frequency level in simple declarative sentences and negative sentence forms, but not in the passive sentence structure. Assuming that the passive form is syntactically more complex than the other two forms (in support of which Ronson cited McNeill, 1970, and Slobin, 1966), his findings would contradict the supposition that stuttering is some function of greater syntactic complexity.

A study by Tornick and Bloodstein (1976) was undertaken in reference to the evidence that stuttering is influenced by word length. Tornick and Bloodstein inferred that if it is motor planning that makes word length a factor in stutter occurrence then sentence length should also be a factor.

These authors had 14 young adult stutterers read a list of 40 sentences, consisting of 20 short and 20 long sentences, in which the long and short items appeared in 14 different randomizations. The short sentences, three to five words in length, also made up the first part of the long sentences, which were 11 or 12 words long. For purposes of testing their inference these authors compared the frequency of stuttering on words of the short sentences to stutter occurrence in the identical sections of the long sentences. The difference between group means was significant at the .025 level of confidence. However, four of the subjects stuttered more on the short sentences, and one subject showed no difference.[23] Also, although more stuttering did occur on the early words of the long sentences, stuttering on the long sentences tended to be divided between the initial (short sentence) part and the remainder (added part) in about the same proportion as the number of words in each part. The authors recognized that this finding might be due to the fact that their long sentences were composed of what was actually two separable sentences.

Tornick and Bloodstein interpreted the higher incidence of stuttering on the long sentences as being "caused by something we would have to refer to as the subjects' perception of, or preparation for, the greater length of the long sentences" (p. 654). However, one should also consider that longer sentences are potentially more demanding relative to several other influences, such as grammatical complexity, word frequencies, stress pattern, and other features.

Wells (1979) investigated the influence on stuttering of sentences containing varying numbers of clauses. She had 20 moderate to very severe adult male stutterers tell a story to each of five cards of the Thematic Apperception Test. From the resulting protocol she chose from each subject's corpus two groups of six active declarative sentences; each sentence in the group contained only one relative clause, the sentences of the second groups contained two or more relative clauses.

Wells found that the frequency of stuttering was significantly greater in the sentences containing two or more clauses. Additionally, this finding was positively related to rated severity of stuttering. She viewed these findings as suggesting that increases in transformational demands tend to be related to stuttering. Contrary to her statement that Ronson's findings corroborate this suggestion, his results, reviewed above, actually contradict it.

A study by Wall (1980) was addressed to the comparison of syntactic structures in the speech of child stutterers and normally speaking children. Wall obtained sizeable spontaneous speech samples from four children of each category who were approximately six years of age. The samples were analyzed for frequency of: complex sentences; main, coordinate, relative and complement clauses; and three types of "and" clause. (The several "and" clauses were included as separate categories because of the excessive number of "ands" occurring in the stutterer samples).

Results indicated that the stutterers used simpler and less mature language than the normally speaking children. One clear feature of this immaturity was their excessive use of "and," but the stutterers also used immature types of clauses more often than the normals, used fewer complete clauses, and showed less syntactic complexity in their utterances.

Wall, Starkweather, and Cairns (1981) reported a study designed to identify where stuttering occurs relative to the syntactic structures of sentences. They were interested in determining whether stuttering varies relative to sentence complexity, type of clause, and locus in a clause structure. Individual recordings, approximately 45 minutes in length, were made of the spontaneous speech of nine stutterers between four and six-and-a-half years of age. The extensive samples (809 to 1,780 words) obtained from each child were subjected to conventional constituent structure analysis after which stutter occurrences were noted relative to the structural dimensions of simple or complex sentences; relative frequency in 10 clause types; and position in clauses.

As expressed by the authors, the single most important factor that emerged from their analyses was the finding that stuttering occurs predominantly at clause boundaries (i.e., in clause-initial position). Stuttering occurred with significantly greater frequency on the first uttered word of a clause, whether that word was a "filler" (such as "well") or the actual syntactic beginning of the clause. Among the clause types the "and" clauses were more likely to be associated with stutter occurrence. No significant difference in stuttering frequency was found between simple and complex sentences.

The authors hypothesized that the apparent effect on stuttering of clause boundaries might reflect organizational activity at clause boundaries, as proposed in Garrett's (1976) suggestion that sentence planning is organized in syntactic units roughly equivalent to surface clauses.

The main purpose of the study reported by Bloodstein and Grossman (1981) was to explore further the influence of "word-bound factors" on early stuttering. However, they also sought information about the prevalence of word repetitions and the extent of their occurrence at the beginnings of syntactic units. This interest extended from the supposition that "whole word repetition reflects hesitancy in the initiation of entire syntactic units" in the same way that "part-word repetition or prolongation may represent hesitancy in the initiation of words" (p. 299).

Note first that these authors say that part-word repetitions and prolongations may be only "hesitancy." Second, note that whole-word repetitions are accorded the same status relative to large portions of an utterance (syntactic units) as part-word disfluencies are for small ones (words). Thus word repetitions are construed as being the same in nature as are part-word repetitions and prolongations; they are considered to be simply different forms of the same process. In the quotation just discussed, the sameness of the two forms is said to be that they reflect "hesitancy;" later, in the heading of the article's table 1 (Bloodstein & Grossman, 1981, p. 300), both forms are identified as "disfluencies;" then in the actual table entries they are listed as "instances of stuttering."

The inconsistency revealed in the preceding paragraph characterizes Bloodstein's treatment of disfluencies. His contention that the stuttering of early childhood differs from later stuttering is based on a policy of simply counting disfluencies rather than attempting to identify stutters.[24] The data he reports can thereby be made to show several differences in the "stuttering" of young children, because those data include many items that are not stutters. This bias is particularly inflated by including word repetitions as "instances of stuttering."

As discussed earlier, in several places, a word repetition may mark a stutter event, which immediately succeeds it, but the word repetition is not properly identified as the stutter. On the other hand, many word repetitions are not associated with a stutter event, but represent a normal nonfluency. Further, word repetitions occur frequently in the speech of young children, and evidently they occur more frequently in the speech of young stutterers than of normal youngsters.[25] In fact, the data in the report presently under review show that almost half of the "instances of stuttering" consisted of word repetitions. The fact that word repetitions occur more frequently in the speech of stutterers (adults as well as children) is certainly of interest and has some significance for the eventual understanding of stuttering vis-a-vis normal nonfluency. However, it is necessary to keep in mind that word repetitions are associated with two different kinds of events in the flow of speech—one that is normal and one that is not.

As noted earlier in the chapter, the policy of counting word repetitions as instances of stutter also distorts the description of other language factors in early stuttering, such as the content-word/function-word proportions, the consonant/vowel ratio, and word length. It is then no surprise to find Bloodstein and Grossman reporting that the grammatical class, initial phoneme, and word length factors in their data were different from those typically reported for older stutterers. It is of considerable interest that their data regarding position[26] is the same as that reported in all of the language factors research for stutterers of any age. Word (and phrase) repetitions, "almost without exception" occurred at the beginning of sentences, clauses or phrases. In presumed contrast, "17.8% of *other types of stutterings* [sic][27] (part-word repetitions, prolongations, and hard attacks) were observed at loci other than the beginnings of syntactic units" (p. 300). This means that 83.2% of the kinds of disfluency typically identified as stutters occurred at the beginning of sentences, clauses, or phrases.

Bernstein's (1981) study of syntactic factors in the speech of stuttering and normally speaking children is similar in many respects to the earlier study of adults reported by Hannah and Gardner (1968). Like the results obtained by Hannah and Gardner, the significance of Bernstein's findings for the study of stuttering per se is not clear. First, she did not differentiate between stutters and normal kinds of disfluency. The kinds of disfluency she recorded and analyzed were "hesitations, repetitions [revealed later as full- and part-word], prolongations, and filled pauses." Second, the speech samples actually analyzed are not likely to have been representative of the individual subjects' productions, inasmuch as they consisted of "only full sentences."[28] It seems clear that her findings, like those of Hannah and Gardner, are relevant only to a comparison of overall disfluencies occuring within a special and circumscribed type of speech sample from the respective groups.

Within these limitations it is of interest that she reported that "the major difference between the two groups appears to be in the strength and quantity of constituent-initial disfluency." At the same time, for both the normal speakers and stutterers, the major locus of disfluency was the first noun phrase (i.e., at the beginning of an utterance). The next most frequent locus, for both groups, occurred relative to the linking conjunction "and." There was a difference between the two groups, however; the stuttering youngsters had a significantly greater frequency of disfluency at another locus—the initiation of the verb phrase.

Bernstein pointed to evidence from the study of normal language function that spoken language is evidently processed in clauses. She interpreted her findings as indicating, contrary to Bloodstein's claim, that the occurrence of disfluencies is due, not to "attributes of syntactic structures that cause their [stutterers] motor planning to be more difficult," but to the planning of syntactic strings and the process of integrating such structures into meaningful wholes. In other words, the occurrence of disfluencies is related to higher level sentence planning processes, rather than to motor-gesture processes.

Bernstein's interpretation of her findings was evidently in reference to disfluency in general, which she noted as "a common childhood process." Significantly, she concluded that "differences between stuttering children and normal children may end up best explained in terms of *the manifest form of the disfluency,*[29] and not in terms of its precipitation" (p. 350).

A study of the influence of sentence length and clause position reported by Jayaram (1984) is particularly valuable for several reasons. First, it yielded pertinent information for two languages, English and Kannada.[30] Second, it is of special significance to the focus of this section that the two languages differ syntactically as well as in other ways. Third, the design of the study permitted actual comparisons on the dimension of clause position.

Jayaram pointed out that the findings reported by Tornick and Bloodstein (1976) could not give an adequate indication of the relative contribution of sentence length and clause position because their design made no provision for assessing the influence of clause position. To resolve this problem Jayaram constructed 20 sets of sentences, each set containing three declarative sentences of the following forms. One sentence in each set was a short sentence; another was a long sentence in which the short sentence appeared as the initial clause; and in the third member of the set the short sentence appeared as the final clause of a long sentence. The design also permitted assessing the influence of the relative lengths of the two clauses in the long sentences.

The 60 sentences were constructed in English and then translated into Kannada. The short English sentences contained 6 to 12 words, the long sentences were 14 to 23 words in length. In Kannada the short sentences contained 5 to 8 words, the long sentences had 10 to 15 words. The words used in the sentences were among the 1,000 most frequently occurring words in the respective languages.

Twenty young adult male stutterers served as subjects. Ten were monolingual speakers of Kannada; the other 10 were bilingual in English and Kannada.

Jayaram's results indicated that the frequency of stuttering is related to both sentence length and clause position, that these influences are similar in both languages, and are independent of whether the speaker is mono- or bilingual. In both languages the frequency of stuttering on early words in long sentences was greater than on the same words when they appeared in an isolated short sentence, reflecting an evident influence of sentence length. However, the findings regarding clause position were even more compelling. For both Kannada and English the frequency of stuttering was significantly greater (.01 level) in a clause appearing as the initial part of a long sentence than when the same clause appeared alone as a short sentence. In turn, the frequency of stuttering on the same clause, isolated as a short sentence, was significantly greater than when the clause occurred as the final part of a long sentence. As Jayaram noted, these consistent findings, showing a significantly higher frequency of stuttering associated with words occurring in early sentence positions, concur with previous reports, from many varied sources, that stuttering occurs more frequently early in an utterance.

Synopsis

Evidently neither stutter events nor the occurrence of disfluencies in general are related directly to syntactic structures per se. The findings of the research reviewed in this section are variable and, at best, equivocal in regard to a relationship between disfluencies, of any kind, and grammatical structures. In particular, there is no consistent evidence that stuttering is related to syntactic complexity, type of syntactic unit, length of unit, or syntactic relationships. It would appear then that syntactic structures themselves, or relationships among syntactic structures, are inadequate bases from which to attempt an interpretation of stuttering.

At the same time, the findings point in two seemingly different directions. On the one hand, there are grounds for inferring that the overall significance of these varied data is that they reflect demands placed on higher level language processing; the "organizational activity" mentioned by Wall et al. (1981) or the "integration into meaningful wholes" suggested by Bernstein (1981). In this vein, it is germane to recall the concept of propositionality and its applicability to stuttering. It is curious that this concept was not mentioned in any of this recent research.

The second apparent direction was expressed through the clearest result found regularly and repeatedly in all this research, namely, that stuttering, or disfluency in general, occurs in early position regardless of the syntactic structure in focus. These studies thus concur in indicating that, relative to disfluencies of any kind, the most notable feature of syntactic structures is that they have a beginning.

The most impressive finding of this research, then, is the evident significance of early-constituent position. It is especially pertinent to make the point, though it should be obvious, that words constitute the beginnings of syntactic structures. A comment by the authors of the earliest study in this line (Hannah & Gardner, 1968) seems particularly a propos. They observed that their findings revealed that the linguistic relationship with stuttering/disfluency is "not a simple matter of increased level of grammatical complexity" because of the evidence of a significant positive correlation between stuttering/disfluency and "the most elemental" of verbal segments, namely, one word.

I mentioned previously that the two general findings from this area of research might seem to point in different directions, in that one is oriented to the abstracted level of language processing while the other is tied to the seemingly lower stratum of individual words. However, one must not lose sight of the fact that words are the crucial focus in language processing, and that grammatical structures are created on the foundations of words and their significances. The two general findings devolving from this line of research are therefore intimately related, and both pertain ultimately to the language dimension of words.

Although much of the research in this area has dealt with stuttering, an appreciable portion of it has dealt, either knowingly or in error, with all kinds of disfluency. It is of considerable interest that both stutters and disfluencies of other kinds occur in early-constituent position. This finding has significance for any explanation of disfluency in general, and of stuttering in particular, and the difference between the two. I will defer discussion of this matter to appropriate sections of Chapter 5 (those addressed to early position, grammatical class, and stress). For the moment it is important to note that this finding does not signify a basic identity of stutters and other types of disfluency, nor does it indicate that they are on a continuum or are simply degrees of the same thing. As qualifications requiring immediate note, attention is directed to the evidence from this research that: (1) stutterers have more disfluencies of all kinds (in early position) than do normal speakers; (2) disfluencies of stutterers occur in early position of more kinds of constituents than do those of normal speakers; and (3) stutters, though occurring most often in early position, occur elsewhere as well.

Early Sentence Position

The research reviewed in the preceding section, although designed to provide information relative to syntactic factors and stuttering, turned out to yield impressive evidence of the importance of early position. It would be redundant to review those studies again for this section but their contribution deserves special mention. There are many other sources that also give clear indication of the extent to which early utterance position is associated with the occurrence of stutters.

In passing, mention should be made of the evidence contained in the earliest relevant study (Milisen, 1937) and in those early studies that yielded corroboration of Brown's factors (Cohen, 1952; Egland, 1938;

Hahn, 1942a; Meissner, 1946; Oxtoby, 1946; Trotter, 1956) of which early sentence position was one of the four factors assessed.

Supporting evidence from a slightly different direction is found in the findings of Johnson's early (1942, 1955)[31] study of 46 stuttering children. Information regarding position was obtained from parental report about the children's early stuttering. Parents reported that, from the beginning, stutters "evidently involved the first words of sentences, or of phrases, the first phrases of sentences, and the first syllables of words" (Johnson, 1955, p. 64).[32]

Similar evidence is found in Johnson's major publication on children (Johnson and Associates, 1959) in which many comparisons were made of 150 stuttering and 150 normal children. Statements obtained individually from each parent of each child revealed that significantly more of both the mothers and the fathers of stuttering children, in contrast to control parents, reported that the child's disfluencies occurred on the first word of utterances. It is pertinent to mention that these parents also (significantly) more often reported their child's disfluencies to evidence force or "more effort than usual." In contrast, significantly more parents of the normally speaking children reported, individually, that they had noticed, in the speech of other children, the same kinds of disfluencies evidenced by their child.

The significance of early position has been revealed consistently in all of the pertinent research published since the resurgence of interest in language factors in stuttering. In one of the two initial studies of this era, Quarrington et al. (1962) found that evidence for the importance of early position was the most impressive of the variables they set out to investigate. In fact, the prominence of early position led them to consider that their notion of a grammatical gradient "may well be, in part, a function of positions which grammatical forms commonly assume in English prose" (Quarrington et al., 1962, p. 393).

The salience of position was emphasized in the results of the next study in this line (Conway & Quarrington, 1963), in which the positional effect was prominent for all three levels of sentence "meaningfulness" (contextual constraint). In fact, finding that stuttering occurred so much more frequently in early sentence position, regardless of the level of sentence meaningfulness, led Conway and Quarrington to suspect that the position effect in stuttering might be more appropriately interpreted as reflecting the stutterer's efforts to organize the material to be spoken.

The subsequent study by Quarrington (1965) also found stuttering to be significantly associated with early position, and again this relationship was independent of "meaning," in this case meaning being construed as word information value.

Although a number of studies reviewed in the section on syntax found that normal disfluencies also occur at constituent-initial positions, several studies addressed to the investigations of Brown's factors in stuttered and normal speech have yielded evidence that stuttering is associated more frequently with early sentence position than are normal disfluencies.

Two of these studies contrasted speech samples from stutterers and nonstutterers. F.H. Silverman (1965) compared instances of disfluencies occurring during the reading of a 1,000-word passage by 15 young adult male stutterers and 24 normal speakers of comparable age and sex. He found the stutterers to have significantly more disfluencies on early position words than did the normal speakers. Williams and colleagues (1969b) obtained the same results with children. They had 76 stutterers and 76 matched normally speaking children, from kindergarten through grade six, perform speech tasks appropriate to their ages. They found that, in contrast to the stutterers, early sentence position had "the least influence on loci of disfluency" in the speech samples from the normally speaking youngsters.

Two other studies investigated the concurrence of Brown's factors and disfluencies in the speech of normal speakers only. Silverman and Williams (1967a) recorded all disfluencies occurring while 24 young adult males read the same 1,000-word passage used by Brown. They found that disfluencies occurred most often on words characterized by "Brown's factors" *except for* the factor of early sentence position. Chaney (1969) collected similar data from speech samples of 24 young adult college females. She obtained the same results as Silverman and Williams, namely that disfluencies were associated with words characterized by Brown's factors, except for the variable of sentence position.

One could well have expected that research would consistently show stuttering to be significantly associated with early-utterance position. As Brown (1938b) noted, stutterers frequently report having difficulty "getting started," a testimony that has been corroborated often, over a long period of time, by direct observation. For instance, almost 400 years ago Sir Francis Bacon (1627) observed in his *Sylva Sylvarum*[33]: "And so we see, that they that Stut, doe Stut more in the first offer to speake, than in Continuance."

Summary and Discussion

One can speak of several trends or directions of inquiry in the research reviewed in this chapter, trends that have somewhat differing foci even though they are also interrelated, in various ways, around a central theme of the four language factors in stuttering identified by Brown (1945).

One dimension was the corroboration of Brown's findings through work done with other adult stutterers speaking in various circumstances different from those of Brown's. A second dimension was the extension of

Brown's work to younger age levels, which resulted in the evidence that those four language factors apply equally to stuttering in children, including very young children. Another trend is found in the efforts to expand Brown's findings beyond the variables he identified, as reflected in the excursions into information load, short-term cycles, and syntactic influences; endeavors that bore little fruit. A fourth trend is represented in the application of Brown's work to the comparison of disfluencies in stuttered speech with those found in normal speech. The comparisons made via the research undertaken so far are, at best, grossly incomplete; first, the research has been based on the limited "disfluency" list constructed by Johnson, and second, it has been mounted in respect to only four of the six variables investigated by Brown. The findings of this research thus have an uncertain value. Ironically, the least that can be said for them is that they are contradictory to the "theoretical" position on which this trend was based (see the discussion that follows).

Threading through several of these trends is the theme of a search for the most important of the four factors emphasized by Brown, and at the core of this theme lies the concept of "meaning," especially meaning as related to words. This theme surfaces pointedly in the preoccupation with information load, in the attention to contextual constraints, and in Bloodstein's effort to present the grammatical factor as a feature only of "well developed" stuttering. This interest in establishing the relative importance of the four factors has precluded a consideration of the interrelationships among them, and what this might suggest.

Overall, the research published subsequent to Brown's work has consistently corroborated his findings regarding the concurrence of stutters with the four language factors he considered to be sufficient in accounting for instances of stuttering. Brown's findings, established for young adults, have been found applicable to stutterers of all ages.

There is, within this post-Brown research, a serious complication that, fortunately, has positive as well as negative dimensions. This complication centers in the confounding of stuttering and disfluency introduced from Johnson's (1959, 1961a) publications that obscured the distinctiveness of stuttering. The complication is represented in the findings of studies done since the early 1960s through the fact that this research has not been addressed consistently to what is properly identified as stuttering but, instead, has incorporated all of the kinds of disfluency contained in the Johnson list. This practice has not represented an intent to investigate stutters and nonstutter disfluencies jointly but, instead, as undifferentiated.

I will briefly consider first the negative aspects of the foregoing complication. The central detriment is that stutters and normal kinds of disfluencies are melded together. There is, therefore, no way to discern possible differences in loci of occurrence, or in any other variables, between stutters and nonstutter disfluencies. Fundamentally, it is at least pretentious to contend that, in adopting this approach, one is studying stuttering.

A positive aspect of this complication derives from the indications that, in certain respects, overall disfluency in the speech of stutterers (including stutters) follows the same pattern relative to Brown's factors as that established for instances of stutter. A related benefit is that, with appropriate reservations, the loci of overall disfluency in the speech of stutterers can be compared to the loci of overall disfluency in samples of normal speech. This opportunity has yielded some interesting comparisons, namely, that the disfluencies of normal speech seem to be related to the same four factors found to be associated with stutterers' disfluencies (and stutters considered separately), with the notable exception that early-utterance position is evidently more critical in stuttered speech.

The indications that the other three (of Brown's) factors show an apparent similarity in disfluency loci in stuttered and normal speech, does not, as proponents of Johnson's position claim, demonstrate the kind of similarity, or continuum, of stuttered and normal speech that they wish to establish. That is, it does not demonstrate a similarity along the lines of explanation they espouse. According to any particular version of an "evaluation," "anticipation," or similar account, stuttering represents an excessive (and unwarranted) reaction to imagined circumstances in the act of speaking. This characterization implicitly separates stutters from nonstutter disfluencies even in a stutterer's speech, because presumably stutterers' nonstuttered disfluencies are not reflections of unwarranted and excessive reaction. Certainly this characterization of the nature of stutters separates them from the nonfluencies of the normal speaker.

It seems evident that the nature of whatever similarity exists must be some function of the variables through which the similarity is expressed, namely, the language factors. The common dimension, therefore, is most likely to be linked to the process of oral language production. Exploration of this dimension requires that the matter be approached from a knowledge of research based in normal speech, and particularly knowledge of the normal speech research addressed to "hesitation phenomena." Typically, reference to research on normal nonfluencies is not to be found in the publications reviewed in this section. However, some citation of research in normal speech began to appear in more recent sources, and included mention of the evidence, from some hesitation phenomena research, that normal nonfluencies reflect aspects of expressive language formulation. It is in respect to such evidence that the findings obtained from comparing overall disfluencies of stutterers and normal speakers, gross though these comparisons are, can make some contribution to an understanding of stuttering.

Because the (post-Brown) disfluency research has obscured stutters by blending them with other kinds of disfluency, it is not clear from this research that stutter events are involved in the language processes that are hypothesized here as possibly subtending certain kinds of irregularity in fluency. On the other hand, the research done before the 1960s (Brown's work and the early corroborations), which established and confirmed the "language factors," evidently did limit observations to actual stutters. There is good reason, then, to consider that stutters also, in some way, reflect a facet of the oral language production process. In view of the observable character of a stutter event, it seems appropriate to deduce that stutters are an *anomalous* facet of the processes; that is, they have a unique, different connection with those processes than do normal nonfluencies.

One must bear in mind two important features of all of the published research on language factors in stuttering that qualify any efforts to relate the disfluencies of stuttered speech, particularly the stutters, to the nonfluencies of normal speech. First, this research has consistently used the Johnson list of disfluencies, which has a special bias and is limited in scope. Second, the language factors that were the foci of this work were limited to the four that Brown (1945) emphasized. All of this research has excluded the other two language factors identified by Brown, each of which had a highly significant and consistent association with stutters: word-initial position and stress. This second feature has critical significance for the research attempting to compare stuttered and normal speech. Not only were these factors not included in the comparisons made; one might well expect that they would yield dramatic differences.

Word-inital position and stress are dimensions of a different order than grammatical class, word length, word position, and even phoneme type. Word-initial position and stress are syllabic phenomena; in literal designation they translate to "syllable-initial position" and "stressed syllable." These two factors occur at the level of stutter events; most likely that is why each of them is so highly correlated with stutters in Brown's research. As pointed out in Chapter 3 these two factors, almost perfectly correlated with stutter events, were each more surely associated with stutters than any of the other four factors, or all of them combined.

Word-initial position and stress, unlike the other language factors, represent basic aspects of the speech production process. Although all seven language factors represent aspects of the structure of the language, word-initial position and stress are more intimately involved with the speech production process. In view of their intimate association with stutters it would seem that we have found further significant clues to the nature of stuttering. This important point comes into special focus in subsequent chapters, especially in Chapters 6 and 9.

Footnotes

[1]This study by Van Riper and Hull is hardly ever mentioned in the extensive literature on stuttering "adaptation" although actually it was in this study that the "adaptation effect" was first noted. The publication by Johnson and Knott (1937) is acknowledged, erroneously, as reporting the first study dealing with that phenomenon. The adaptation literature, following Johnson's bias, has carried the unwarranted assumption that adaptation reflects learning (see Wingate, 1986a, 1986b). Van Riper's account of this phenomenon, that he discovered, was quite different.

[2]It is of some interest that this article appeared in the *Journal of Speech Disorders* in the pages immediately sequential to the final article in the Brown series (Brown, 1945).

[3]Whether length is measured in letters, phones, or syllables.

[4]The data were obtained in conjunction with another study that required the subjects to talk continuously, except for rest periods, 10 hours a day for 5 consecutive days. The speaking was essentially soliloquy, although the subjects were most likely aware that the experimenter, and perhaps others, were probably listening. These unusual circumstances do not seem to materially qualify the fact that the samples were self-formulated speech. The total corpus consisted of 248,806 words, of which 17,143 were stuttered.

[5]The frequency distribution of initial phones in his random sample of the total corpus (Hejna, 1955, table 29) correlates .90 with a composite ranking of word-initial phones based on several extensive studies of normal speech (see Chapter 5, Table 5.7).

[6]Word frequency values are based on large samples of *written* English.

[7]Although "information load" undoubtedly had appeal from the standpoint that it seemed to offer some quantification of "meaning," it seems likely that a substantial dimension of its appeal lay in it being semantically captivating.

[8]Even though Schlesinger et al. (1965) related sentence position, grammatical class, and word length to predictability in their introduction.

[9]To justify her contention that consonants are unpredictable, Taylor cited Sumby and Pollack (1954) as having reported that "the uncertainty of prediction is about 1.5 bits greater for the initial *letter* than for the mean of all the remaining *letters* in monosyllabic words." (The italics are mine.) Stutters relate to phones rather than letters. At the same time, similar findings are reported for phones (Bruner & O'Dowd, 1958; Miller, 1963). However, this emphasis on the initial phone misses the point that the stutterer is not having trouble with (or "on") the initial phone. (See Chapter 1, pp. 11 ff.)

[10]But no effect for "difficult" versus "easy" consonants, which were also incorporated into the design.

[11]Possibly the information load concept had already biased the reading of Brown's account.

[12]One should take note here of a crucial difference between word meaningfulness and utterance meaningfulness.

[13]This ratio is closer to the usual *overall* distribution of content and function words. See Chapter 5.

[14]A good description of Kannada is presented in Schiffman (1983). See also McCormack (1966).

[15]This percentage ratio of content words to function words is comparable to their usual overall distribution in the language. See pertinent data and discussion in Chapter 5.

[16]It is appropriate to note that in Brown's own data a careful separation of the

grammatical classes in terms of actual percentage-of-stuttering values would place adverbs with function words. See Table 3.3.

[17]Note that the grammatical factor is equated with content words, which are presumed here to be the words "crucial for the meaning" and therefore, presumably, are evaluated as important, difficult, requiring special effort, likely to be stuttered, etc. This account is a restatement of the Johnson conjecture, implicit in Brown's work.

[18]It is of considerable interest that four other children "were eliminated as subjects because their recorded speech was unintelligible or did not contain an arbitrary minimum of five nonfluent words." In itself this statement makes a cogent commentary on the claim that all children are disfluent, and supposedly in about the same proportion.

[19]Once again word repetitions were counted as instances of stuttering, a distorting and misleading practice.

[20]"Cycles" does not necessarily imply a regularity of recurrence.

[21]Said to resemble Hockett's (1955) macrosegment, "a unit commonly considered to exist between two terminal juncture points" (p. 854).

[22]In addition to these two reservations, it is also curious that: (1) there is a preponderance of verbalization in the postverbal phrases, (2) more content words occur in these phrases, and (3) there is a higher correlation between function words and "stuttering" in all three units.

[23]Possibly the difference may have been minimized by some amount of familiarity and practice (i.e., adaptation). In this case randomization may have operated to confound rather than objectify.

[24]As found also in his other publications reviewed here, Bloodstein is not alone in this claim. There are many others who subscribe to this position, notably E. M. Silverman, F. H. Silverman, and D. E. Williams. However, Bloodstein has made the greatest issue of the purported difference in childhood stuttering.

[25]See the relevant tables in Chapter 2 (Tables 2.4 through 2.10). Why they occur so much more frequently in the speech of young stutterers is a question that remains to be answered.

[26]Because of the issue being drawn here, it seemed appropriate to report this information regarding position at this point rather than deferring it to the section on Position.

[27]Italics mine. This statement indicates that word and phrase repetitions are also "types of stutterings."

[28]A constraint imposed by constituent structure analysis which, possibly defensible for purposes of some kinds of study, creates an artificiality and clear bias relative to the study of spontaneous speech.

[29]Italics mine.

[30]The salient features of Kannada are described earlier in this chapter.

[31]The 1955 publication is an expanded version of the 1942 report.

[32]Forty two of the 46 children evidenced "brief repetitions;" the other four youngsters evidenced prolongations at these loci.

[33]Cited by Rieber and Wollock (1977, p. 7).

5
Normal Language: The Necessary Reference

The objective of this chapter is to reanalyze the language factors considered in previous stuttering research, bringing into focus: (1) interrelationships among the several variables; (2) consideration of matters overlooked in previous research; and (3) appropriate attention to the two variables that have been largely disregarded—word-initial position and word stress. Developing this analysis will require, as the necessary reference, relevant data from research in the structure of normal language use; a reference that has been routinely neglected.

The research on language factors in stuttering that began in the 1960s proceeded in reference to S.F. Brown's work and concerned itself mainly with five factors: the four that represented Brown's emphasis, namely, the "phonetic factor," grammatical class, word length, and sentence position of words; and a fifth factor, word frequency, that was introduced within a few years after the revival of interest in this area of research.

A prevailing objective of this subsequent research effort seems to have been to isolate the most important of these five factors, or at least to establish a ranking of their relative importance. As will become evident in the latter part of this chapter, it would have been more profitable to direct attention to the interrelationships among all of the variables that had been found to be related to stutter occurrences. Although one can find, in the literature on language factors, occasional mention of possible relationships between certain of the language factors identified,[1] such matters were not explored or developed further. Most likely such neglect was due to the preoccupation with explaining stuttering as a psychological (reactive) problem, in which stutter events were presumed to be essentially surface phenomena overlaid on a basically normal language function. The possibility that stuttering might reflect some essential disorder in oral language processing seems not to have been considered.

Interest in exploring interrelationships between the language factors was dependent on an interest in, and knowledge of, relevant data from the study of normal speech. As discussed in Chapter 2, the literature of stuttering has shown very little evidence of interest in the findings from research based in the study of normal speech. As noted there, this disinterest reflects a presumption that stuttering is known to be behavioral in nature; that it is a functional problem originating from environmental pressures and expressed through acquired motor acts. In contrast, recognizing the importance of reference to normal speech follows readily from a position that makes no assumptions about the cause of stuttering but, instead, approaches it at an observational/descriptive level, from which stuttering is viewed at its face value, as a disturbance in oral language expression.

Structural Features of Ordinary Oral Language

Especially in consideration of what has been found regarding language factors and stuttering, the most relevant normal language data are those that describe major structural characteristics of the language, particularly as it is spoken in ordinary discourse. Here the syllable is the basic reference. The syllable, identifiable as the minimum unit of phonological structure (O'Connor, 1977; Studdert-Kennedy, 1975) is, on one hand, the structural unit that can account for all larger units and, at the same time, is the largest unit necessary to explain how phonemes, the smallest units, combine in a language. The core, or nucleus, of a syllable is the vowel, and although a syllable may consist of only a vowel, most often the syllable is "a functional unit compounded of a consonant and a vowel, each fulfilling some syllabic function." (Studdert-Kennedy, 1975, p. 114). In English these "functional units" range from the simplest form, a vowel only (V), to structures of considerable complexity in which the vowel is preceded by up to three consonants and followed by up to to four consonants—CCCVCCCC (Jesperson, 1960; O'Connor, 1977, p. 200).

The syllabic structure of the English lexicon is represented in analyses such as those of Moser, Dreher, and Oyer (1957) and Trnka (1968). Similar data that are more pertinent to actual language use are contained in comparable analyses made by French et al. (1930) and Roberts (1965).

The analysis by French et al. was based on a corpus of almost 80,000 words sampled from 1,900 telephone conversations that were mostly business calls between two adult males. The method of sampling did not record complete conversations; it focused, over successive weeks of sampling, on each of the several grammatical classes of words constituting the traditional "parts of speech." All instances of one grammatical class, for example, nouns, were recorded over a specified number of conversations, then all items of another grammatical class were recorded, and so on.

The original source of the corpus analyzed by Roberts was Horn's (1926) frequency count of over 15 million running words obtained from various written sources, one-third of which consisted of personal letters. Horn's compilation was carefully selected by Roberts as the material best suited to meet a number of criteria that would ensure a large corpus that also adequately represented "everyday living English." Although the original material had been recorded in standard English orthography, Roberts derived the basis for his phonemic analysis by having a native speaker, who spoke "a North Central variety of General American dialect," speak the different words of the Horn material in normal sentence frames.

Table 5.1 presents the results of a syllabic analysis of the words constituting the corpus of each of these two studies. In their analysis French et al. reduced all words to syllables; the analysis by Roberts is based on words per se but is limited to the 21 most preferred canonical forms of the 1,790 forms he identified. Though few in number, these 21 forms accounted for 75% of the frequencies of occurrence of the many different canonical forms found in this extensive corpus.

Even though the sources of the data in the two displays of Table 5.1 differ in terms of origin and, in some sense in treatment, the data are remarkably similar. Independently, and jointly, they indicate that, in actual language usage, a certain limited number of canonical forms are predominant, in contrast to the potentially extensive variety of such forms.[2] The differential frequencies of the various structural patterns—the "favored" canonical forms—are much the same whether analysis is made in terms of syllables (French et al.) or of words (Roberts).

It is also clear that the most frequently occurring forms are also the simplest. In both French et al. and Roberts (and others; see, for example Denes, 1963), about 95% of word usage consists of words of two syllables or less (Table 5.2). Further, both sources show a preponderant use of

TABLE 5.1. Phonetic structure of English words as used in connected oral and written expression

Canonical	French et al.	Roberts
Monosyllabic		
V	9.7	2.3
VC	20.3	19.5
CV	21.8	11.1
CVC	33.5	26.1
VCC	2.8	2.4
CCV	0.8	0.0
CVCC	7.8	8.6
CCVC	2.8	1.5
CCVCC	0.5	0.6
Polysyllabic		
CVCVC	—	2.2
CVCCVC	—	0.8

TABLE 5.2. Proportional frequencies of occurrence of English words of various lengths

Source	Number of words in corpus	Word length in syllables					
		1	2	3	4	5	6
French et al.	79,390	82.0[a]	13.8	3.2	0.86	0.15	0.01
Roberts	15,465,010	76.9	17.1	4.6	1.14	0.31	0.006
Denes	23,049	77.2	17.2	4.4	1.0	0.16	—

[a]Note the considerably higher percentage of single-syllable words in this sample, which is the only one of these three that is of actual spontaneous speech.

single-syllable words: 82% and 77% respectively (Table 5.2). Denes' data yield a similar value.

It is evident from Table 5.1 that the structural complexity of syllables is not conditioned by word length (measure in syllables); a notable structural complexity is to be found even in one-syllable words. Still, simple forms predominate. This, too, is evident from the distributions presented in Table 5.1; most of the words contain three phonemes or less.

This predominance of simple forms is represented more dramatically in Table 5.3, reproduced from Roberts (1965). The values bracketed in the lower left corner of Table 5.3 account for 80% of the use-frequency of one-syllable words. What is even more impressive is the fact that these short words account for 62% of the use-frequency of the total corpus. These values indicate that the bulk of connected speech consists of words having three phonemes or less.

The findings just presented are corroborated by data from a number of other sources that yield values reflecting average word length in ordinary language use, for both spontaneous speech and "spoken prose." The values presented in Table 5.4, obtained from such sources, show consistently that the average word length in a corpus of connected expression is about three phonemes. In general, the data for written material is similar to that for sources based on spoken language. Only the Dewey data, based entirely on formal written sources, diverges somewhat from the evident standard.

As a body, the data presented in the foregoing tables concur in indicating that, for much of the actual use of English, "word" is equivalent to "syllable."

The data presented in Table 5.1 reveal another important fact about the structure of English, namely, a relative predominance of consonants over vowels. Both of the data sources in Table 5.1 yield an overall C-V ratio of 3:2. Other sources providing structural statistics of English yield similar C-V ratios, as shown in Table 5.5. The arrangement of entries in Table 5.5

TABLE 5.3. Joint frequency distribution of word length by numbers of syllables and phonemes[a]

Syllables	1	2	3	4	5	6	7	Total
15				294	811	81		1,186
14				5,884	3,401	695	14	9,994
13			16	4,576	11,663	81		16,336
12			4,699	15,437	19,229	155		39,520
11			11,344	42,166	9,206			62,716
10		1,479	51,143	36,920	3,084			92,626
9		13,920	166,725	40,630	983			222,258
8		82,302	221,035	30,875				334,212
7	1,371	429,032	200,676	160				631,239
6	42,721	915,837	48,503					1,007,061
5	559,554	777,834	67					1,337,455
4	1,733,258	366,148						2,099,406
3	4,461,932	51,010						4,512,942
2	4,738,940							4,738,940
1	359,119							359,119
Total	11,896,895	2,637,562	704,208	176,942	48,377	1,012	14	15,465,010
Percent	76.9	17.1	4.6	1.1	0.3			

[a]Reproduced from Roberts (1965, table 3).

separates works based on informal speech from those based on "spoken prose" and from those representing actual prose (written material). The sources representing these three categories are placed in that order, from top to bottom of the table. The sources listed in the middle section are neither ordinary spontaneous speech nor prose. The samples from Denes (1963) and Fry (1947), though included in this section for "spoken prose," are most likely to be very close approximations of ordinary speech. Both Denes and Fry used phonetic readers[3] as the corpus for their analyses. As described by Denes (1963, p. 893) the phonetic readers "contain conversation and simple narrative in the manner, and with the pronunciation, that the skilled compilers of these books consider spoken English is produced by native speakers" (p. 893). The C-V ratios in Table 5.5 show a clear correspondence to the type of material from which the data were derived, being lowest for those speech samples drawn from conversation and becoming higher as the samples become more like real prose.[4] These differences again call attention to the matter of differences between spoken prose and spontaneous speech. Abercrombie's (1963) remarks on such differences were introduced in Chapter 2; the matter has also been discussed, from different points of view, by Berger (1967), Carterette and Jones (1974), Denes (1963), French et al. (1930), and others.

TABLE 5.4. Average length of words, in number of phones, in a variety of language samples

Source	Nature of corpus	Number of words	Average word length in phones
Carterette & Jones:			
1st graders	Small group conversations	20,030	2.93
3rd graders	Small group conversations	21,368	2.95
5th graders	Small group conversations	27,072	2.99
Adults	Small group conversations	15,694	3.10
French et al.	Adult telephone conversations	79,390	2.87
Denes	Phonetic reader	23,049	3.13
Berger	Adult conversations	3,418	3.09
Roberts	Mixed written[a]	15,465,010	2.66
Miller, Newman, & Friedman	Several written sources[b]	36,299	3.12
Dewey	Mixed written	100,069	3.65

[a]For these sources the corpus size was originally given as number of phonemes.
[b]For these sources the corpus size was originally given as number of consonants.

Carterette and Jones (1974) and Wang and Crawford (1960) computed correlation matrices for the data of studies included in both parts of Table 5.5. Correlation values between pairs of data were generally high (.70 to .99), but highest for data based on sources closest to natural speech (.89 to .99). Our immediate interest in these data is in the evidence that the overall C-V ratio for ordinary verbal expression is consistently of the order of three consonants to two vowels.

There are several other important dimensions of consonant-vowel differences that are necessary to include in an adequate analysis of language structure. One of these dimensions is the fact that the various consonant and vowel phonemes are not distributed equally in the canonical forms listed in Table 5.1, nor do they contribute equal weighting to the overall ratios recorded in Table 5.5. Differences in the frequency with which the various phonemes occur, in actual use, are presented in Table 5.6. The rank order of consonants is shown in the first column, and a similar ranking of vowels in the second column. These rankings are composites, based on several different studies of language in ordinary use.[5]

Rank ordering, without evidence of rank differences, gives an incomplete representation of relative frequency of occurrence. Therefore, the

TABLE 5.5. Overall consonant:vowel ratio found in several studies of the language in use

Source	Nature of the corpus	Number of words	C:V Ratio
Carterette & Jones:			
1st graders	Three-person group discussion	20,030	60:40
3rd graders	Three-person group discussion	21,368	60:40
5th graders	Three-person group discussion	27,072	60:40
Adults	Three-person group discussion	15,694	60:40
French et al.	Two-person (adult) telephone conversations	79,390	60:40
Denes	Phonetic reader	23,052	61:39
Fry	Phonetic reader	3,292[a]	61:39
Voelker	Radio announcements	130,830[a]	62:38
Hayden	University lectures	21,707[a]	63:37
Roberts	Mixed written[b]	15,465,010	60:40
Dewey	Newspapers	100,069	63:37
Whitney	Modern prose	2,740[c]	64:36
Fowler	Modern prose	2,792[c]	68:32

[a]For these sources the corpus size was originally given as number of phonemes.
[b]Half of this written material was correspondence; a third of the total corpus consisted of personal correspondence.
[c]For these sources the corpus size was originally given as number of consonants.

tables include the relative frequency values for each phoneme. These values reveal the actual extent of the large differences in frequency of occurrence among both consonants and vowels. Clearly, some phonemes occur very often, others are relatively rare.

Another important dimension of the distribution of consonants and vowels is that the consonant-vowel ratio changes as a function of phoneme locus, specifically, word-initial and word-final positions. The C-V ratio for each of these positions differs from the overall C-V ratio of 3:2, identified previously. For both initial and final positions the C-V ratio is notably higher, 2:1 or greater (see Tables 5.1 and 5.8).[6] Further, the relative frequency of occurrence of the various phonemes also varies considerably in relation to word-initial and word-final position. This differential distribution of phonemes as a function of word position reflects certain important grammatical aspects of the language, which will be identified shortly. It so happens that the data on phoneme frequency distribution for both initial and final positions, particularly word-initial positions, are

TABLE 5.6. Rank order, frequency of phoneme occurrence in ordinary language usage

Consonants[a]		Vowels[b]	
Rank	Frequency	Rank	Frequency
n	7.6	e	10.8
t	7.5	ɪ	6.6
r	5.0	ɛ	3.0
d	4.5	aɪ	2.7
s	4.3	i	2.4
l	4.0	æ	2.0
ð	3.4	o,ou	1.9
k	3.3	e,eɪ	1.8
m	3.2	ɑ	1.6
w	2.8	ʌ	1.6
z	2.6	u	1.6
b	2.2	ɔ	1.5
v	1.9	ɜ,ɝ	1.0
f	1.7	au	0.8
h	1.7	u	0.8
j	1.7	ɔɪ	0.1
p	1.7		
g	1.4		
ŋ	1.2		
ʃ	0.8		
θ	0.6		
tʃ	0.4		
dʒ	0.5		
hw	0.3		
ʒ	0.1		

[a]This ranking is a composite of data obtained in seven separate studies of ordinary spoken language use (Wingate, 1985).
[b]This ranking is a composite of data from five separate studies of ordinary spoken language use (Wingate, 1985).

also of particular significance to our ultimate objective of applying these structural analyses to an understanding of stuttering.

In presenting data relative to differential frequency of occurrence of phonemes as conditioned by locus, our major emphasis will be on consonants for several reasons. First, again for several reasons, much more attention has been paid to consonants in the relevant literature (see compilations by Voelker (1937) and Wang & Crawford (1960)). Second, in those publications that consider locus, most often only the consonants are analyzed (Berry, 1953; French et al., 1930; Henrickson, 1948; Mader, 1954). Most likely this bias is occasioned partly by the fact that consonants predominate in both initial and final positions; but also, as noted by several authors, because there is a certain amount of variation in vowel usage, and transcription. A third reason for the emphasis on consonants is that they are a major focus of interest in descriptions, and explanations, of stuttering.

Data on consonant distributions in both final and initial positions provide important and useful information. However, since our primary interest is in the word-initial position comparatively less attention will be paid to final-position consonants. Consequently, it seems appropriate to deal with this briefer content first. Table 5.7 presents the ranking and relative frequency values of word-final consonants as found in the several sources concerned with the language in ordinary use. The rank order of final consonants shows certain similarities to the overall consonant ranking (cf. Table 5.6), particularly among the highest ranks, yet some differences are evident. As noted earlier, such differences reflect certain gram-

TABLE 5.7. Rank order, frequency of consonant occurrence in word-final and word-initial positions in ordinary language usage[a]

Word-Final position		Word-Initial position	
t	.186	ð	.115
d	.112	w	.083
n	.106	t	.071
z	.089	s	.071
r	.088	h	.069
l	.057	b	.052
s	.055	m	.049
v	.043	k	.046
m	.041	d	.044
ŋ	.037	j	.039
k	.032	g	.037
p	.013	f	.036
f	.011	p	.036
ð	.008	l	.031
tʃ	.006	n	.030
θ	.003	r	.024
dʒ	.003	hw	.015
g	.003	ʃ	.014
ʃ	.002	θ	.013
b	.002	dʒ	.012
ʒ	.001	v	.010
		tʃ	.004
		z	.003
		ʒ	.002

[a]Data from Wingate (1985).

matical features of the language. For example, /z/ is found at a higher rank level in the word-final list than in the overall ranking, reflecting its occurrences as a possessive and plural marker. Similarly /ŋ/, which never occurs initially in English, occurs frequently in the word-final morpheme used to create present participles and verbal nouns.

Turning now to word-initial position, let us first consider the general C-V ratio in initial position and its difference from the overall C-V ratio. For both sources of data represented in Table 5.1 (French et al., 1930; Roberts, 1965) the *initial* C-V ratio is 2:1, notably higher than the overall C-V ratio of 3:2. This higher C-V ratio for word-initial position is also found in other sources of structural analysis for which such a statistic is available or can be computed. Table 5.8 lists the ratios in percentage and ratio form; all of the values can be expressed as ratios of 2:1 or larger.

The word-initial C-V comparison is of considerable value simply for what it reveals about the extent to which consonants occur in initial position. However, there are other aspects of the relationship between phoneme type and word-initial position that are important to identify. One notable feature of the word-initial C-V ratio is that it varies as a function of word length, becoming gradually lower as word length increases. Documentation of this relationship is revealed in direct analysis of individual words. The data in Table 5.9 summarize an analysis of word-initial C-V ratios for words of increasing length, measured in syllables. The data were compiled from word lists tabulated for four separate studies of oral language expression that vary in respect to source. Actually, because these data are based on the (approximately) 1,000 most frequently occurring words in each study, they provide limited evidence of the fact

TABLE 5.8. Ratios of consonants to vowels in word-initial position[a]

Source	Nature of the corpus	Number of words	Percent initial C:V	Word-Initial C-V ratio[c]
Berger	Adult conversations	25,000	83:17	4.9:1.0
Berry	Adult telephone conversations	24,781	72:28	2.6:1.0
French et al.	Adult telephone conversations	79,390	67:33	2.0:1.0
Denes	Phonetic readers	23,052	73:27	2.6:1.0
Dewey	Mixed written	100,069	70:30	2.4:1.0
Roberts	Mixed written	11,598,757[b]	68:32	2.1:1.0

[a]Data from spontaneous speech and written language sources.
[b]Represents 75% of his total corpus. (See Roberts 1965, table 5.)
[c]Similar ratios are found in sources addressed to the study of stuttering. (See Table 5.17.)

TABLE 5.9. Percentage of consonant-initial words, relative to word length, occurring among the most frequent words in samples of spontaneous speech[a]

Source	Number of words	Word length in syllables 1	2	3	4/+	Overall Percent C:V	C-V Ratio
Berger	1,202	92	80	65	59	85:15	5.7:1
French et al.	737	80	70	57	45	73:27	2.7:1
Howes	1,002	91	77	66	52	84:16	5.3:1
Horn	1,000	92	76	70	50	88:12	7.3:1

[a]Data from Wingate (1985).

that the C-V ratio decreases as a function of word length. Nonetheless, the trend is clear. Note that the C-V ratio becomes progressively lower as word length increases until, at word lengths of four-or-more syllables, initial consonants are no more frequent than initial vowels. For our purposes the important point is that the word-initial C-V ratio is very high among words that are used most often, and especially so for the shorter, frequently occurring words. Thus the word-initial C-V ratio is also related directly to frequency of word usage as well as to word length.

This relationship between type of word-initial phone, word length, and word frequency will be found, in turn, to be intimately bound to another structural dimension of the language, namely, the grammatical class of words. The words that occur with greatest frequency in language use are words from the various grammatical classes identifed as function words: articles, prepositions, conjunctions, auxiliaries, and pronouns.

Function words, though few in actual number, make up approximately half of the corpus in samples of ordinary speech. Howes and Geschwind (1969), for example, reported that normal speakers use 42 to 50% function words in the course of a 5,000-word interview. Comparable values are reported by Blankenship and Kay (1964), Denes (1963), and Fairbanks (1944). Even higher percentages of function words were found by French et al. (1930) and Miller, Newman, and Friedman (1958). The pertinent data are presented in Table 5.10; all of these data are based on large, complete samples.

There is one further aspect of the word-initial C-V ratio that is of considerable importance to a general description of the language as used; it is also of particular importance for application of the analyses presented here to an understanding of stuttering. This particularly valuable information derives from identifying the relative frequencies of occurrence with which the individual phoneme types, essentially the various consonants, occur in word-initial position.

TABLE 5.10. Proportions of content and function words occurring in various language samples

Source	Nature of corpus	Number of words	Percent	
			Content	Function
Howes & Geschwind	Interviews	5,000[a]	54	46
H. Fairbanks	Interviews	30,000	55	45
Blankenship & Kay	"Speeches"	(extensive)[b]	54.5	45.5
French et al.	Telephone conversations	79,390	43	57
Miller, Newman, & Friedman	Various prose	36,300	41	59

[a]The authors refer to average samples of this size obtained from normal speakers.
[b]The corpus consisted of "5 hours and 54 minutes of American-English speech."

Table 5.7 includes the rank order of initial consonants, and their relative frequencies of occurrence, in ordinary language use. This is a composite ranking based on several sources, including adult and child conversations, spoken prose, and actual prose. Although certain differences in the rankings from the several sources were apparent, overall agreement was very good as reflected in correlations between .95 and .99.

The rank order and frequency distributions of consonants in word-initial position is considerably different from the overall consonant ranking (see Table 5.6). There is a striking shift in rank of several consonants: /ð/, /h/, /w/, /hw/, and /j/. The prominence of /j/ in word-initial position is occasioned largely by the words "you" and "yes," and their variants. Note particularly the extent of this predominance in the data from samples of actual spontaneous speech. The dramatic shift of the other four consonants is occasioned by two facts of English structure. The first fact is that these phones occur predominantly in initial position, as documented in data from several sources presented in Table 5.11. A second, and closely related, fact is that these phonemes "overload" in words of certain grammatical classes. These markedly frequent initial consonants are ones that occur extensively as the initial sound in a number of words that are vital to the structural organization of utterances: those words identified as function words—articles, conjunctions, prepositions, and auxiliaries; and it is the function words that occur so frequently in actual language use, as documented in Table 5.10. Further, the function words used most often are also predominantly short words, as shown in Table 5.12: almost 95% of the "minor" words are one syllable in length, and occurrences of a word of more than two syllables are rare.

TABLE 5.11. Frequency, in percent, with which the phonemes /ð, h, w, hw, j/ occur in word-initial position

Source	Nature of corpus	Number of words	ð	j	w	hw	j
French et al.	Adult telephone conversations	79,390	90	100	100	100	100
Mader	Interviews with children	77,300[a]	93	99	94	98	98
Henrickson	Interviews with children	7,200[a]	90	99	88	97	95
Denes	Phonetic reader	23,052	85	98	86	—	77
Dewey	Various written	100,069	89	99	71	—	75

[a]The number of words is estimated from the original data, reported as total number of consonants.

Also, as noted previously, most function words begin with certain consonants that, with two exceptions: (1) occur predominantly as word-initial consonants (see Table 5.11), and (2) routinely top the word-initial consonant lists (see Table 5.7). The exceptions to be noted are /t/, which does not occur predominantly in word-initial position, and /hw/, which does not rank high in the initial-consonant lists. In contrast to /t/, which occurs in all positions and in many word classes, /hw/ occurs almost exclusively in word-initial position and, as noted earlier, predominantly in frequently used function words.

The interrelationship between function words, initial consonants and word frequency is revealed dramatically in Figure 5.1, and its accompanying notes, taken from French et al. (1930). These figures show the changes in relative occurrence of initial consonants in respect to what words of the corpus are retained for the analysis. It is important to mention that the definite article is not represented in any of these figures. Because both the

TABLE 5.12. Syllabic structure of conversational vocabulary[a]

	Percent of words having number of syllables shown						Average number of syllables
Parts of speech	1	2	3	4	5	6	
Nouns	53.3	33.8	9.7	2.7	0.47	0.03	1.63
Verbs	81.9	15.0	2.8	0.3	—	—	1.21
Adjectives and adverbs	57.8	30.7	8.0	2.8	0.66	0.02	1.58
Minor	94.8	4.7	0.6	0.1	—	—	1.06
All words	82.0	13.8	3.2	0.86	0.15	0.01	1.23

[a]From French et al. (1930, table VI).

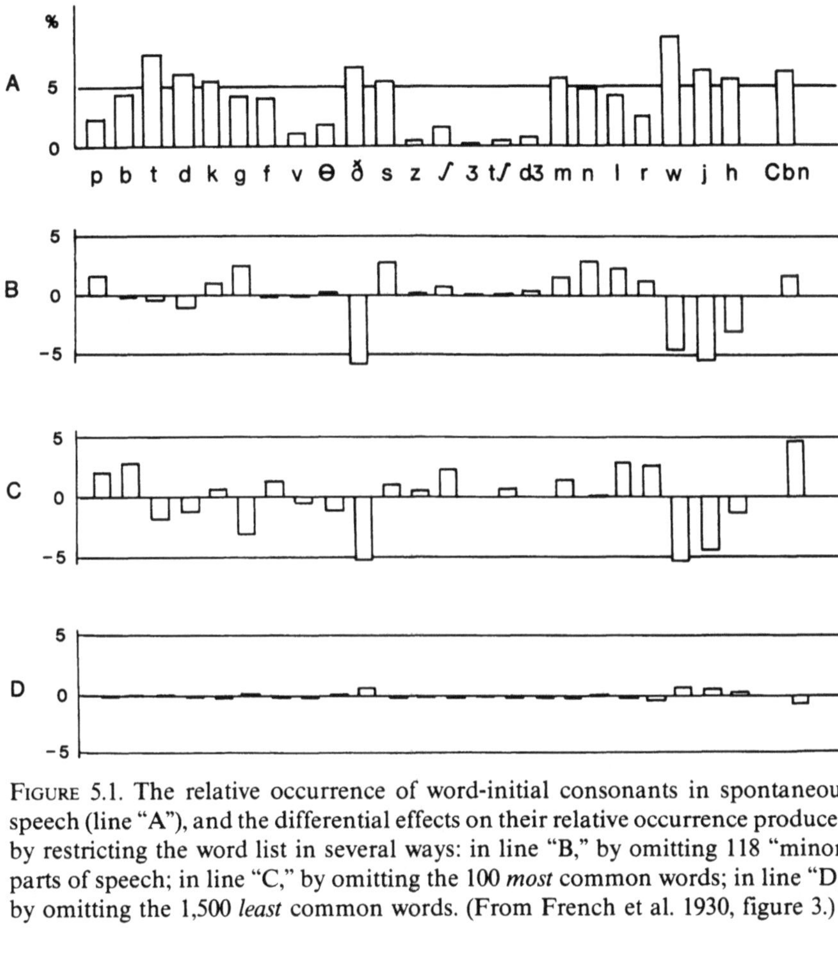

FIGURE 5.1. The relative occurrence of word-initial consonants in spontaneous speech (line "A"), and the differential effects on their relative occurrence produced by restricting the word list in several ways: in line "B," by omitting 118 "minor" parts of speech; in line "C," by omitting the 100 *most* common words; in line "D," by omitting the 1,500 *least* common words. (From French et al. 1930, figure 3.)

definite and indefinite articles vary in pronunciation, French et al. excluded them from their detailed analyses. Since "the" is one of the most frequently occurring words in English, the phoneme /ð/ is thus very substantially underrepresented in this figure.

Each line in the figure shows the relative occurrence per 100 for each consonant in initial position. The top line (A) represents this distribution for the complete corpus. The second line (B) shows the *changes* in relative occurrences of these initial phonemes after exclusion of (only 118 different) function words. The third line (C), similar to (B), shows the changes in distribution after exclusion of the 100 most common words, which includes both content and function types in equal proportion. Note particularly the marked decreases in frequency of occurrence of /t/, /ð/, /w/, /j/, and /h/ in both the second and third lines. French et al. noted that these decreases were due largely to the exclusions of " 'they,' 'this,' etc.; 'will,' 'would,' etc.; and 'you,' respectively." In contrast to lines (B) and (C), the last line (D) shows only negligible changes in distribution resulting from exclusion of the 1,500 least common words, which are predominantly content-type words.

It is well to recall here that, although not indicated in these figures, word length and word frequency are also represented in this material, because function words are predominantly short words that occur very frequently.

Of course, not all short words are function words. However, short content words have two major features in common with longer content words that differentiate them from the function word classes. First, the most common initial consonants of content words differ from those that characterize function words. Second, and of at least equal importance, in connected utterance words of the content classes, regardless of length, will receive stress; in contrast, function words, of any length, will not be stressed (except under rare and unusual circumstances). The latter feature is another dimension on which content words contrast dramatically with words of the function classes. This feature of English language structure was expressed succinctly and cogently by H.L. Smith (1959):

> It is necessary to bear in mind that the various classes of words in the language can appear only with certain stresses and not with others. For instance, excepting "compounds," nouns, adjectives, adverbs, and main verbs never occur with less than secondary stress; auxiliary verbs, prepositions and conjunctions never appear with more than tertiary. Articles almost always occur with weak stress—never more than tertiary—and personal pronouns regularly with no more than tertiary though they quite frequently are 'nominalized' by virtue of being said with secondary. Of course, any word can be said with primary stress when a higher degree of pitch is shifted to it for reasons of emphasis, in which case the word that would normally carry the primary stress in the sequence is reduced to secondary. These are *facts* of the structure of the language, internalized by all native speakers outside of awareness (p. 3).

In view of certain relationships identified previously, one might deduce that the occurrence of stress is related to word length. Such a relationship is documented in several sources. Denes (1963) identified the length, in syllables, of 10,699 stress-bearing words and 12,350 words spoken without stress in the corpus he analyzed. The comparative data are presented in Table 5.13. Most of the words, 77%, are short words, whether stressed or unstressed. However, as the data show, the preponderance of unstressed words are short words; a full 92% of all unstressed words are one-syllable in length. A substantial majority of stress-bearing words are also short words; 60% are one syllable in length. However, stress-bearing words clearly tend to be somewhat longer; 27% of the remainder are words of three-or-more syllables. In contrast, 99% of the unstressed words are words of two syllables or less.

TABLE 5.13. Relationship of stress to word length and frequency of occurrence[a]

Syllables per word	Total words	Cum. percent	Stressed words	Cum. percent	Unstressed words	Cum. percent
1	17,798	77.2	6,401	59.8	11,397	92.3
2	3,969	94.4	3,130	89.1	839	99.0
3	1,004	98.7	904	97.5	100	99.9
4	240	99.8	230	99.7	10	
5	38		34		4	
	23,049		10,699		12,350	

[a]Data from Denes (1963, table VI).

Stress is also clearly related to frequency of word occurrence. Berry (1953), from his analysis of a corpus of 24,781 words from telephone conversations, provides evidence of the direct relationship between stress and word frequency. Figure 5.2, reproduced from Berry, shows that "practically all the commonest words are unstressed, while practically all the least common ones are strongly stressed" (Berry, 1953, p. 396). These curves show that as the frequency of occurrence of individual words decreases, the proportion of unstressed words also decreases, in a direct

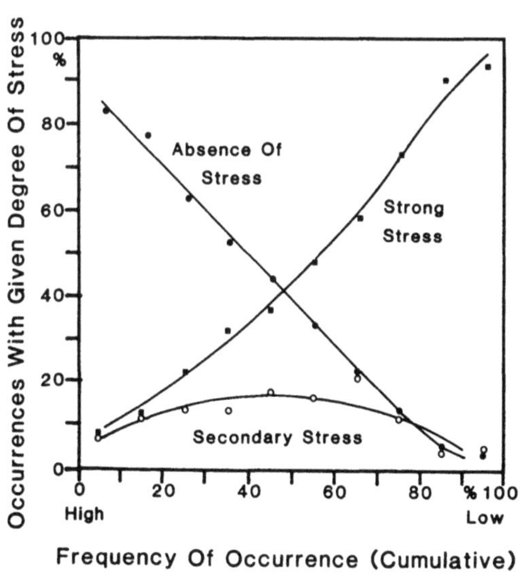

FIGURE 5.2. Percentage of occurrence of words with various degrees of stress as a function of cumulative occurrences when words are arranged in descending order of frequency. (From Berry, 1953.)

linear relationship. In contrast, the proportion of strongly stressed words steadily increases, almost linearly, as word frequency decreases.

Stress is also related to the consonant-vowel distinction. Denes (1963), in his analysis of phonetic readers, found that about 66% of all phonemes in stressed syllables are consonants as compared to 56% consonants in unstressed syllables. Berry's (1953) analysis of the spontaneous speech of telephone conversations found consonants to be the initial phoneme in 87% of the syllables bearing primary stress as compared to 59% of unstressed syllables.

Stress is also related positively to word-initial position. Most often, in polysyllabic English words, the stressed syllable is the first syllable. The data presented in Table 5.14, derived from several studies of spontaneous speech, show this relationship clearly.[7] Even though there is some tendency for primary stress to "move" rightward as words increase in syllabic length, stress falls predominantly in early-syllable, largely initial-syllable, position.

Analysis of the word-initial phoneme of the words described in Table 5.14 reveals that consonants occur considerably more often than vowels as the initial phoneme in these stress-initial polysyllabic words; see Table 5.15. This finding corroborates the reports of Berry (1953) and Denes (1963), cited previously, regarding the concurrence of consonants and stressed syllables. This evidence of direct relationship between stress in initial position and consonants as word-initial phonemes is augmented in-

Table 5.14. Location of stress in polysyllabic words

Source	Nature of sample	Number of different polysyllabic words[a]	Word length, in syllables, and percent of syllables bearing stress: 2		3			4			
			1	2	1	2	3	1	2	3	4
French et al.	Adult telephone conversations	362	71	29	57	38	5	34	29	37	0
Berger	Adult conversations	552	79	21	58	37	5	24	56	20	0
Howes	Adult interviews	440	80	20	58	37	5	39	25	28	8
Horn	Kindergarten talk	334	87	13	60	35	5	75	25	0	0
Delattre	Written	2,610	74	26	55	39	6	33	36	29	2

[a]Data for the first four sources are based on the approximately 1000 most frequently occurring words in the respective samples. The data from Delattre were derived from short stories. This larger—and therefore presumably more representative—sample gives values very consistent with the other samples from adult speech.

TABLE 5.15. Location of stress in the most frequent[a] polysyllabic words as related to type of word-initial phone

Source	Nature of corpus	Number of different words	Phone type	Percent having stress on syllable 1	2	3	4
Berger	Adult	414	C	72	26	1	1
	conversations	132	V	46	47	6	1
French et al.	Adult telephone	231	C	73	23	4	0
	conversations	129	V	48	45	7	0
Howes	Adult	320	C	82	16	2	0
	interviews	116	V	49	44	6	1
Horn	Kindergarten	260	C	90	10	0	0
	talk	67	V	61	37	2	0

[a]Words contained in the approximately 1,000 most frequently occurring words according to the sources cited. (From Wingate, 1985.)

directly by the fact (see Table 5.9) that among longer words, wherein stress is more likely to be on a syllable other than the first syllable, words become more likely to have a vowel as the initial phoneme.

In view of the evidence, presented in the foregoing material, regarding the relationships between content versus function words, initial phoneme, word length, and occurrence of stress, it is of some interest to find evidence that content words occur proportionately more often than function words in early positions of sentences, assuming written prose to be representative of language usage on this dimension. Table 5.16 shows the frequency with which words of different grammatical classes occurred in the first 3 positions of 200 sentences sampled from ordinary prose. The data represent an analysis of the first 20 sentences in 10 articles, selected at random, 1 from each of 10 different popular magazines.[8] Although, as might be expected, articles and pronouns occur most often as the first word of these sentences, nouns, verbs, and adjectives (stress-bearing words) predominate in the other two early sentence positions.

TABLE 5.16. Grammatical class of words occurring in the first three positions of sentences from ordinary English prose[a]

Position	Noun	Adj.	Verb	Adv.	Pron.	Aux.	Prep.	Conj.	Art.
1st	13	21	4	20	60	3	21	17	41
2nd	57	31	37	12	23	17	10	4	9
3rd	36	31	53	22	20	11	13	3	11

[a]The data were obtained from analysis of the first 20 sentences in 10 articles, selected randomly, one each from: *Better Homes and Gardens, Ebony, Ladies Home Journal, Life, McCalls, National Geographic, Newsweek, Popular Mechanics, Reader's Digest, The New Yorker.*

Speech research having a physiological focus yields evidence that stress prominences usually occur early in ordinary sentences. Figures 5.3 and 5.4, from Lieberman (1967), show pertinent physiologic and acoustic records from speech samples of the same person saying a declarative and an interrogative version of a short sentence. The curve representing subglottal air pressure is the tracing that is of most interest here. Lieberman discussed the subglottal air pressure contour as encompassing a "breath group," a basic pattern in connected speech that is analogous to what, in more traditional terms, is identified as a phonemic phrase or phonemic clause. Following Lieberman's use of subglottal air pressure as a major indicator of stress prominence, it is clear that in both declarative and interrogative forms of the utterance the major prominence occurs very early in both forms of the sentence. The stress prominence may shift, however, to a word occurring later in the utterance if that word is, for some reason, the word emphasized. Such shift in prominence is represented in Figure 5.5, which shows the tracings for the same speaker saying the sentence now emphasizing the last word.

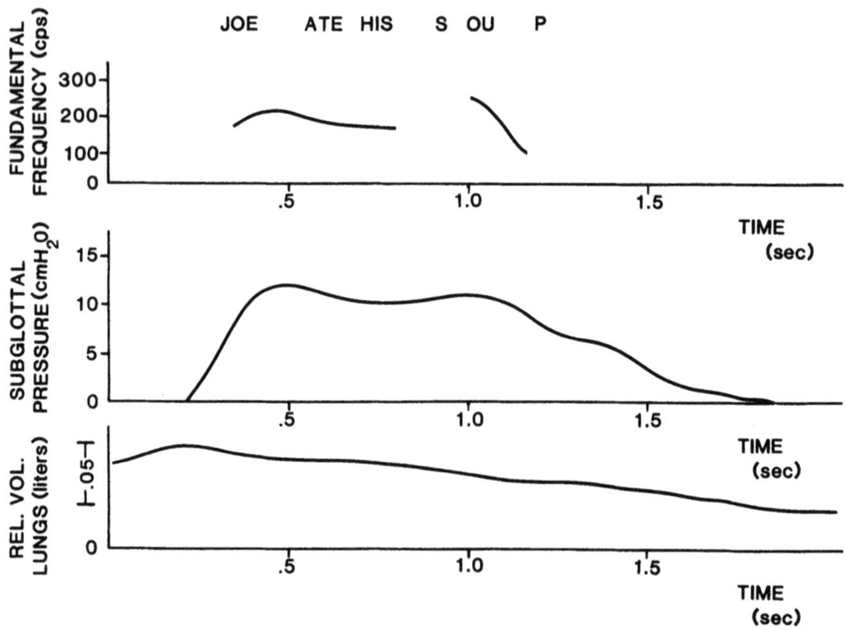

FIGURE 5.3. Acoustic and physiologic data for a normal speaker reading the declarative sentence, "Joe ate his soup." (From *Intonation, Perception, and Language* (p. 67) by P. Lieberman, 1967, Cambridge, MA: MIT Press. Reprinted with permission. Figure 4.10.)

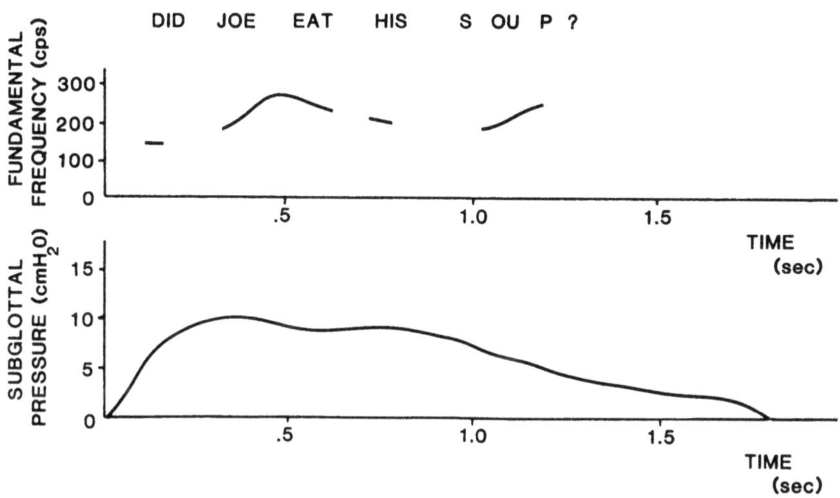

FIGURE 5.4. Acoustic and physiologic data for a normal speaker reading the interrogative sentence, "Did Joe eat his soup?" (From *Intonation, Perception, and Language* (p. 73) by P. Lieberman, Cambridge, MA: MIT Press. Reprinted with permission. 1967, figure 4.13.)

Synopsis

The foregoing analyses reveal that in English, particularly as it is spoken: (1) there is a clear predominance of short words; that (2) have a simple phonetic structure; in which (3) consonant phonemes predominate.

In typical samples of English usage one can identify two broad categories of words, roughly distinguishable in terms of grammatical roles, that comprise grossly comparable proportions of the corpus. One group, called function words: (1) are few in actual number, (2) recur with great frequency, (3) are typically unstressed, and (4) are characterized by a fairly limited set of initial phonemes. The other group, known as content words: (1) consists of many different words, (2) vary greatly in the frequency with which they occur, (3) typically bear stress, and (4) have many different, and varying frequencies of, phonemes in initial position.

This brief summary of structural features of English, as it is used, does not reveal the many details of these features and the nature of their relationships to each other. A succinct composite statement describing such a matrix is probably best presented graphically, as in Figure 5.6.

The remainder of this chapter will present an appraisal of the language factors reported to be associated with stuttering, developing the appraisal in reference to the foregoing analyses of normal speech samples.

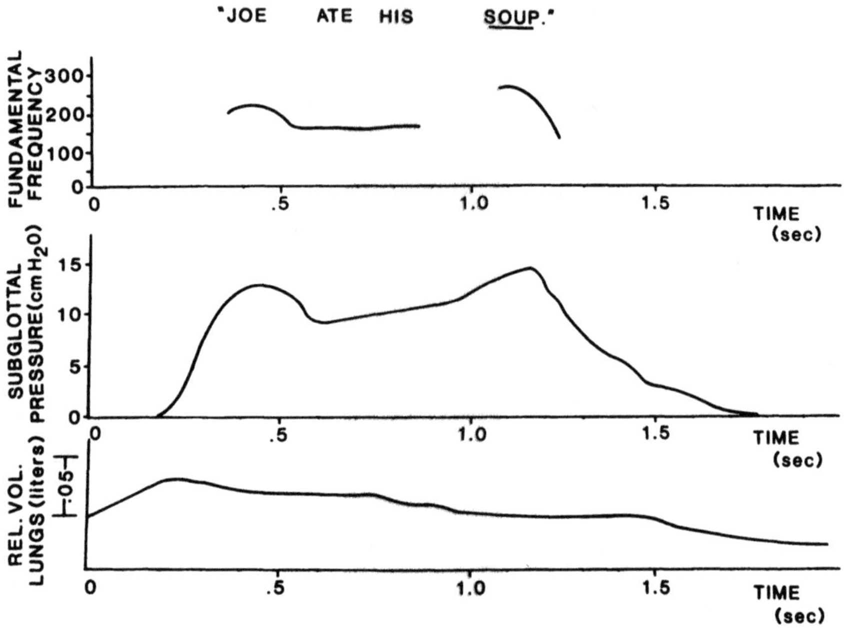

FIGURE 5.5. Acoustic and physiologic data for a normal speaker reading the declarative sentence, "Joe ate his *soup*." (From *Intonation, Perception, and Language* (p. 70) by P. Lieberman, 1967, Cambridge, MA: MIT Press. Reprinted with permission. Figure 4.12.)

Language Structures and Stutter Events

As discussed in Chapters 2 and 5, a proper analysis of language factors in stuttering requires that the analysis be undertaken with reference to what is known about pertinent features of the language in ordinary normal use. Such an analysis will not only be objective and realistic but will lend itself to a more broadly based psycholinguistic analysis of research findings in stuttering that, in turn, should lead to a better understanding of the disorder. It also holds promise for contributing to our understanding of how oral language is organized and produced.

At the outset of this reanalysis of language factors in stuttering it is important to make the point that the findings of relevant research have indicated only that stuttering is *more likely* to occur in association with most of the language factors identified in that research. This fact, evident since early in this area of research, is clearly revealed in S.F. Brown's (1945) report that his subjects stuttered on less than 20% of the occurrences of words having all four of the attributes he studied (consonant type, grammatical class, word length, sentence position) and that, at the same time,

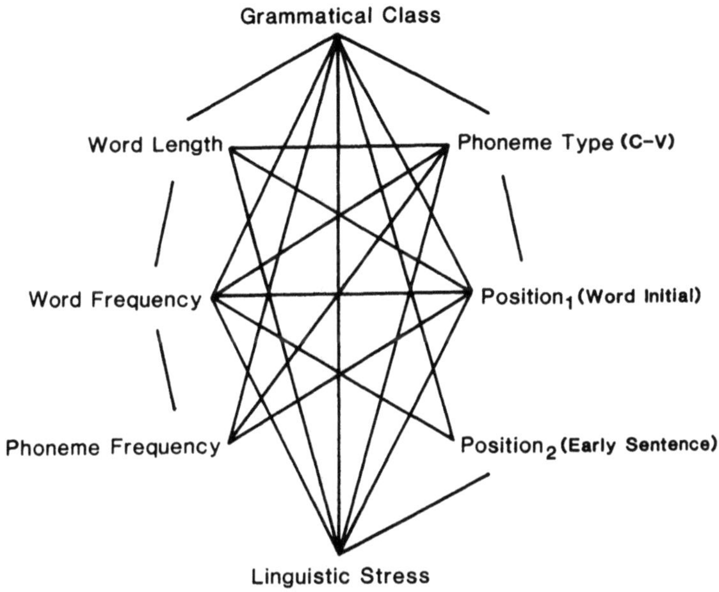

FIGURE 5.6. Interrelationships among various attributes of spoken words.

they stuttered on many words having none of these features (Brown, 1945, p. 187). A similar point should be made relative to the factor of linguistic stress, in spite of its strong association with stutters; that is, many stressed words are not stuttered and, occasionally, some unstressed words are stuttered. On the other hand, syllable-initial position is the one language factor that is consistently associated with instances of stutter.

Thus the association of the several language factors with stuttering, although impressive, is not complete. A point is made of this fact because it contradicts any assumptions to the effect that there is something about these factors that causes stuttering. Instead, it does encourage a logical deduction that the language factors should be recognized as important clues to understanding the nature of stuttering.

In undertaking a reanalysis of language factors reported to be associated with stuttering, it is appropriate to consider first the "phonetic factor," not only because this dimension served as the original precipitant of this area of research but also because it has been, for such a long time, a prominent feature in conceptions of stuttering.

The Phonetic Factor

As used in the relevant literature of stuttering, the "phonetic factor" means stuttering "on" consonants, with special reference to consonants other than those that Johnson and Brown (1935), and many others, reported to be "easy" consonants. The idea that consonants are the difficult phonemes for stutterers has been widely accepted for a long time. As noted earlier, stuttering has been reported frequently, for many years, to occur principally on consonants, and explanations of stuttering have continued to emphasize their significance. As pointed out in Chapter 3, Brown's interpretations of his data reflect the persisting belief that consonants play a significant negative role in stuttering. More recently, Taylor (1966a, 1966b) claimed that, compared to the factors of word length, sentence position, and grammatical class, consonants play the greatest role in stutter occurrences.[9]

Although reports of a predominance of stuttering on consonants have been made many times, one rarely finds a statistical statement of the extent of this predominance. However, pertinent data are available from several sources. Sheehan (1974) reported a consonant-to-vowel ratio for stutter occurrences, and similar ratios can be computed from the data reported in several other sources. These ratios, along with pertinent related information, are presented in Table 5.17. Two of the entries in the table do not give data regarding the initial C-V ratio of the corpus itself and thus might not be adequately representative samples. However, the reference values for samples for ordinary speech (see Table 5.8) suggest that these missing ratios could be expected to be somewhere between 2:1 to 3:1. It is of interest that three of the four word-initial C-V ratios given in Table 5.17 are also in this range. Further, it is pertinent to note that the C-V ratios for stuttering from each of these two sources are so comparable to the other stutter C-V ratios.

TABLE 5.17. Consonant-vowel ratios of stuttering relative to word-initial C-V ratio of the corpus

Source	Nature of corpus	Number of subjects	Total number of words	Word-Initial C-V ratio	Stutter C-V ratio
Johnson & Brown (1935)	Oral reading	32	311,903	2.0:1.0	5.8:1.0
Taylor (1966a, 1966b)	Oral reading	9	7,803	Not given[a]	5.4:1.0
Wingate (1979a)	Oral reading	35	12,670	3.3:1.0	7.4:1.0
Hejna (1955)	Spontaneous speech	18	15,061	1.8:1.0	2.7:1.0
Sheehan (1974)	Spontaneous speech; paraphrasing	20	Not given	Not given[a]	4.6:1.0
Wingate (1988)[b]	Spontaneous speech	20	2,206	4.7:1.0	8.3:1.0

[a]In terms of reference values (see Table 5.9), one could estimate these ratios as most likely being between 2 and 3 to 1.

[b]Data from the research to be reported in Chapters 7 and 8.

Keeping in mind that the C-V ratio for stutters implies word-initial position, these ratios are to be compared to the word-initial C-V ratios obtained form normal speech samples. The comparison reveals the C-V ratio for stuttering to be considerably higher than the word-initial C-V ratios of reference data; in fact, about twice as high, speaking in terms of approximate averaged values. These data thus provide some statistical support for the frequent statement that stuttering is associated more often with consonants than with vowels.[10] However, this does not necessarily imply that consonants are "more difficult" for stutterers than are vowels. The nature of the differential association of stuttering with consonants and vowels remains to be explored.

The first matter to consider is that these data regarding C-V ratios and stuttering do not support the claim that stuttering occurs "on" consonants. Second, they also do not indicate that stuttering occurs predominantly with consonants. Moreover, to find that stuttering is more often associated with (initial) consonants than (initial) vowels does not mean, as has been so regularly presumed, that consonants are therefore inherently more "difficult" than vowels. Actually there are a number of reasons to question whether consonants, per se, are more difficult than vowels.

One very cogent reason to doubt that consonants themselves present the difficulty is to be found in the regularly observed, and well-documented, fact that stuttering does not occur in word-final position.[11] The significance of this fact to the matter of stuttering "on" consonants is augmented substantially by the fact that consonants typically occur more frequently in word-final position than in word-initial position. The data supplied in French et al. (1930) reveal that 68% of final positions are occupied by consonants. Roberts' (1965) figures show this frequency to be 62%, a value almost identical to the 63 percent figure to be found in Denes' (1963) data. (Dewey's [1923] analysis of written material yields a figure of 82% final consonants.) This evidence suggests strongly that the higher incidence of stuttering associated with consonants is some function of the word-initial position of these consonants, rather than of the consonants per se. In other words, something about word-initial position is the more potent feature.

A second reason to question the inherent difficulty of consonants per se is that the same consonant that might be involved in a stutter when it occurs in word-initial position will not be stuttered in word final position: for example, the /m/ in /met/ but not in /tem/.[12] Again, this fact also indicates that the more important factor is word-initial position.

A third reservation is supplied in an observation, introduced earlier, that has been mentioned only occasionally in the literature at least since the 19th century: namely, that it seems a misinterpretation to say that the stutterer has difficulty with, or "on" (initial) consonants since, most clearly in the clonic expressions of stuttering, he makes the supposedly "stuttered" sound repeatedly. Clearly, if the stutterer produces a phoneme, particularly repeatedly, one should question how the sound itself can be "difficult." Again, it seems evident that the problem is not the sound itself, but that the obvious difficulty has something to do with the site where the difficulty occurs.

Fourth, it must be considered that if consonants are inherently difficult phonemes then there should be evidence of increased levels of stuttering when consonants are compounded, as in consonant blends or clusters. Yet blends are not found to be more difficult than single consonants; in fact, there is no evidence that being in a blend increases the difficulty level of even purportedly "difficult" consonants. This finding has recurred since it was originally reported by Brown (1938a). Brown reported that for all his subjects the percentage of stuttering was different for any single sound compared to one or more blends of that sound. In fact, for 71% of his subjects, statistically significant differences were found between the percent stuttering for a consonant occurring singly and the percent stuttering for one or more blends of that sound. Further, in 60% of these instances significantly *less* stuttering occurred on a blend than on the single sound initial to that blend. Such data indicate an influence associated with syllables, not phonemes.

Another matter to consider relative to stuttering and blends is that, when a consonant blend is involved in a stutter, the marker of the stutter event typically involves more than the first consonant of the blend; for instance, if a stutter event occurred on the word "study," "student," or "stutter," the event is typically marked by apparent difficulty with the blend itself, /st/, not with just the /s/. This phenomenon is particularly evident in clonic stutters, in which cases the iterations afford more opportunity to observe the character of the marker.

One additional consideration relative to blends is that, as is the case for single consonants, the involvement of a consonant blend in a stutter is absolutely conditioned by position: that is, stuttering may involve consonant blends in initial position but not in final position. And again, as with single consonants, consonant blends occur more often in word-final than in word-initial position. Additionally, the structure of blends is more complex in word-final position. These features of the language structure are documented in Table 5.18; the entries from R.M. Williams (1960) list only the common blends of English, the data from Dewey (1923) and Roberts (1965) reflect the sizable corpus analyzed in each of these studies. In spite of the clearly heavier consonant loading in word-final position shown by these data, stutters do not occur in final position. Once again it seems evident that initial position is the more critical factor than either phoneme type or particular phone.

Fifth, it must also be considered that the reported rank order of stuttering "on" consonants is not related to type of consonant. If stuttering were

TABLE 5.18. Number of consonants in consonant clusters of various sizes as found in word-initial and word-final positions

		Number of consonants per cluster					
	Number of different words	Word-Initial			Word-Final		
Source		2	3	4	2	3	4
Williams[a]	Lexicon	24	5	0	48	—[a]	4
Dewey	10,119	28	6	0	77	76	7
Roberts[b]	10,065	33	5	0	73	53	2

[a]Williams did not include final clusters resulting from the use of inflectional /s/.
[b]The 38 initial clusters comprise approximately 9% of all initial consonants. The 128 final clusters comprise approximately 14% of all final consonants.

related directly to a true consonant-vowel distinction, to an inherent difficulty of consonants versus vowels, then one should expect to find increasing levels of stuttering as the consonant type becomes more distinct from vowels. Consonants have been "scaled" in this way in reference to the constriction of the upper airway, a scale in which plosives appear at the top of the range and semivowels at the bottom.[13] If plosives epitomize consonantism (as defensibly claimed) one should find the highest incidence of stuttering on plosives and a gradually decreasing stutter incidence on other consonant types, consistent with the "consonantism" scale. However, the rank order of difficulty of phonemes does not follow such a sequence. In fact, several phonemes high in the consonantism scale (especially /t/, but also /h/ and /hw/) are among the "easy" consonants.

The five points of analysis just presented indicate that, in essence, the phonetic factor cannot be rationalized on either phonetic or phonemic grounds.

Results of the study by Soderberg (1962a) are particularly relevant to the point just made. Although a procedure that has subjects read lists of words has certain major limitations for broad applicability to the study of language factors in stuttering, it was appropriate for demonstrating that several types of consonant did not differ from vowels in their frequency of association with stuttering.

Fairbanks (1937) identified certain groups on which "the phonetic factor" might be linked to stutter occurrence; namely, "systematic variations in physiological difficulty." In reference to the Johnson and Brown (1935) data, Fairbanks observed that "the sounds upon which stuttering most often occurs are ... those sounds which, in general, necessitate the most extreme and active use of the speech mechanism" (p. 68). The suggestion that consonants are more difficult because they make greater articulatory demands has, of course, also been made by others. In all cases the explanation of greater articulatory demand has been made with the assumption that stuttering occurs "on" consonants. Only a general reference to other sources is necessary here. Special reference to the Fairbanks analysis is made for several reasons: its vintage; the fact that it has been cited frequently; his inclusion of attention to vowels; and, probably most important, because of what he reported regarding the relationship between the rank order of stuttered phonemes and their reported frequency of occurrence in the language.

Fairbanks obtained a rank order correlation of .43 between sound difficulties for stutterers and initial-sound difficulty for two-year-old children. He also showed that stuttering was inversely related to the intensity and duration of speech sounds; this inverse relation, of course, reflects primarily the finding of less stuttering on vowels. At the same time he found a positive correlation between stuttering and pitch, revealed in a rank difference coefficient of .66 between the difficulty of vowels reported by Johnson and Brown and the fundamental pitch of English vowels.[14]

Fairbanks' attention to vowels was rare in this literature, and the suggestion carried in his data was not pursued. The preoccupation with consonants as the difficult phonemes has led investigators to disregard implications from Fairbanks' data regarding vowels, and as well, the implications of another relevant study of the same era, a study that still merits replication. This other study, by Robbins (1936), included an oral reading task in which subjects were instructed to omit the initial consonants of words; that is, to read each word in the sequence as though it began with the first vowel. Robbins found that stutterers had much more trouble with this task than did the normally speaking control subjects.

The idea that the difficulty in stuttering lies, not with the (initial) consonant but, with the immediately sequential vowel has been suggested several times (Bluemel, 1913; Kussmaul, 1877; Wingate, 1969b, 1976).[15] Bluemel (1913) contended that the initial consonant is prolonged or repeated because the vowel is "delayed." He conceived this "delay of the vowel" to reflect a momentary inability to generate the correct "vowel color" or "vowel quality." This led him to explain stutter events as "transitory auditory amnesia:" the stutterer is temporarily unable to recall the auditory image of the vowel he must produce.

Bluemel maintained that the difficulty in stuttering involved vowels, not simply phonation. He reasoned that the difficulty in stuttering could not be simply a problem in phonation. He noted that there are many circumstances in which stutterers readily produce voiced sound spontaneously or voluntarily. (Actually, the most compelling observation along these lines is that, even in the course of a stutter, the stutterer often produces a voiced consonant or the so-called neutral vowel.[16]) Bluemel concluded that, since the stutterer can produce voice but not the appropriate vowel, the stutter event must reflect a temporary inability to re-auditorize the correct vowel sound. As support for this idea Bluemel noted that a stutterer can almost always say the (difficult) word as soon as someone pronounces it for him, an observation that has been reported often by others, too. Bluemel also offered as support his observation that stuttering occurs much more often on short vowels than on long vowels, because short vowels are "least definite and tangible in their coloration." He cited certain other sources that concurred in his observation regarding long and short vowels, but the additional sources he mentioned were, at best, equivocal. This claim has received only very limited support from later sources, including those based on casual observation; it does not concur with the rank order of difficulty for vowels in the Johnson and Brown data.

It seemed that some evidence for this hypothesis—that stutter events are some function of the vowel immediately sequential to an initial consonant—might be found by comparing the vowels following the "easiest" and the "most difficult" consonants as identified in the rank order of the Johnson and Brown list. Therefore the Iowa Oral Reading Test for Stutterers, the material used by Johnson and Brown (1935), was analyzed (by author) to identify the first vowel in all words beginning with the five "easy" consonants and in all words beginning with the five "most difficult" consonants. It was reasoned that if consonants at the extremes of that ranking of "difficulty" were followed by different vowels, or sets of vowels, some clue of a bona fide phonetic factor might emerge, along the lines suggested by Bluemel's position. The analysis revealed that, for the consonants at both extremes of the "difficulty" ranking, the most frequent immediately sequential vowel was /ɪ/. Since /ɪ/ is the most frequently occurring stressed vowel in English, this result could have been predicted purely in terms of probabilities. While this finding suggests that stutters are not connected to specific vowels any more than to particular consonants, it does not actually discredit Bluemel's "amnesia" hypothesis,[17] since the occurrence he posits could be an ad hoc event, unrelated to any particular vowel. Similarly, the finding also raises no reservation about the general idea that inquiry into stutter events should direct attention beyond the initiating consonant (or consonant cluster).

It is relevant, at this juncture, to consider another dimension of a possible relationship between stutters and vowels. This dimension can be addressed through a correlation of the rank order of stuttering "on" the vowels reported by Johnson and Brown (1935)[18] with the frequency with which various vowels occur in word-initial position in the language. The pertinent data are presented in Table 5.19. As noted earlier in this chapter, the literature on ordinary, normal language addresses relatively little attention to rankings of vowels, particularly in regard to their relative positions in words. Studies reported by Dewey (1923) and Denes (1963) are

TABLE 5.19. Comparison of rank orders, frequency of word-initial vowels in ordinary language usage with "difficulty" of vowels for stutterers

Word-Initial vowels[a]	Vowels associated with stuttering[b]
ə	ɜ
ɪ	ɛ
ɑ	ɪ
aɪ	ɔɪ
ɛ	i
ɔ	ou
æ	ʌ
ʌ	eɪ
o	aɪ
a	ɔ
au	ɑ
e	au
i	æ
ɔɪ	ə
ɜ	

[a]Composite, based on several sources (Wingate, 1985).
[b]As reported in Johnson and Brown (1935, table IV).

unique in this regard, having supplied data regarding the frequencies with which the various phonemes occurred in word-initial and word-final positions, as well as in overall distribution. Although these two studies were based on considerably different language samples, the rankings they give for word-initial vowels agree well, as reflected in a significant rank order coefficient of .66. A composite of the Dewey and Denes findings regarding the rank of word-initial vowels is presented as the first column of Table 5.19, and is used here as the reference rank, representing ordinary language use. The second column of the table reproduces the rank order of vowel "difficulty" reported by Johnson and Brown (1935). The two ranks show a clearly inverse relationship, expressed in a significant negative correlation of −.61.[19]

These data constitute evidence that a relationship does exist between stuttering and word-initial vowels. However, there is no indication of a relationship to any particular vowel nor even to any vowel type (i.e., front, high, rounded, tense, etc.). One might well have expected that the more frequently a vowel occurs in initial position the more it would be stuttered. However, the data show the opposite; that is, that the more frequently a vowel occurs in word-initial position the less likely it will be stuttered.

As mentioned earlier, Fairbanks (1937) concluded that phoneme difficulty for stutterers, as reflected in Johnson and Brown's (1935) data, is not related to the frequency of occurrence of sounds in the language. Fairbanks' conclusion was based on a correlation of .08 that he computed between Dewey's (1923) data on the relative frequencies of phonemes and the data reported by Johnson and Brown. Fairbank's report was cited in several of Brown's articles (Brown, 1937b, p. 212; 1938b, p. 116; 1938c, p. 225), and his conclusion has been accepted routinely in the subsequent relevant literature. In fact, it was thought to have been corroborated recently by Soderberg and MacKay (1972), who used as their reference for initial phoneme occurrence an estimate derived from the tables of transitional frequencies of English phonemes compiled by Hultzen, Allen, and Miron (1964).

The relationship between stuttered phonemes and phoneme frequencies reported in both of these sources is inaccurate. Since there is less reason to be concerned with the report by Soderberg and McKay, their contribution will be discussed first. There are several serious limitations to the Soderberg and McKay data. First, the speech samples from which the stutter events were tabulated were highly artificial: the stutters were recorded in the course of an experiment in which subjects said pairs of words or nonsense syllables five times in succession at maximum rate. Such performance is a considerable departure from ordinary speech, or even oral reading. Second, their identification of initial phonemes is highly questionnable. Their reference for occurrence frequencies of initial phonemes was simply an estimate derived from a corpus that also is an unlikely representation of ordinary everyday speech. The corpus was a fragmented sample of "spoken prose;" it consisted of the sequential juxtaposition of 11 one-page selections, 1 selection from each of 11 different plays for young people (Hultzen et al., 1964, p. 5).[20] Also, the tables of phoneme frequencies in this source are not based on natural word boundaries, a particularly pertinent matter. As revealed earlier in this chapter, word-initial phoneme frequencies regularly differ considerably from the overall phoneme frequencies in the same speech samples (see especially Tables 5.6 and 5.12). Estimating one set of frequencies from the other would be, at best, not only a complex procedure but also one most likely to yield unreliable values.

The data from Hultzen et al. have also been criticized in analyses mounted from a different perspective. In his formal review of the Hultzen et al. publication, Wang (1965) described the data as not representative of ordinary speech. Later, Carterette and Jones (1974) showed that the findings were indeed "very different from natural speech."

Returning now to Fairbanks' conclusion that the Johnson and Brown ranking of sound "difficulty" is not related to the frequency of occurrence of sounds in the language, it seems clear that this conclusion was based on a crucial error in selection of data. The correlation value reported by Fairbanks expresses the relationship between the Johnson and Brown ranking and the *overall* frequency of phoneme occurrences reported by Dewey.[21] But the overall ranking is not appropriate for this comparison. Evidently Fairbanks neglected to consider a most basic feature of stutter events: namely, that they involve word-initial phones. A rank-order correlation between the entire Johnson and Brown list and the frequency of occurrence ranking of all *word-initial* phones in Dewey's data yields a significant negative correlation (rho = −.34). If one considers consonants and vowels separately, an inverse relationship is even more clear-cut. The data relative to vowels were presented earlier (Table 5.19 and pertinent text). Comparable data for consonants are presented in Table 5.20; a highly significant rank order correlation of −.83 expresses the extent of this inverse relationship.

These significant negative correlations involving both consonants and vowels indicate that the more frequently a phone occurs in initial position, the less likely it will be associated with stuttering. The full nature of this

TABLE 5.20. Comparison of rank orders, frequency of word-initial consonants in Dewey's (1923) corpus with "difficulty" of consonants for stutterers[a]

Word-Initial consonants[b]	Consonants associated with stuttering
ð	d
h	z
s	g
w	tʃ
t	dʒ
b	v
f	k
m	θ
k	l
p	r
d	m
n	p
r	s
l	b
j	ʃ
g	n
ʃ	f
θ	j
v	t
tʃ	hw
dʒ	w
z	ð
	h

[a]Data from Johnson & Brown (1935).
[b]Dewey did not record /hw/.

relationship is not adequately revealed in these data alone. Reference to some of the other, closely related, data on language structure suggests a more complex relationship. Before proceeding to look at such data it is pertinent to direct attention to some relevant findings from the speech error ("tongue-slip") research. Comparably to stuttering, most speech errors involve initial consonants. However, in contrast to stuttering, the frequency with which these phonemes are involved in errors is proportional to their frequency of occurrence in the language (Shattuck-Hufnagel & Klatt, 1975, 1979). Of related interest is the evidence that the frequency of phonological errors in aphasia corresponds to the the frequency of phoneme distribution in the language (Blumstein, 1973).

Returning to a consideration of the inverse relationship between stutters and initial phonemes, we should begin by noting that this relationship is higher for consonants than for vowels. Next, note that, with two exceptions (/hw/ and /s/, to be examined presently), the consonants that are found to be "easy" for stutterers (/ð/, /h/, /w/, and /t/) are also the most frequently occurring initial consonants. Attention should be directed now to the material presented in Figure 5.1, and its accompanying narrative. Clearly, the same "easy" consonants (/ð/, /h/, /w/, and /t/)[22] are not only the most frequently occurring initial consonants, they are also the initial phonemes of the most frequently occurring words. Here several other structural dimensions enter the picture. These most frequently occurring words are also predominantly: (1) short words, that are also (2) function words, that are (3) almost always unstressed.

We can now return to consideration of /hw/ and /s/, which were apparent exceptions to the pattern of a close relationship between easy consonants and most frequently occurring initial consonants. The phoneme /hw/, though an easy consonant, is not one of the most frequently occurring initial consonants; the /s/ phoneme has just the opposite description. These inconsistencies can be resolved by noting the kinds of words for which each of these sounds is the initial phoneme. The /s/ phoneme is initial to words of varying lengths and frequency, representing various grammatical classes—except that few function words begin with /s/. In contrast, proportionately few words begin with /hw/ but most of them are short, unstressed, function words that occur with great frequency. Thus /s/and /hw/ also fit into the pattern identified for /ð/, /h/, /w/ , and /t/.

Two details of the results reported by Hejna (1955) are especially pertinent here. As noted in the earlier review of his work Hejna's treatment of stuttered phones occurring in spontaneous speech took into account the frequency with which the various phones occurred in word-initial position in the total corpus. He found that both /s/ and /ð/ were among the most frequently occurring initial sounds *and also* among the most frequently stuttered. However, comparison of their relative occurrences in the two distributions revealed significantly *less* than expected stuttering on /ð/ and significantly *more* than expected stuttering on /s/.

The interrelationships described in the preceding paragraphs lead directly into consideration of the grammatical class of words: the content word/function word distinction, and related matters.

Grammatical Class

Brown (see Chapter 3) found that the relationship of stutters to the grammatical class of words was much more substantial and stable than that manifested by the phonetic factor. As reviewed in Chapter 4, subsequent research has often corroborated this relationship, although there also have been certain apparently equivocal findings that raised at least some question about the essential validity of the "grammatical factor" in stuttering. Nonetheless, "kinds of words" has continued to have explanatory appeal, on dimensions reflecting the same theme originally expressed by Brown—namely, word meaningfulness. In more recent times, this theme has been expressed in such terms as "information load," "transition probability," or "uncertainty," all of which retain the essential notion that certain types of words are more important than others and, for that reason, are more often involved in stutter events. Reservations about the information load concept have already been expressed in Chapter 4.

Although at the present time grammatical class is not so widely mentioned as an explanation of stutter loci, the content word/function word distinction remains an important consideration in efforts to understand stuttering. Therefore, it is relevant to consider here certain issues that have always been, and remain, pertinent to any effort to account for stuttering in terms of word type and word meaning. These issues center in the distinction drawn between content words and function words in terms of their importance in an utterance. Content words have standardly been considered the *important* words in a message, with function words (either by implication or actual statement) treated as subsidiary. Brown drew this distinction clearly in his interpretations. Years later, the same bias was expressed in the fact that the concept of a "grammatical gradient" in stuttering encompassed only the four content word classes (see Chapter 4). Also, in the subsequent "information load" type of explanation, only content words were considered to carry the load; an assumption based on the notion that content words are the important words.

This assumption regarding the comparative importance of word class categories was unwarranted. Actually, Brown's own published data did not support it. His ranking of the "eight parts of speech" on the basis of frequency of associated stuttering (see Table 3.3) shows that, in respect to the numerical values on which the rankings are based, verbs are more appropriately classed with function words.[23] But it was the word-class concept, not the actual data, that determined the direction of analysis. The persistence of this view regarding word importance represents another instance of the limitations that pervade the literature of stuttering; limitations that are based in a preconception of the nature of the disorder and a concurrent disinterest in pertinent, broadly based information on normal speech and language function.

Brown (1937b) invoked the "telegram argument" as evidence that content words are the important words in a message, and this claim evidently has been accepted thereafter. The crux of this contention is that telegrams and newspaper headlines use only those words (i.e., content words) that are "necessary" to convey a message and omit the "unimportant" (function) words. But such examples provide a misleading criterion of word importance. Francis (1958, p. 236) and others have pointed out that both headlines and telegrams are prone to ambiguity largely because they omit function words. For example, either of the two possible meanings of the ambiguous message, "Ship sails today," is quickly clarified by proper placement of the most frequently occurring function word, "the." Many of the unintentionally humorous headlines featured in the bimonthly *Columbia Journalism Review* result from the omission of some function word. The following headlines are three of many examples; in each case the ambiguity could have been avoided by appropriate placement of "and," a common function word. "Man shot in back, head found in street." "Grover man draws prison term, fine for sex acts." "Garden Grove resident naive, foolish judge says."[24]

There are many other sources of evidence that function words are by no means unimportant. The Stanford-Binet Intelligence Tests contain, at the 12-year and Superior Adult I levels, items from a previously devised measure of intelligence, the Minkus Completion test. These items consist of sentences in which certain words have been omitted; success requires that the examinee supply the correct word to appropriately complete the sentence. The specific relevance of this task to the present discussion is that the omitted word is always a function word. In discussing the attributes of this test and its suitability as a measure of intelligence, Terman and Merrill (1937) noted: "The idea is a clever one, for no other part of a complex or compound sentence is so crucial in the correct comprehension of the whole as the relational elements" (p. 271). The crucial role of "the relational element" can also be illustrated in incomplete sentences for which, unlike the Minkus items, a number of different function words may be used correctly. For example, in the sentence "The woman ran ______ the man," a correct insertion could be any of the following words: *to, from, after, before, with, against, beside,* or *by.* Each of these words is critical to the meaning of the sentence; in fact, each word creates a significant change in the meaning of the entire sentence, in some cases to a direct opposite.

A simpler, but nonetheless powerful example of the importance of function words is the significant difference in meaning between the two most commonly occurring function words: the definite and the indefinite articles (which are also regularly found to be the least stuttered).

Function words simply cannot be dismissed as having little meaning. Fries and Traver (1950, p. 86) point out that "it is to be expected that the most frequently used words will develop a very wide range of meaning" which they illustrate by noting that, according to the *Oxford Dictionary*, the words *at*, *by*, *in*, *of*, and *with* each have 40 or more separate meanings. Along similar lines, Zipf (1935) gave examples of how the words *it* and *did* (pronoun and auxiliary) often refer to very extensive concepts:

> An example of the complexity of meaning of a simple word is offered by a few obvious sentences: 'It must have been funny when John dropped the eggs,' 'It was.' In the sentence 'it was,' the subject *it* does sole but adequate duty for the several concepts contained in the words 'when John dropped the eggs.' In the conversation, 'Why didn't you go to the store and buy the things I wanted,' 'I did,' the verb *did* performs similar duty for 'go to the store and buy the things I wanted.' That *it* and *did* make specific sense only because of the elaboration of the context in the preceding sentences does not alter the fact that *it* and *did* are simple subject and verb and that each represents a highly articulated concept (p. 235).

One must also bear in mind that many of the words typically designated as function words often are used as a grammatical form that crosses over the content/function distinction. For instance: *in* and *under* may be either a preposition, adverb, or adjective; *will* may be an auxiliary, a noun, or a verb; *on*, *out*, and *over* may be a prepostion, adverb, adjective, or noun; *when* and *where* may be pronoun, conjunction, adverb, or noun; and so on. Content and function words are not absolute or natural categories, as revealed by the foregoing examples and, as well, by the fact that there is more than one system for differentiating them. As Long (1961) put it: "Attempts to distinguish 'function words' and 'content words' in modern English have been made by many grammarians . . . [and] have never been successful. The truth is that almost all words have both grammatical and semantic value" (p. 86).

At the same time there are certain respects in which this (imperfect) categorization has utility, a utility well exemplified in the present analysis. The content/function distinction has served to highlight, in the study of stuttering, a language-related dimension of stutter occurrence. As shown in the foregoing discussion, this dimension is not realistically described in terms of word meaningfulness. Also, data from certain studies of language factors in stuttering (Soderberg, 1967; Taylor, 1966a) raise some question as to whether this dimension is defensibly expressed in terms of the content/function distinction itself. Nonetheless, the relationship of stutter events to the content/function distinction is a bona fide and reliable finding; further, it provides a focus that helps to illuminate those language factors that can be reasonably posited as being central to the occurrence of stutters.

The review of findings relative to "the Phonetic Factor," in the preceding section, and those relative to "the Grammatical Factor," in this section, reveals that these two factors are intimately interrelated with each other and with the factors of word length, word frequency, and stress. These interrelationships could be anticipated in view of the facts regarding the interwoven ties among these variables, shown in Figure 5.6, which reflects the analysis developed in the first section of this chapter.

Early Sentence Position

The variable of early sentence position is unique among the "language factors" associated with stuttering. The other factors, except for stress, apply to words alone; the sentence position factor transcends the level of words. At the same time, sentence position is also interrelated with the other factors, principally through the variable of grammatical class.

In the first study reporting an association between stuttering and sentence position (Milisen, 1937) the association seemed to be independent of words, and their several features. In that study 25 adult stutterers read 79 four-word sentences in which each of 61 different words appeared once in each of the 4 sentence positions. The results showed a steady decrease in frequency of stuttering from the first through the fourth sentence position. Thus it seemed evident that stuttering was associated with the positions the words occupied in the sequence, rather than with any particular words per se.

Years later, one of the major findings in the study reported by Conway and Quarrington (1963) also showed that the association of sentence position and stuttering maintained a certain level of independence from the actual words of the "sentences" spoken. In that study the 23 adult stutterers read aloud three groups of 7-word sequences. Each group of items had been constructed to represent three different levels of approximation to the structure of English, with the lowest level being meaningless as a sentence. The authors hypothesized that the positional effect on stuttering is dependent on the organization of the material, and that, therefore, a positional gradient of stuttering would not appear in "sentences" that were not grammatically correct.

The amount of stuttering in that material was found to vary directly with the level to which the "sentences" approximated standard English, indicating an influence of sentence "meaningfulness." At the same time, a positional gradient was still evident throughout; concurrence of stuttering and sentence position was proportionately the same at all three levels of approximation to English structure, indicating an influence of early word position independent of sentence meaningfulness.

The significance of the findings from both of the foregoing studies is qualified by the fact, regularly overlooked, that none of the specially constructed sentences in the two studies were typical English sentences; they contained unusual proportions of content words, particularly in initial position. This fact is of considerable importance for interpreting the association, with stuttering, of early sentence position because, as it turns out, there is evidence that the grammatical class of words is involved in the effect associated with early sentence position.

Although function words occur about as often, in overall language use, as do content words (see Table 5.10) the latter occur more often as the early words of sentences in written prose—particularly among the first three words, which is the range embraced by the sentence position factor in its reported association with stuttering. The data in Table 5.16, taken from several sources of ordinary prose, provide a reference. These data show that content words occur considerably more often than do function words in early sentence positions. Expressed in percentage form, the values of Table 5.16 show that 61% of words in the first three sentence positions are content words.

Actually, the prose material that yielded the data for the series of articles by Brown (reviewed in Chapter 3), which established the sentence position factor, has an even higher frequency of content words in early sentence positions; the first three positions in the material used by Brown contain 67% content words. This apparent confounding of sentence position and grammatical class led to research (Wingate, 1979a) designed to investigate the relative influence of these two variables on stuttering.

Position and Grammatical Class

The most feasible means of manipulating the variables of word position and the grammatical class of words was to obtain speech samples from stutterers in which the proportions of content and function words in the first three sentence positions were substantially altered. To this end a special passage was constructed that essentially inverted the usual proportions of content and function words in early sentence positions. In this special passage function words occupied 73% of the first three positions. This special passage, read by 33 stutterers, yielded results that are summarized in Table 5.21. The relative proportions of stuttering on content and function words are presented in ratio form.

There are several important features of these results. First, overall the data show the usual finding of a greater incidence of stuttering on content words (7.1 to 2.8). This finding is due primarily to the fact that content words are stuttered substantially more than are function words in sen-

TABLE 5.21. Frequency of stuttering on content and function words relative to sentence position[a]

Word class	First three positions			Other positions			Total		
	N[b]	Stutt	Ratio	N	Stutt	Ratio	N	Stutt	Ratio
Content	17	64	3.7	189	1,393	7.4	206	1,457	7.1
Function	46	237	5.1	110	198	1.8	156	435	2.8
Combined	63	301	4.8	299	1,591	5.3	362	1,892	5.2

[a]Data from Wingate (1979a, table 2).
[b]N = number of words.

tence positions other than the first three (7.4 to 1.8). Second, contrary to the typical findings regarding frequency of stuttering in early sentence positions, the relative amount of stuttering on the first three words in this special passage is essentially the same as for the other sentence positions (4.8 and 5.3). Third, also contrary to typical findings, stuttering occurs more often on function words—in the first three positions (5.1 to 3.7). Moreover, except for articles, stuttering on function words in these positions is much greater than on function words in other sentence positions. It is of some interest that stuttering on articles, infrequent as usual, was evidently unaffected by the position placement.

The results identified in the second and third items of the preceding paragraph are opposite to what previous research would lead one to expect relative to the association of stuttering with both grammatical class and early sentence position. These results reveal an interrelationship between sentence position and grammatical class of words, and suggest an interaction of these factors in their association with stuttering. The second item indicates that grammatical class evidently qualifies the apparent influence of early sentence position. On the other hand, the third item demonstrates an influence of early sentence position on grammatical class. These findings indicate that the two variables are not separate factors influencing the occurrence of stuttering, as posited by Brown and accepted subsequently. Rather, these results suggest: (1) that some other feature of the language, represented in the distinctions within the variable of grammatical class, is the fundamental dimension associated with stutter occurrences; and (2) that this dimension ordinarily is compounded, or elaborated, by an influence associated with early sentence positions.

Therefore it can be deduced that the "fundamental dimension" just mentioned is to be found in the prosodic aspects of oral language, especially in regard to the expression of linguistic stress. Because a relationship between stress and grammatical class is the more comprehensive association, this connection will be discussed first before proceeding to consider the expression of stress in early utterance position.

Grammatical Class and Stress

As discussed in the first section of this chapter, on the structure of ordinary oral language, linguistic stress is directly related to grammatical class. The relationship is described clearly in Smith's (1959) succinct statement regarding the occurrence of stresses in English. As Smith pointed out, stress is usually determined rather narrowly by the grammatical class of words. In general, words of the content classes are those likely to be stressed; function type words are not. At the same time, some amount of variation is associated with certain subcategories within these classes and, as well, with words of any class as a function of their role in any particular utterance.

The association of stuttering with linguistic stress is clearly reflected in the data of Table 3.2 which shows the relative amounts of stuttering associated with subcategories of grammatical class. The ranking indicates that the frequency of stuttering is not related consistently to grammatical class, per se, but to word types in proportion to the level of stress they are likely to receive in connected speech. Note the concurrence of the rank order of word types in Table 3.2 with the description contained in the quotation from Smith. Nouns, gerunds, adjectives, adverbs, main verbs, and root verbs—the word types stuttered most—are also the classes most likely to be stressed. However, auxiliary verbs, prepositions, articles, conjunctions, and pronouns—word classes least stuttered—are the types most likely not to be stressed. The variable of stress can also account for differing frequencies of stuttering among several function word classes. Possessive pronouns, which are stuttered less than personal pronouns, are typically unstressed, whereas personal pronouns are much more likely to be, in Smith's words, "nominalized," in which case they are stressed. Similarly, subordinating conjunctions, which are stuttered more often than are coordinating conjunctions, are much more likely to be stressed than are coordinating conjunctions.

Articles, at the bottom of this ranking, are the word types that are almost never stressed. Recall that, in the research previously discussed, in which early sentence positions were intentionally loaded with function words, stuttering on articles was not only infrequent, the usual finding in all languge-factors research, but also did not show the influence of position that was found for the other categories of function words that were placed in the early positions.

It is pertinent, and of considerable interest, to mention here that Brown, citing a study by Steer and Tiffin (1934), noted evidence of a direct relationship between the "relative physical intensity" of the (eight) parts of speech and the extent of their involvement with stuttering. He reported a rank difference correlation of .92, and went on to say:

> This is apparently in contradiction with Fairbanks' (1937) finding that a significant negative correlation exists between the rank of difficulty of sounds for stutterers and the physical intensify carried by the sounds. However, it should be pointed out that the Steer-Tiffin ranking is based on the peak phonetic power of the *words*, which depends upon the intensity of the loudest vowel sound, whereas the Fairbanks correlation was based on data containing only the relative frequency of stuttering on initial sounds of words. Only rarely were these latter identical with the loudest vowel sounds of the words (1937b, p. 212).

Brown did not pursue the significance of this strong relationship but, instead, continued to concern himself with the potential psychological significance of grammatical classes and phonemes. However, his data and description, presented in this paragraph, are integral with the analysis developed in this section regarding the significant role of stress in stutter occurrences.

It would seem, then, that the likelihood of a word being stuttered is largely some function of the extent to which it is likely to be stressed. Although stuttering is clearly related to grammatical class at a descriptive, or phenomenal, level, this relationship appears to be, in substantial measure, a surface expression of the association of stuttering with linguistic stress. At the level of words, stress is also related, through grammatical class, to the factors of initial phone, word length, and word frequency.

A graphic illustration of the concurrence of stuttering and linguistic stress is presented in Figure 5.7. The two curves in the figure represent two sets of data generated in reference to the first two sentences of the special passage, described earlier, which read, "From within the small ship the passengers felt the movement of the heavy swells, though now the ship was riding well. On through the stormy night they had struggled over huge waves, in constant danger of swamping" (Wingate, 1984c).

Curve A is taken to represent a typical stress pattern of a normal speaker saying these two sentences. The curve is a graphic level recorder tracing that reflects variations in intensity of the speech signal. Intensity, a major dimension of stress, is accepted here as an adequate representation of stress. The tracing was made from a tape recording of a reference speaker saying the two sentences; the sample was chosen by a linguist, expert in English prosody, as being a typical example.[25]

The thin vertical lines identify, in curve A, the loci of the syllable nuclei in the sentences, recorded in phonetic transcription at the base of the figure. These vertical lines, extended upward, served as the framework for plotting curve B, which represents frequency of stutters that occurred when these sentences were read by 35 young adult stutterers. The peaks of curve B indicate the frequency of stutters occurring at each locus iden-

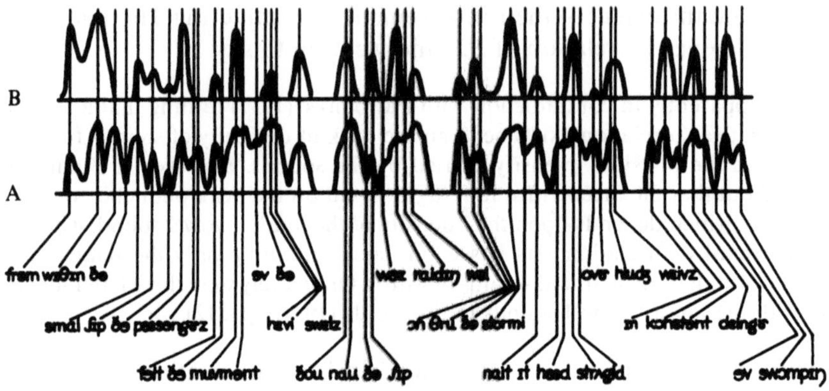

FIGURE 5.7. Concurrence of stutter events and linguistic stress. (From Wingate, 1984c.)

tified by a vertical line. The actual curve was drawn to connect these points smoothly.

The two curves of Figure 5.7 show a clear correspondence between stress prominences and stutter events. Note that most of the stress prominences, and most instances of stutter, are associated with content type words. However, also note that, in this special passage, function words participate in this correspondence of stress prominences and stutter events. The stutter-stress correspondance is not, of course, one to one, which should not be expected. As noted earlier, except for syllable-initial position, it seems most appropriate to consider the "language factors" as dimensions that tag where stutters are most likely to occur. At the same time, linguistic stress is one of the two dimensions most consistently associated with stutters; the only dimension more consistent is syllable-initial position.

Evidence of the association between linguistic stress and stutters is also contained in research conducted with native speakers of German. Bergmann (1986) used a procedure in which 16 young adult male stutterers independently read each of a group of relatively short sentences (average length, 6 words) as an answer to questions. The questions were phrased in various ways so as to induce changes in the stress pattern of the sentence given in appropriate answer. The changes in stress pattern resulted in certain words being stressed at some times but unstressed at others. This procedure isolated the stress variable for analysis, because comparison was made of the same words in the same sentence positions. Bergmann found a highly significant difference in frequency of stuttering on words when they bore sentence stress than when the same words were unstressed.

Early Position and Stress

Certain aspects of the research just reviewed (Wingate, 1979b, 1984c) reveal the involvement of stress in early sentence positions and the joint connection with stuttering. The curves of Figures 5.7 indicate that the inversion of stuttering frequency on function words, resulting from their placement in early sentence positions, was evidently due to the fact that in these positions they were—atypically—stressed. In other sentence positions the relation between stress and content or function words was more consistent with the standard pattern described by Smith (1959).

The occurrence of stress in early sentence position is one of the features of ordinary oral language expression, presented in the first part of this chapter, that have particular significance for understanding the nature of stuttering. Lieberman's (1967) work yielded evidence, presented in Figure 5.3, that stress prominence typically occurs early in ordinary declarative utterances (and as well, in interrogative versions of such utterances, Figure 5.4).

Looking again at the rankings of word categories in terms of extent of stuttering, presented in Table 3.2, several items reflect the involvement of stress in early position as expressed through grammatical class. As noted earlier, there are differences in rank among certain categories of pronouns and conjunctions. Personal and relative pronouns are stuttered more often than are possessive pronouns. The former are pronoun types that are much more likely to be stressed than the latter. They are also the types that frequently occur as early words in utterances; in fact, it is in large measure because of such position occurrences that these types are more likely to be stressed. The rank difference between subordinating and coordinating conjunctions express this same relationship between stress and early utterance position.

Thus the "prominence" of early sentence position is best understood as *stress* prominence, which regularly occurs early in what Lieberman identified as the "breath group." Following Lieberman's description earlier in this chapter, of the breath group as equivalent to what is standardly identified as the phonemic clause, certain findings reported by Soderberg (1967) become particularly relevant. Soderberg analyzed stutter occurrences in reference to phonemic clauses. He found more stuttering on earlier words of phonemic clauses and, also, that an unexpectedly high incidence of stuttering on function words probably reflected the frequency with which such words occurred in early clause position.

As discussed in Chapter 4, it has been widely recognized for a long time that utterance initiation is evidently a site of special difficulty for stutterers, reflected in the fact that stutters occur there so often. Normal nonfluencies also occur at utterance initial loci, in the speech of stutterers and normal speakers. But early position presents special difficulty for stutterers, as revealed in the comparative research reviewed in Chapter 4, pages 106–108, 122–124. In those studies, which compared the "disfluencies" in speech samples from stutterers and normal speakers relative to Brown's four factors, the position factor was significantly more evident in the speech of stutterers.

The findings of a study by Shapiro (1970)[26] bear pointedly on the special significance for stuttering of early word position and its relationship to linguistic stress. Shapiro used intensity of the speech signal as the dimension for comparing the stress patterns of several brief *fluent* utterances of 15 young adult stutterers and matched normal speakers. Shapiro obtained recordings of several identical spontaneous utterances from all subjects by asking carefully phrased questions about cartoons. Graphic level recorder tracings were made from these recordings and all individual tracings were replotted to a common form by quantifying successive points on each curve as percentage values of each axis (amplitude and time.) Composite stress patterns, representative of each subject group, were then computed from these data. A graphic display of these data for the several utterances are reproduced in Figure 5.8.

It is apparent that, for each subject group, the stress patterns for the two three-syllable and the two five-syllable utterances are similar, reflecting intra-group consistency in these samples. Statistical analysis confirmed this consistency, and also indicated significant differences between the curve pairs on both time and amplitude dimensions.

The patterns for the two speaker groups are clearly divergent. For the three-syllable utterances the normal speakers' curves suggest a phrase spoken as a connected utterance; the stutterers' curves appear more like a sequence of separate syllables. Differences between the two groups on the four- and five-syllable phrases are even more dramatic, particularly in reference to the relationship of stuttering to early position. In contrast to the normal speaker's curves, which show well-defined peaks representative of the stress-bearing syllables, the curves of the stutterers show a marked prominence associated with the first stress-bearing syllable[27] but a rapid decay of the curve thereafter. Another comparison of particular relevance to early position is that, in all of the displays, the normal speakers' first syllable peak occurs with a temporal consistency regardless of utterance length. This consistency contrasts pointedly with the stutterer curves, in which initial peaks vary directly with utterance length.

The departures from the normal pattern that are reflected in the stutterers' patterns, for these fluent utterances, imply some anomaly in the manner in which these subjects dealt with the "point of attack" represented in early utterance position.[28] These apparent anomalies would seem to shed some light on the role of early utterance position in stutter occurrences.

It is important to recognize that, although the position effect is regularly

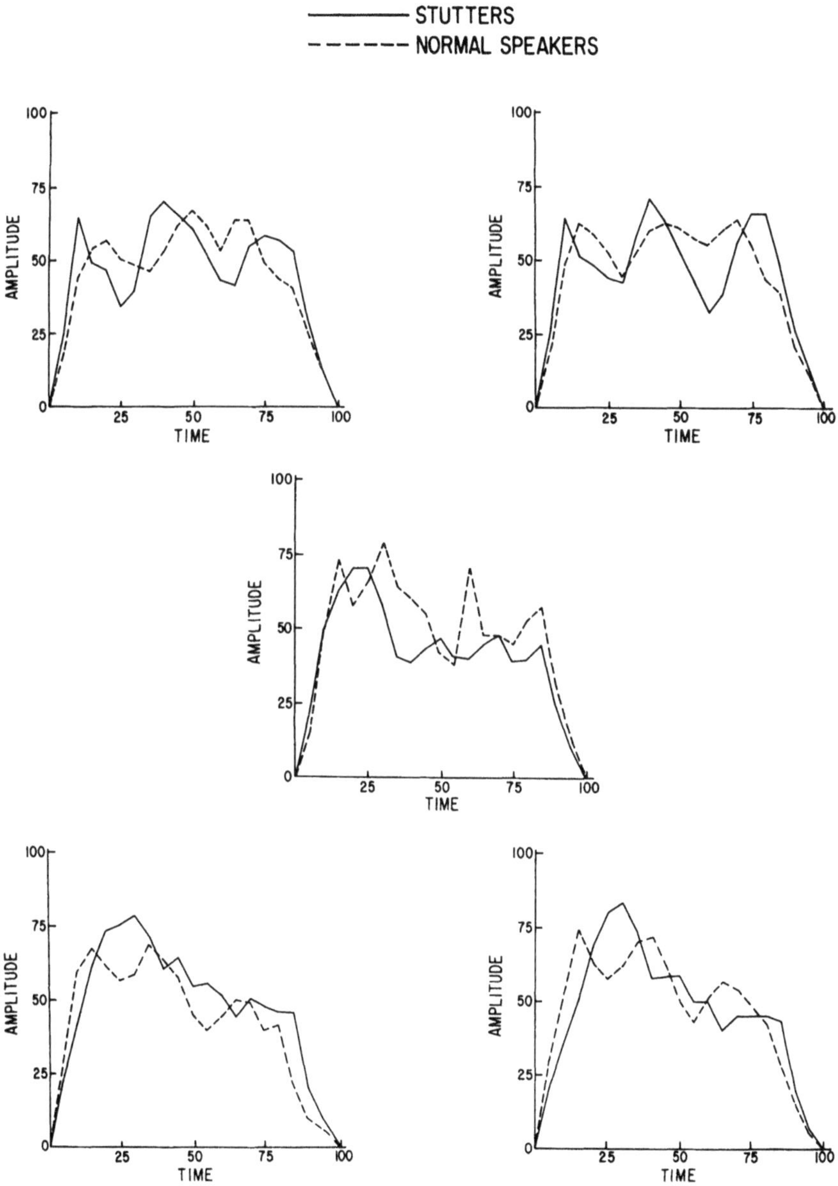

FIGURE 5.8. Averaged stress patterns of 15 stutterers and 15 normal speakers for 5 phrases of three different lengths. (From C.W. Shapiro, 1970.)

referred to as early *sentence* position, there is evidence that the position effect operates at the level of the phrase. Certain findings in the 1960s, which prompted speculation about "cycles" of stuttering (see Chapter 4, p. 111–114), evidently reflected stutter occurrences at the beginning of phrases. Certainly the study by Soderberg (1967) yielded clear evidence of stutter events in phrase initial position. Also, Bloodstein (1974) reported stutters to occur at the beginning of "syntactic structures" which, in the final analysis, are equivalent to phrases.

One important qualification needs to be introduced regarding the well-documented fact of higher frequency of stuttering in early utterance position. The literature supporting this fact has tended to carry the implication that the extent of stuttering is greatest on the first word and then gradually decreases. Very likely this implication is based on certain reports in which stuttering on words in initial position was actually greater than in other positions, and this finding was emphasized in one way or another (e.g., Brown, 1938b; Conway & Quarrington, 1963; Milisen, 1937; Taylor, 1966b). As noted earlier, these results were confounded by the disproportionate occurrence of content words in first position. However, stuttering does not routinely occur with greatest frequency on the first word of utterances. In Hejna's (1955) study of the spontaneous speech of 23 stutterers the frequency of stuttering associated with words in sentence initial position was only 67% of that occurring with words in second position. In Wingate (1979b), the study that focused on early position, the incidence of stuttering on first words was less than 80% of that for words in second position.

Stutter occurrence in first position seems to depend on whether the word appearing there participates in the stress prominence typical of early position. To some appreciable extent this variation involves the *type* of word appearing in first position—basically, whether it is a content or a function word. Content words are likely to be an integral part of the early position stress prominence; they are also likely to be stuttered in that position. The same can be said for certain pronouns, particularly personal pronouns, in utterance-initial position where they are likely to be "nominalized." On the other hand, other function words often found in initial position, particularly articles, are not likely to be stressed—and also are not likely to be stuttered.

The idea that word type contributes to the probability of stutter occurrence in first word position is supported by considering the structure of the material used in those studies that found a higher frequency of stuttering associated with first words. In the research reported by Milisen (1937) and Conway and Quarrington (1963), the first words were always content words. Similarly, the material used by Brown (1938b) has an unusually high loading of content words in sentence-initial positions; 52% of sentence-initial words in the *Iowa Oral Reading Test for Stutterers* are content words. In contrast, data from sources that can be assumed to represent typical prose selections show that *function* words predominate as first words in sentences. Pertinent data (Table 5.18) from a random sample of 200 sentences taken from 20 current lay magazines reveal that only 29% of the words in sentence-initial position are content words. Martin and Strange (1968) found that content words occupied only 18% of the sentence-initial positions in the corpus analyzed by Miller et al. (1958; see Table 5.11), which consisted of over 36,000 words from 6 prose selections.

Linguistic stress can also be seen to influence those instances in which stutters occur in positions other than, and instead of, utterance-initial or even early utterance positions. Bergmann's (1986) work, cited earlier, yielded pertinent data. Bergman's subjects were induced to stress specific words in their answers, which resulted in a higher frequency of stuttering on those words. Although stutters also occurred at sentence beginnings, both absolute and relative values of stuttering frequency were higher for the words specially stressed than for words at the beginning of the utterances. Findings very similar to these results were reported by Kaasin and Bjerkan (1982). These authors, working with 26 teenage stutterers who were native speakers of Norwegian, created circumstances in which subjects were required to convey specific information to certain other members of the group. Accurate communication of the message hinged on the use of certain words, identified by the authors as *critical* words. Their results showed that the critical words were stuttered significantly more often, proportionately, than the remainder. Relative to position, the authors found that stuttering occurred significantly more often in ending positions—which was also where significantly more of the critical words occurred. In Norwegian and German, as in English, the critical words in an utterance are likely to be emphasized; and the emphasis is expressed as a stress prominence (as reflected in Figure 5.5). Thus, in the findings of both studies just reviewed, a shift in frequency of stuttering can be accounted for in terms of changes in relative stress prominence.[29]

Distillation

Four of the language factors associated with stuttering—initial phoneme, grammatical class, word length, word frequency—are attributes of words. A fifth factor, sentence position, transcends the level of words, but its relevance is expressed in terms of words. The other two factors—syllable-initial position and linguistic stress—are attributes of syllables.

The research presented in the first part of this chapter has shown that all of these factors are interrelated in the structure of the language, as summarized in Figure 5.6. The research reviewed in the second section has shown that the same interrelationships exist relative to the association of these variables with stuttering. At the same time, syllable-initial position and linguistic stress can be said to have the more fundamental relationship to stutters, for several reasons.

Like the first five factors listed, stress is not always associated with stutters. However, its relationship to stutters is higher than that for any of the other five. In addition, the apparent influence of other factors often can be shown to actually reflect the effect of linguistic stress. Moreover, stress is the one factor that evidently can alter the usual realtionship to stutters of any of the other factors, except syllable-initial position. That is, the influence of stress has been shown to modify the evident influence on stuttering of word position, and of grammatical class (and, by extension, of the remaining factors, which are closely connected to grammatical class). In contrast, there is no evidence, and one could not expect to generate any, that would show the opposite effect.

Syllable-initial position is the most special of all these factors. It is the one factor that is always present in a stutter, and its expression is not modified by any of the other variables. Unlike the other factors, one cannot speak of it as "contributing to the probability" of stutter occurrence. Syllable-initial position is always involved; it is, in fact, the essential phonemenal feature in the locus of a stutter event.

Thus, from the network of structural features of the language that are evidently related to stutter events, there are two that surface as the truly significant dimensions: linguistic stress and syllable-initial position. Identifying these two features as the crucial dimensions is not equivalent to saying, simply, that they are the most important of the language factors that have been discovered to this time. It seems that evidence from a variety of sources points to these dimensions as being *focal* in stutter events, focal in the sense of: (1) describing the locus of a stutter event; (2) identifying a channel through which features represented in the other factors contribute to the occurrence of stutters, and (3) centering on certain basic features of language structure that point to the essential nature of stuttering.

A detailed consideration of these two dimensions is the topic of Chapter 6.

Footnotes

[1]Both Brown (1938c) and Hahn (1942b) noted a certain level of relationship between initial phone and grammatical class. Some others, for example Schlesinger et al. (1965), remarked on several interrelationships.

[2]Studies of the lexicon (as compared to actual language samples) also show that most words of the language are represented in a very limited number of canonical forms. For example, Trnka (1968) found that 78% of the words of "standard English" have one of only three canonical forms. Similarly, Moser, Dreher, and Oyer (1957), in their analysis of "all socially accepted monosyllabic words in the

English language" (p. 4) found that 80% of the words had one of only four canonical forms.
[3]The phonetic readers, used for teaching English to foreign students, were: *Phonetic Readings in English*, by D. Jones, and *English Conversations*, by N. C. Scott. Fry (1947) also used the Jones reader.
[4]The 60:40 percentage in Roberts' analysis might be due to the very large corpus and the extent to which it included personal correspondence.
[5]The phoneme rankings in Tables 5.6 and 5.7 are composite rankings constructed from pertinent data presented in a number of different studies of the structure of the language, many of them cited at various places in this chapter. Not all of the sources contribute to each of the several rankings, because some of them did not report data pertinent to each ranking. However, for each ranking all pertinent data were incorporated; the object being to establish the broadest possible base for each list.
[6]The data from French et al. yield a 2:1 C-V ratio in both initial and final positions. Roberts' data yield a word-initial ratio of 2:1 and a word-final ratio of 5:1. Similarly, Dewey's data give a word-initial ratio of 2.4:1 and a word-final ratio of 5.2:1.
[7]A clear relationship between stress and word-initial position is also evident in data derived from analysis of the lexicon. Trnka's (1968) figures show 2,451 actual bisyllabic monomorphemic words, of which 2,221, or 90%, are stressed on the first syllable.
[8]*Better Homes and Gardens, Ebony, Ladies Home Journal, Life, McCalls, National Geographic, Newsweek, Outdoor Life, Readers' Digest,* and *The New Yorker.*
[9]Taylor's data present a problem for at least certain dimensions of analysis, inasmuch as the data were derived from a 237-word passage read 5 times in succession.
[10]Since the issue here is the reported difficulty of consonants per se, the source of the data (whether spontaneous speech, paraphrasing, or oral reading) is not a relevant qualification.
[11]This important fact is considered in Chapter 6.
[12]The /m/s in these two positions are not phonetically identical, due to contextual influences. However, it is highly unlikely that such allophonic variation makes any difference in what is being considered here. Certainly there is every reason to doubt that the individual speaker is aware of any difference.
[13]The "sonority (or sonorance) hierarchy." See Chapter 9.
[14]All of these correlations were reported to be significant.
[15]My own focus on the sequential vowel has been addressed to its suprasegmental role.
[16]The focus on phonatory control that is found in much of the recent research in stuttering overlooks this reasoning.
[17]Nor does it discredit his later hypothesis of "temporary mutism." (See Bluemel, 1957, p. 40 ff.)
[18]The Johnson and Brown list contains the only ranking of stuttered vowels.
[19]All correlations are significant at the 0.1 level of confidence.
[20]The tables constructed by Hultzen, Allen, and Miron were derived relative to a rationale based on the notions contained in Shannon and Weaver's *Mathematical Theory of Communication.*
[21]Dewey presented and discussed the overall rank order of phonemes in the text of his book. The rank orders of the phonemes in different positions are the substance of his table 17.
[22]If the mean value of the Johnson and Brown data had been a little higher, /j/ would have been among the "easy" consonants (see Table 3.1).

[23]The difference between verbs and pronouns is *less than half* the difference between verbs and adverbs. Moreover, the latter difference is over twice as large as any of the other differences between categories.
[24]From, respectively: the *Richmond* (Virginia) *Times-Dispatch*; the *San Luis Obispo* (California) *Telegram-Tribune*; the *Orange County* (California) *Register*, in 1985.
[25]The linguist was H. L. Smith, author of the quotation reproduced earlier in this chapter. It is relevant to note that, having made his selection, Smith indicated that any one of a majority of the 10 samples from which he chose could have been defended as a good choice (although each differed in certain ways from the others).
[26]The Shapiro study is reported in considerable detail in Wingate (1984c).
[27]Note that, in the five-syllable sentences stress falls on the *second* word, the first being the unstressed definite article.
[28]Replication of the Shapiro study (Doyle, 1981) yielded very similar results.
[29]Here we find evidence of stuttering being related to meaning, but *utterance* meaning, not simply word meaning (especially word meaning as conceived in stuttering research).

6
The Fault Line

Stuttering is routinely described as a difficulty in saying words or sounds. Although stuttering obviously does involve sounds and words, characterizing the disorder in either of these terms misleads in opposite directions. Stuttering is most appropriately identified as a *syllabic* phenomenon, an intra-syllabic event—essentially because it is expressed at the level of the syllable. The denouement of the analyses presented in Chapter 5 was the isolation of syllable-initial position and linguistic stress as the focal "language factors" associated with stuttering. Syllable-initial position and linguistic stress are syllabic phenomena.

Focus on the Syllable

It has been previously noted that although the fact of stutter occurrence in initial position is probably the most widely known feature of the disorder, it is typically taken for granted and has hardly received the attention it deserves. The extent to which this standard feature of stuttering is disregarded finds clear expression in the fact that no list of the "facts" about stuttering even mentions it (Andrews, Craig, Feyer, Hoddinott, Howie, & Neilson, 1983; Bender, 1943; Bluemel, 1913; Karlin, 1959; Reid, 1946; Travis, 1933; West, 1943, 1958). This is a truly critical oversight, especially if one considers that the other "facts" listed in these sources do not approach the universality of occurrence that is a hallmark of initial position. There is, in addition, a corollary to the fact of initial position that has special relevance to a descriptive characterization of stuttering as a syllabic phenomenon. The corollary is that stuttering does *not* occur in syllable-final position (usually identified as word final). This is a widely observed, and amply documented, feature of stuttering (Bluemel, 1913; Emerick, 1963; Froeschels, 1961; Hahn, 1942b; Robbins, 1936). However, with the single exception of Bluemel's (1913) coverage, this feature, too, is not mentioned in any of the lists of facts about the disorder; a companion critical oversight. The fact that stuttering does not occur in syllable-final position complements and emphasizes the significance of stutter occurrence at syllable-initial position.

Intermittently over the past 100 years or so a few authors writing on stuttering (see Chapter 1, p. 12) have recognized that "syllable initial" does not necessarily mean the initial phone of the syllable. This insight has repeatedly been ignored, as evidenced in the persistence of the notion of "difficult sounds" (or "feared sounds"), in which the stutter is conceived as occurring *on* a particular (word-initial) sound. However, contrary to superficial outward appearance, and to routine description in the literature, there are very good grounds (as discussed in Chapters 1 and 5) for realizing that stutters do not occur *on* the first phone—which most often happens to be consonantal. The stutter event is more properly conceived as reflecting some anomaly in the transition from initial phone to the sequential phone—which is invariably a vowel form and, as well, also the syllable nucleus. Moreover, it so happens that very often the syllable involved in a stutter is the nuclear (i.e., stressed) syllable in the syllabic sequence. Thus the nature of a stutter event is revealed through the two cardinal features of initial position and linguistic stress: *a stutter represents a failure of the usual relationship between initial phone and syllable nucleus.*

The evidence that stutters do not occur *on* any particular phone is entirely consistent with the evidence, reviewed earlier (Chapter 4), that stutter occurrence is not firmly related to any specific phones, nor directly to any particular group or types of phones. It thus seems clear that there is actually no "phonetic factor," as such. Instead, the pertinent evidence indicates that the relative involvement or, more properly, lack of involvement, of certain phones must be explained in other terms; namely: (1) the position of phones in a word, (2) word type, and (3) word frequency. The one surviving residual of the presumed phonetic factor is the evidence that stuttering does occur much more often with *consonant*-initial syllables than would be expected statistically, that is, in reference to the proportional occurrence of consonant-initial syllables in the language. However, this evidence should not be construed as meaning simply that consonants are "more difficult" than vowels; consider, for instance, all those syllable-final consonants that are never stuttered. Nonetheless, the consonant-vowel distinction is very meaningful for stuttering, in several ways.

It is not certain whether one can properly contend that consonants, in general, are more difficult to produce than are vowels. However, it is well established that consonant production is more complex, is executed more rapidly, and requires more precise timing than does the production of vowels. In respect to such differences one could reasonably describe consonant production as more difficult than that for vowels. However, the more fundamental point is that the two classes of sounds are physiologically different. In general, it appears that different types of muscles are involved in production of the two sound classes; yet, at the same time, many of the differences between the two classes result from the same parts of the speech system acting in different ways. (Fowler, 1980, Kozhevnikov & Chistovich, 1965; Ohman, 1966; Perkell, 1969). There is no need to attempt to summarize the extensive literature dealing with the processes of speech production at the level of motor commands, but it is pertinent to restate the point made by Liberman (1970) that the relationship between articulatory gesture and sound is very complex, and to emphasize that, in large measure, this complexity is due to substantial differences between the production of consonants and the production of vowels.

Consonants and vowels are also different linguistically. They perform different roles in the structure of the language, occasioned by and reflected in their differential function as constituents of the basic unit of language, the syllable. The most straightforward difference is that consonants serve to initiate and terminate syllables. Vowel forms, on the other hand, constitute the major substance of the syllable, its nucleus. An additional, and unique, feature of the vowel form is that it is the vehicle through which the prosodic dimension of language is expressed.[1]

There are certain other important matters, involving the consonant-vowel distinction relative to syllabic structure, that are particularly pertinent to understanding the nature of stuttering. These matters embrace certain findings in the literature of linguistics and psycholinguistics that are specific to the structure of syllables. These findings are especially pertinent to stuttering because they converge in pointing up the uniqueness and importance of the initial part of the syllable.

Osgood and Sebeok (1954) noted that, in most languages, the syllable-initial phone is more distinct than the phone in syllable-final position. This suggestion of asymmetry of the syllable later received support from work such as that reported by Peterson and Lehiste (1960) and Pelc and Leeper (1976) who found evidence of different internal relations between the vowel nucleus of a syllable and the initiating and terminating consonants. There is a great deal of phonological evidence that indicates syllable-initial position to be universally stronger than syllable-final position (Hooper, 1976; Selkirk, 1984; Venneman, 1972a, 1972b).

Although consonants and vowels have a certain clear psychological reality they lose much of their individual identity in the composition of a syllable, and of course in longer sequences. It has been known since at least the work of Ohman (1963, 1966) that the phones of connected speech are not unit sounds, strung together like series of beads but, instead, are coarticulated; their forms show the influence of neighboring phones, which effect varying modifications in their production.[2] Ohman's work (1966), and later that of R. D. Kent and Moll (1969), drew particular attention to the effect of such influences at syllable-initial position, noting that production of an initial consonant usually involves making simultaneous adjustments for that consonant and for succeeding sounds. In contrast, evidence from other sources (MacNeilage & DeClerk, 1969) indicates that production of syllable-final consonants does not require such anticipation of other speech sounds. The asymmetry of the syllable described in these sources also emphasizes the uniqueness of the initial part of the syllable.

These findings regarding production of the syllable-initial consonant indicate that it has a special relationship to the syllable nucleus, the succeeding vowel form. Delattre (1958) suggested that it would be impossible, in direct speech, to separate the initial consonant from the rest of the syllable and that even on a tape recording it would be very difficult to separate the initial consonant "with the certainty that the burst is entirely cut off or the transition entirely left in." Some years later Liberman (1970), using patterned playback technique, demonstrated that indeed the initial consonant cannot be separated out[3] and that, in fact, the acoustic clues to its identity are contained in the character of the formant transitions of the succeeding vowel.

In terms of the process of speech production, then, the syllable is appropriately described as asymmetric, with the special character of the initial position being that the initiating consonant and the succeeding vowel nucleus are inseparable; they are merged into one continuous flow of action.

In comparison to the foregoing account of syllable structure from the standpoint of speech production (i.e., the programs leading to the motor sequence), it is of considerable interest that a *linguistic* analysis of the syllable yields a very different picture of syllabic structure, particularly in respect to syllable-initial position. The next few paragraphs review how the characterization of the syllabic structure from a linguistic analysis is based on evidence that the initial consonantism of a syllable (word) is *separable* from the rest of the syllable (word).

Hockett (1967) proposed that syllables have an internal constituent structure consisting of two elements: (1) initial consonantism (even if zero) and (2) all that follows. Hockett's "initial consonantism" includes consonant clusters as well as single consonants. In later writings[4] other terms for Hockett's two elements have been suggested. In this later work there is an evident preference for the simple yet appropriate terms that refer to these two syllable constituents as "onset" and "rime," respectively. Certain expansions of the rime have been suggested[5] but the value of such expansions remains uncertain (at least they are not important to the present discussion). The hypothesized elements of onset and rime have proven to be very useful in discussions regarding the nature of speech organization and production, and have found support in a number of investigations (e.g., Claxton,1974; Fudge, 1969; Halle & Vergnaud, 1980; Harris, 1983; MacKay, 1972, 1974, 1978; Shattuck-Hufnagel, 1983; Treiman, 1983, 1985).

Hockett developed his characterization of the internal constituent structure of the syllable in reference to monosyllabic words in English,[6] and he offered four sources of evidence as support for the hypothesis. The first line of evidence comes from the substantial literature on "slips of the tongue."[7] The research in this area has shown that the most common speech errors are ones in which the initial consonantism (individual consonant or consonant cluster) of two words are transposed, each of them being "joined to" the remainder of the other word of the pair (e.g., /ʃel/ and /jaut/ instead of /jel/ and /ʃaut/). A second source of evidence for the onset-rime structure of the syllable is contained in the common practice of creating verse by rhyming monosyllabic words that differ only in respect to initial consonantism. Third, one finds evidence of the same internal constituent structure of the syllable in language forms that have the direct opposite of rhyming verse; namely, in alliteration, wherein the initial consonantism of several syllables is kept the same while the remainder of each of the syllables is changed.[8] A fourth line of evidence is provided in the structure of the "secret" language used by children, known as "Pig Latin," in which the coding system consists of separating the initial consonantism from the remainder of the word and inserting it at word end.

There is other evidence that the initial consonantism is uniquely separable from the remainder of the syllable (word). A vernacular, but impressive, dimension of evidence is the standard, basic organization of language dictionaries. Although irregularities and vagaries of orthography have introduced certain complications, particularly during the time when dictionaries were first compiled, dictionary entries are organized, fundamentally, in terms of word-initial sounds. This line of evidence coincides with the fairly common human experience in which, when searching for a word, one attempts to use the initial sound/letter of the word as the clue to identifying what is "on the tip of the tongue." A reference study by R. Brown and McNeill (1966), which created an experimental analogue of this phenomenon, yielded results indicating the importance of the initial phone in the organization of the mental lexicon. Later work by Tweney, Tkacz, and Zaruba (1975) and by Stemberger (1983) have yielded support for the findings reported by Brown and McNeill. Shattuck-Hufnagel (1981, 1983, 1987) has provided other compelling evidence that word onsets play a critical role in lexical retrieval.

Asymmetry of the syllable is also revealed by linguistic analysis. Halle and Vergnaud (1980) point out that in English any initial consonantism can occur with any vowel nucleus but that, in contrast, there are severe constraints on which final consonantisms can occur with any particular vowel nucleus. With greater latitude of C-V combinations in syllable initial position there is also greater latitude for error, and presumably greater demands are thereby placed on the system. Linguistic analysis of syllable structure also points to another significant dimension; namely, that the rules for stress assignment apply only to the syllable nucleus, or the rime.

Analysis of the syllable is of significance to linguistics because, first, it reveals an internal structure between the level of phonetic segments and the level of the syllable as a unit. Beyond this, the identification of a structure within the syllable contributes importantly to the understanding of speech production. Awareness of the influence of these syllable constituents at the level of production enlarges this understanding.

Synthesis

Analyses of the syllable from the standpoint of both speech production and of linguistic structure point to the special nature of the initial portion of the syllable, and recognize the unique relationship between onset and rime—between initial consonantism and vowel nucleus. At the same time, although the two analyses direct attention to the same locus, and its special features, their characterization of the circumstances at that locus differ considerably. At the linguistic (lexical) level, onset and rime are intrinsically separable; they are interchangeable parts that evidently retain their idealized phonological representation. In contrast, at the level of signal production, onset and rime are "unitized"; speech performance of onset and rime represents an intricate blending of the complex muscle systems[9] involved in the differential production of consonants and vowels, such that the identities of consonant and vowel are merged and blended. This dramatic contrast, which can be said to characterize syllable-initial position, suggests that the relationship of onset to rime can be considered a "fault line" in speech production. This fault line, which is the site of errors in verbal expression—as evidenced in "slips of the tongue"—is also evidently vulnerable to the more dramatic breakdown that is represented in the occurrence of stutters.[10]

The inference from this analysis is that breakdown at the fault line is the critical feature, the crux, of a stutter event. It appears to be no coincidence that the focal language features involved in a stutter event are precisely those that are highlighted in the analyses of syllabic structure. Also although the stutter event finds expression as a breakdown at the level of execution, that is, in motor performance, it seems likely that the fault extends from higher levels of the hierarachy of neural organization for language expression, through several stages of the process that extends from the plane of verbal formulation to the level of final motor execution. This analysis will be developed further in Chapter 9.

Footnotes

[1]These, and other, important distinctions between consonants and vowels will be incorporated in the discussion in Chapter 9.

[2]One implication of coarticulation is that, contrary to long-standing belief, stutters cannot be associated with phones as invariant entities because phones are produced as part of a sequence. Evidently this is particularly true of syllable-initial phones—which are the phones that are involved in stutters.
[3]Even though, holistically, the initial consonant(s) have a perceptually and psychologically real independent identity.
[4]For instance, MacKay used "initial consonant group" and "vocalic group."
[5]The following terms have been used to specify sequential parts of Hockett's "all that follows:" peak or vowel nucleus; coda or final consonant (or cluster); and appendix or inflectional suffix. See MacKay (1972); Halle and Vergnaud (1980).
[6]Justifiable on, among other grounds, the fact of the frequency with which monosyllabic words occur in ordinary discourse.
[7]See, for example, Fromkin (1973b, 1980).
[8]Hockett's example: "Let us flee, said the fly, so they flew through the flaw in the flue."
[9]Partly different, yet evidently partially duplicating.
[10]This characterization of a "fault line" is borrowed from the field of geology where it refers to a crack in the earth's crust, not always evident at the surface, that penetrates deep into the underlying structure.

[illegible]

Part III: Enlarging the Scope

A Comparative Study of Language Dimensions in Stuttering

The investigation to be reported in Chapters 7 and 8 was undertaken to explore certain dimensions of stutterers' actual word usage and of their skills in dealing with words, as compared to similar function in normal speakers.[1]

This research was basically exploratory in nature although, at the same time, it was closely linked to certain hypotheses regarding language function differences between stutterers and normal speakers. The dimensions explored in the research were derived from ideas based on work reported prior to 1968 and on intuitions I had developed by that time relative to likely problem areas in the language function of stutterers. In particular, several of my investigations that were published about this time (Wingate, 1966a, 1966b, 1967a, 1967b, 1971) were precursors to this considerably more extended study of language function in stutterers. Although the research was completed several years prior to the development of the language analyses presented in Chapters 5 and 6, the findings articulate well with those analyses.

The measures used in the research to be reported here are ones that lend themselves to analyses that center on words and word usage. The word has always figured prominently in accounts and discussions of stuttering; as

---

[1]The research was initiated in 1967 and collection of data extended over a period of approximately three years. This rather lengthy period of data collection was occasioned primarily by the demands of subject matching and appropriate scheduling of the various measures at a time when I was in the process of changing locus of employment. Due to subsequent demands on my time, I was unable to undertake analyses of the data until 1982, at which time a sabbatical leave for that purpose was granted by Washington State University.

Support in implementing this research was provided through the Agnes H. Anderson Fund of the University of Washington, and by the Research Foundation of the State of New York. A semester of professional leave, granted by Washington State University, provided the necessary opportunity to undertake analyses of the data and begin preparation of this report.

noted in earlier chapters, stuttering is widely recognized as a disorder that is manifested in the attempt to produce words or parts or words, and a substantial literature has accumulated that is organized in respect to words and word usage. Conducting analyses in terms of words is appropriate in spite of the fact that stuttering is best conceived as a syllabic disorder.

The content of Chapter 7 is addressed to the description of: (1) the subjects participating in the research; (2) the measures employed and the rationale for their selection; and (3) the procedures for collecting the data. Chapter 8 is addressed to presentation and discussion of the results obtained in the study.

7
Method and Procedure

Subjects

Experimental Subjects

The experimental group consisted of 20 young adult, Caucasian, male stutterers, ranging in age from 16 to 40 years, with an average age of 23.4 years. They were native-born, monolingual, native speakers of American English who had received their primary and secondary education in the public schools in one of two large metropolitan areas. Those having postsecondary education had pursued their study in a state-supported university. Their educational levels ranged from 11 to 18 years, with an average of 14.1 years of formal education.

All subjects came from homes of middle class socioeconomic level. None had any history of major illness, or complications related to common illnesses; no history of notable accident or injury; and no record or report of any noteworthy problems of personal adjustment.

The subjects' participation in the research was voluntary, enlisted during the course of their enrollment in therapy, for their stuttering, in the Speech Clinic at one of two universities. They represented a wide range of severity level, from very mild to very severe, although the majority fell in the lower limits of the range (Table 7.1). This skew in the distribution of stuttering severity, with most cases in the "mild" range, is typical (Johnson, 1963, p. 252; Soderberg, 1962b). In fact, this group is representative; the mean and median severity values are very comparable, and represent a severity level in the mild-to-moderate range. All of the subjects had had therapy, the extent of therapy correlating roughly with rated severity level.

Control Subjects

The primary criteria for selecting the normal speaking control subjects were the same basic features characterizing the stutterer subjects. Ex-

TABLE 7.1. Stuttering severity level of subjects in the experimental group

Rank		Number of subjects
Label	Value	
Very severe	7	1
Severe	6	3
Moderately severe	5	2
Moderate	4	1
Mild to moderate	3	4
Mild	2	4
Very mild	1	5
	Mean = 3.2	
	Median = 3.0	

plicitly, these criteria were: young adult Caucasian male, native monolingual speaker of American English, middle class socioeconomic origin, and negative medical history. Additionally, each control subject was carefully matched to a stutterer subject on three specific criteria: (1) age, (2) years of formal education, and (3) score on the Vocabulary section of the SRA Tests of Primary Mental Abilties.

The control subjects were selected from among individuals whose original involvement as a potential subject was obtained by informal solicitation through colleagues. They were retained as subjects if they met the three matching criteria listed. The control subjects were paid a nominal hourly rate for their participation in the study.

Measures Used and Rationale

Vocabulary Tests

Some measure of vocabulary is a basic dimension of many types of investigation focusing on language function. It is particularly appropriate when the focus of study is directed at word knowledge and word usage. In this research two measures of vocabulary were included.

PMA Vocabulary

This test is a part of the Primary Mental Abilities test, published by Science Research Associates.[1] It is a measure of recognition vocabulary, an objective test in which the subject evidences his knowledge of each test word by selecting an equivalent from one of five alternatives. This type of test makes minimal demands on the subject; that is, in terms of recall, word search and selection, or formulation of a verbal statement. It could therefore be expected to provide a basic reference or indicator of extent of word knowledge. This measure was one of the three specific criteria on which the stutterer and normally speaking subjects were matched individually.

WAIS Vocabulary Subtest

This test is one of five subtests of the Verbal Scale of the Wechsler Adult Intelligence Scale (1955). It is a definition type measure of vocabulary in which the subject has the responsibility of giving an adequate statement of each word's meaning. An adequate "statement," of course, can be contained in one word, a synonym.

This second measure of vocabulary was included for several reasons. First, it extends the base of vocabulary assessment; it was assumed that the two measures would be highly correlated for individuals. Second, at the same time, it affords a different dimension of vocabulary assessment in that it requires active recall and a statement of meaning equivalence. Third, as an expressive measure, it could be expected to yield several derived measures of word knowledge and use, such as the extent of synonym usage, the total number of words used, and the number of different words used.

Word Fluency

The word-fluency measure used in this research is taken directly from the Tests of Primary Mental Abilities developed by Thurstone (Thurstone, 1938; Thurstone & Thurstone, 1941). The measures constituting Thurstone's tests of Primary Mental Abilities were selected on the basis of factor analyses of a variety of tests administered to large numbers of subjects representing a considerable age range. The factor analyses led to the identification of eight separate factors, six of which were clearly defined by repeated study. Word-fluency, which Thurstone designated "W," was "one of the most clearly defined" of these factors. Thurstone (Thurstone & Thurstone, 1941, p. 3) described word-fluency as the factor that is "involved whenever the subject is asked to think of isolated words at a rapid rate." Significantly, especially for the interests of the present research, word-fluency was clearly a distinct factor from "V," the verbal factor in the Primary Mental Abilities, even though the two factors showed some correlation. As described in the Primary Mental Abilities manual: "Word Fluency is the ability to write and talk easily. It differs from Verbal-Meaning because it concerns the speed and ease with which words can be used, rather than with the degree of understanding of verbal concepts" (p. 2).

The essential feature of a word-fluency measure is that it requires the subject to produce as many words as possible, within a specified brief period of time, that meet certain constraints. For example, words with a specified initial letter, or initial and final letter; words having a certain prefix or suffix; words having four letters; words of a given category; and so forth. Several variations of the word-fluency measures are described in certain literature sources concerned with the neuropsychology of language (e.g., Benton, 1968; Gaddes & Crockett, 1975; Milner, 1964; Perret, 1974). Most of these variations are ones included in Thurstone's analyses.

The test used in the present research replicates the original, which also is the type of word-fluency measure often used in other research. This test requires the subject to write, in a time limit of 5 minutes, as many different words as he can think of that begin with the letter "s." In this particular type of measure there are also certain other pertinent constraints, in keeping with the requirement that the words used be different. For instance, one cannot use simple variations of the same word, such as adding plural or tense endings; proper names are not allowed; and so forth.

At face value, at least, word-fluency performance reflects the ability to retrieve quickly lexical units that meet certain structural constraints. The word-fluency task is a kind of controlled association[2] in which associative activity focuses on certain structural aspects of words; in this case, the focus is on "bringing up" words that meet the single specification of having a particular initial consonant.

Some years ago, at a time when it was becoming more evident to me that stuttering was more than a problem in motor coordination, it occurred to me that stutterers would probably not do well on a test of word-fluency. The findings of a preliminary study (Wingate, 1968), conducted on 16 pairs of subjects, supported the hypothesis: the stutterers performed significantly less well than their controls.[3]

Story-Telling

There were several reasons for including story-telling measures in this research. One reason was to obtain data on language variables, fluency features, and the relations between the two as they find expression in spontaneous speech. Some of the data to be derived from the story-telling protocols would relate to previous work on (1) the "language factors" in stuttering and (2) the nature and extent of irregularities in fluency evidenced by both stutterers and normal speakers. Additionally, there was a need to explore certain dimensions of language use in stutterers that have not been considered previously, such as the extent of free spontaneous expression and certain facets of its composition. Matters of this kind have not been investigated, evidently because of certain implicit assumptions about stutterers' language use, such as that stutterers' language function is not different from that of normal speakers, except that they are inclined to talk less than normal speakers because of their fear of stuttering; or that stutterers have large vocabularies, and know many synonymns, as means of avoiding stuttering.

The "new" assessments to be applied to this story material consisted of a few dimensions of language analysis that might reveal something very useful about the language function of stutterers, namely, the ratio of content to function words, the distribution of word lengths, the total number of words used in a narrative and the number of different words used. The two latter measures, expressed in ratio form, have been used in a variety of studies of language use as an index of diversity of word use.

Several methods have been developed to provide an index of diversity in word usage. The simplest measure of diversity, the number of different words relative to the total number of words, turns out to be a function of the number of words in the corpus. It varies inversely with the size of corpus, reflecting the fact that with increasing length of sample progressively fewer new words are introduced. Recognizing this limitation, Carroll (1938) developed a rather complex formula that would yield an index of diversity that was independent of corpus size. Another early measure, much simpler than Carroll's, is the "segmental Type-Token Ratio" (TTR; Chotlos, 1944). This index expresses diversity directly, as a simple ratio of the number of different words (types) divided by the total number of words (tokens). An overall TTR, of course, tends to vary inversely with length of corpus; the "segmental TTR" offsets this tendency by computing the ratio for sequential segments of equivalent size, ideally every 100 words. Although the segmental TTR is thus somewhat cumbersome to compute and, as well, is a roundabout way of yielding an overall index of diversity in word usage, it has been used in a variety of studies of language use. Carroll (1964) later reported the development of a single index, more easily computed than his earlier formula, yet still relatively independent of corpus size. Most recently Sankoff and Lessard (1975), using very extensive samples of ordinary spontaneous speech, derived a formula that accurately relates the number of different words to total words in a sample. The Sankoff-Lessard formula thus has particular utility as a normative reference base.

Story One

Samples of spontaneous oral expression are central to any study of stuttering that is concerned with language factors. It was particularly important to obtain samples of genuinely spontaneous speech, in which subjects generated their own verbal expression and were free to say as much or as little as they would.

In order to justify making comparisons relative to spontaneous speech samples, it was necessary that the sample from each subject have a circumscribed, common focus yet represent individual freedom of formulation and expression. The simplest and most satisfactory way to meet such requirements is to have subjects tell a story based on a picture.

The picture used for this task was the picture on card number 2 of the Thematic Apperception Test. It was selected primarily because it has essentially neutral content and has been recognized among those using this test as an "easy" card that is likely to yield stories of appreciable length.

Story Two

This task was included to provide a written counterpart of Story One. In view of the many statements made regarding stutterers' negative attitudes about speaking, it seemed pertinent to obtain samples of spontaneous written expression as well, for purposes of comparison. That is, if it is true stutterers avoid talking, one might expect that, if given comparable outlets for self-expression, they would be more expressive in writing than in speaking. Samples of written expression would at least permit certain dimensions of direct comparison to subjects' spontaneous oral expression. Several studies comparing written and oral expression of normal speaking individuals (Bushnell, 1930; Drieman, 1962; Fraisse & Breyton, 1959; Horowitz & Newman, 1964; Mann, 1944; Moscovici & Humbert, 1960) would serve as comparative reference for both subject groups in the present study.

In addition, results of some previous work (Arnold, 1966; Eisenson, 1937b; McDowell, 1928) have indicated certain irregularities in the written performance of stutterers. Although the data from those studies were obtained under different conditions than planned for the present research, reference to those findings seemed indicated.

The requirements for the Story Two task were the same as for the oral counterpart; namely, that the sample from each subject have a common, but circumscribed, focus that nonetheless allowed individual freedom of formulation and expression. Therefore, the task was similar: subjects were asked to write a story about a picture. The picture selected was the "Post Office" story-telling picture from the Stanford-Binet Intelligence Test, Form L. This is another "easy" picture, of neutral content, from which one could expect a story of appreciable length.

Word Association

In regard to word-associative activity, the interests of the present investigation focused primarily on the nature of the subjects associations and reaction times. These variables are the two that had been found in previous research to differentiate the word-association performance of stutterers and normal speakers. Also, in view of the common belief in an emotional basis of stuttering, it seemed appropriate to explore the potential effect of presumed emotional arousal on association activity.

In view of these interests, the Kent and Rosanoff (1910) list of words[4] seemed the most suitable one to use, for several reasons. First, it is a rather large "general content" word list, consisting of a wide range of ordinary words. Second, the list has had wide usage, including many studies addressed to some aspect of language function. Third, appropriate norms of associative responses to the Kent and Rosanoff words are available. Additionally, some previous work with stutterers made use of this list.

A fair amount of research has been addressed to the word associations of stutterers. The objectives of previous research have varied, some of them being simply exploratory. Both Hanes (1950) and Font (1955) used the Kent and Rosanoff list of words with stutterers and a reference group of normal speakers. Hanes compared, to Kent and Rosanoff norms, the associations given by 40 male stutterers and those from 26 normal speakers of comparable age. He found that the stutterers' associations had a significantly greater mean percentage of "individual" responses. (Reaction time was not recorded.) Similarly, Font compared the associations given by 9 college-age stutterers to a comparison group of 49 normally speaking college students. There was no notable difference in reaction time, but the stutterers gave fewer "common" and more "individual" associations than did the normal speakers.

Several word association studies of stutterers have been undertaken with an interest in what the associations might reveal about the presumed affective or psychodynamic aspects of stuttering. For example, Borghi (1955) used the word association method to search for evidence of disturbance in stutterers' associations to words having a sexual or hostile significance. He used a special word association test developed by Rapaport, Gill, and Schafer (1946)[5] to which he added other words selected from clinical records of the stutterer subjects. Borghi found no evidence of disturbed associations to words of this list; his only notable finding was that his 11 stutterers had a significantly longer mean total reaction time than the normal control subjects. Adams and Dietze (1965) used a word association test of their own construction that contained words representing several categories of emotional state (i.e., joy, depression, aggression, fear, guilt) as well as neutral words. Again, the only finding of significance was that their 30 stutterers had longer reaction times to all word categories than did the matched control subjects. Kline (1959) used a word association test of his own design with 23 stutterers, and controls, to probe certain goal-activity drives that included foci on speech and speech difficulty. Comparison of the associations of the two groups yielded equivocal results, except for the finding that the stutterers' mean reaction time was longer than that of the normal speakers.

Henja (1968) reported use of a word association test specifically constructed to yield "highly specific" responses. He found that a group of 35 stutterers gave significantly more "unexpected" associations than did 50 subjects with normal speech. He did not report reaction times.

In general, the findings of the word association research with stutterers does not support assumptions of an emotional basis for stuttering.[6] In particular, there is no support for the beliefs that stuttering is related to certain special areas of emotional involvement, such as anxiety about speech, sexual conflict, latent aggressiveness, and so on. At the same time, it is of some interest that, in the two studies employing a standard word list having many common words (the Kent-Rosanoff), stutterers gave a higher frequency of uncommon associations than did normal speakers. In contrast, in the three studies employing specially devised lists, stutterers had longer reaction times than the normal speakers. Comments on this contrast will be deferred until the results of the present research are discussed (Chapter 8).

Tests of "Soundmindedness"

Tiffany (1963a, 1963b) reported the development and initial use of three measures of language manipulation—*Phonetic Anagrams, Backward Speech,* and *Slurvians*—that he referred to as "tests of soundmindedness." These tests seem to reflect a familiarity with basic structural aspects of the language—phones, phonetic patterns, phonetic sequences, word composition—and a concurrent ability to create and modify such patterns. The first two measures, Phonetic Anagrams and Backward Speech, are addressed to tapping such skills at the level of words. The Slurvians test deals with word strings. Although this test evidently also requires some amount of ability to "manipulate" phonetic and word units, dealing successfully with Slurvians also seems to involve, in addition, some kind of skill with prosodic aspects of the language.

Phonetic Anagrams

This measure, one of two tests of phonetic ability described by Tiffany (1963b), is an oral form of the well-known letter anagram puzzles. In this test the anagrams consist of spoken phones instead of written letters. The test contains 15 items, each of which requires the subject to construct as many actual words as possible from a series of individual phones, spoken separately in measured sequence but in an order that does not make a bona fide word. For example, the phones /i/, /f/, /l/ can be used to make the words "leaf," "feel," "flee," and "flea."

Previous study (Wingate, 1971) found a group of stutterers to be significantly inferior to normal speakers in solving the Phonetic Anagrams.

Backward Speech

This measure, the other test of phonetic ability reported by Tiffany (1963b), consists of 24 items in each of which the task required of the subject is to produce a "target" word that is the exact reversal, in sound, of a spoken "source" word. The target word is always a bona fide English word; however, its reversed form, the spoken source word, may or may not be a true English word. For example, the word "tack" is the correct solution to the (true) source word /kæt/; the word "magazine" is the correct answer to the (nonsense) source word /nizəgæm/.

Previous investigation (Wingate, 1971) found that a group of 25 adult stutterers performed significantly less well than normal speakers on this measure. Perozzi (1970) reported similar findings for 20 stuttering youngsters from the second and third grades, compared to matched normally speaking children.

Slurvians

This test requires identification of familiar sayings from cues embedded in a string of unrelated words. For example, the three-word string, "scene—owe—weevil," represents the familiar expression, "See no evil." In this example the phonetic pattern of the test item is practically identical to the familiar expression target. In most items of the test there is less similarity between the word string and its familiar expression target. The following example is illustrative: "a—feud—rink—toned—rife" is to be identified as, "if you drink, don't drive."

Two comparable forms of the test, used in this research, were modifications of the two original forms reported by Tiffany. The revision was based on research undertaken by Wingate (1970a) to establish comparable forms in which the 15 items of each form increase progressively in levels of difficulty. Having two forms of the test permits presentation in both visual and auditory modes.

Success in solving Slurvians apparently involves language facility having several dimensions. "Translation" of the word strings into standard English seems to require a readiness of word access, flexibility in word choice, and ability to manipulate suprasegmental as well as segmental features of the language while concurrently searching for a familiar linguistic/cognitive pattern that will match the one being constructed. The idea that solving Slurvians involves an ability to deal constructively with prosodic dimensions of the language is supported by evidence that the format of presentation in the auditory mode makes a considerable difference in success rate with Slurvians. Tiffany (1963a) reported that (normal speaker) subjects were more successful in solving auditory, as compared to visual, Slurvians when the items were read to them by a naive speaker, who typically read each word string as a connected utterance, often in phrasal units. In contrast, when each string is presented as a series of isolated words spoken in measured sequence, subjects have considerably more difficulty with the auditory form of Slurvians than with the visual form. The "isolated words" format of auditory presentation gives little, if any, information about prosodic structure or word elisions of the target expression. Of course, this auditory form of the test also places heavier demands on short-term memory.

Previous research (Wingate, 1967a), conducted with 25 young adult male stutterers and a matched group of normal speakers, found that both normal speakers and stutterers are better able to solve Slurvians presented in the visual mode (with the auditory version presented in the standard isolated words format). At the same time that study also showed stutterers to have significantly greater difficulty than normal speakers on both the visual and auditory forms of the test. Recently, Newman, Fawcett, and Russon (1986) employed a procedure in which the Slurvians were divided into an "easy" set and a "difficult" set, both of which were administered by visual mode to 18 young adult male stutterers[7] and matching controls. The difficult set did not differentiate between the two groups[8] but the normal speakers scored significantly higher than the stutterers on the easy set.

Test of Behavioral Rigidity

The Test of Behavioral Rigidity (TBR) (Schaie & Parham, 1975), developed by Schaie (1955, 1960) and described further by him in several places (e.g., Schaie, 1970), resulted from a factor analysis of a variety of tests of psychological rigidity—or its converse, flexibility. The factor analysis isolated three dimensions, identified as *Motor–Cognitive, Psychomotor Speed,* and *Personality—Perceptual.* The Motor-Cognitive and Psychomotor Speed variables are based on different dimensions of two sets of tasks, one called "Capitals," the other called "Opposites." The Capitals task contains two series: in Series A the subject is required to copy, *in writing* (not printing), a paragraph in which lower- and uppercase letters vary unsystematically, for example: "The Duke DREW his sword." In series B of this task the subject is required to do the opposite, that is, to copy the same paragraph but write a lowercase for every uppercase letter and vice versa. The Opposites task contains three series: in Series 1 the subject writes an antonym for each of a list of words; in Series 2 he writes a synonym for each of a different list of words; and in Series 3 he writes, to words taken from both of the preceding lists, an antonym or synonym depending on whether the cue word is printed in lower- or uppercase letters.

The Psychomotor Speed variable represents performance on the Capitals test, Series A, and Opposites, Series 1 and 2. The Motor–Cognitive variable reflects performance on Capitals, Series B and Opposites, Series 3. The *Personality–Perceptual* variable reflects the subject's pattern of answers to a questionnaire.

The relevance of a measure like the TBR in the study of stuttering rests on its pertinence to the hypothesis that stuttering is a form of perseveration. Some years ago Eisenson and coauthors (Eisenson, 1937a; Eisenson & Pastel, 1936; Eisenson & Winslow, 1938) proposed that stuttering is "a manifestation of the phenomenon of perseveration." The results of their work, which employed a variety of sensory measures of perseveration, provided some suggestive evidence for the hypothesis that stuttering reflects some sort of perseveration in central nervous system function. Goldsand (1944), using tests of sensory perseveration with 16 adolescent and young adult subject pairs, also reported evidence that stutterers are less able, than are normal speakers, to make rapid shifts in adjustments. Results obtaining by Gold (1941), using auditory material, and Sheets (1941), who employed visual tasks, showed stutterers to be more perseverative than normal speakers, although the differences did not meet the standardly required levels of statistical significance. Overall, the studies designed to assess sensory perseveration in stutterers have yielded evidence that is strongly suggestive of perseverative tendencies, though not conclusive.

Investigation of perseverative tendencies in motor function of stutterers has generally yielded similar findings: stutterers differ from normals, though not in sufficient magnitude to meet standard statistical criteria. H. Hill (1942) failed to find statistically significant differences between stutterers and normal speakers on tasks designed to reflect perseverative features in motor function. Kapos and Standlee (1958) reported also that the differences they found between stutterers and normal speakers on two tasks of motor function were not statistically significant. Results of studies by R. Martin (1962) and Samson and Cooper (1980) again failed to show significantly greater perseverative tendencies in stutterers on certain motor tasks similar to those used in previous research. However, Green (1967) reported highly significant correlation between severity of stuttering "consistency," and perseveration as measured on four motor tasks.

The most extensive study of perseverative tendencies in stutterers was reported by King (1961). He had a very large subject population consisting of 72 male and 8 female stutterers, and 82 male and 55 female comparison normal speakers. He used a battery of 10 tests that included measures of sensory, motor, and dispositional rigidity. His findings showed stutterers to evidence significantly more perseverative tendencies than normal speakers, especially on specific tests that "demand a contiguous mental, or mental and motor, change of set." At the same time, his overall results did not seem to indicate a general, or "broad underlying" factor of perseveration in stutterers.[9]

A study by Solomon (1951) yielded results most pertinent to the possible involvement of rigidity in language function. She compared the performance of 18 college stutterers with matched normal speakers on tests of motor performance, mental arithmetic, and oral word puzzles. The first two measures did not reveal differences between the two groups. In contrast, the stutterers evidenced significantly less flexibility than the normal speakers in dealing with the word puzzles.

Although the research investigating perseverative tendencies in stutterers has generally yielded little support for the concept of a broad underlying factor of perseveration, of general behavioral rigidity, in stutterers, there is recurring strong suggestion that in certain mental functions stutterers lack the level of flexibility typically found in the normal speaker. In fact, Eisenson (1958, 1975), basing his position on the research reviewed here and certain other data, developed an account of stuttering as perseverative behavior. It is of considerable interest that his explanation of stuttering as perseverative behavior originated with, and continued to center on, the idea that the classical markers of stuttering—the tonic and clonic features—constitute the prima facie evidence of perseveration.

Discussion of rigidity in stuttering is not complete without mention of the concept of "moral rigidity" suggested by West (West & Ansberry, 1968). West contended that stutterers typically give evidence of moral rigidity, hypothesized to be a personality trait manifested in such characteristics as: perfectionism (not limited to speech performance), a tendency to set unrealistic goals, and evidences of a severe conscience. The sources of West's claim are not clear. Evidently the notion was derived from sources in the clinical literature; he did not cite any research that might have contained even suggestive evidence.

The Test of Behavioral Rigidity is particularly well suited to investigation of rigidity in stuttering. The overall substance of this measure is relevant to several dimensions of psychological functioning previously hypothesized to be involved in stuttering. In particular, certain features of the test are especially appropriate to the interests of the present investigation, in that the principal tasks of the TBR involve language-related functions.

A previous study (Wingate, 1966a) comparing 12 young adult male stutterers and controls on TBR performance found the stutterers to evidence less flexibility on language-related functions measured by the test, but no difference on the personality dimension.

Procedure

Overall Procedure

In view of the number of tests to be administered, it was clear that several sessions would be needed. The overall plan of procedure was designed to meet two major considerations: (1) no session should be longer than approximately 45 minutes and (2) the tests administered within any one session should be as dissimilar as could be arranged. Each test was therefore assigned to one of four groups, each group given on a separate day, with at least a week intervening between test days.[10] The tests were given in the same order to all subjects. All tests were administered individually, by the author, in a quiet room.

The test groups, and their order of presentation, is presented in the following list. Because the PMA Vocabulary was to be one of the variables on which the normal speakers were to be matched individually with stutterers, this measure was always given first. The word-fluency measure was given twice, simply to provide a broader base for individual scores on this test. Each of the two equivalent forms of the Slurvians test was given to half of each subject group as the Visual form of the test, and to the other half of each group as the Auditory form of the test.

Sequence of Test Administration
Day 1: Word-Fluency 1; Visual Slurvians, Story One
Day 2: Wechsler Adult Intelligence Scale (WAIS) Vocabulary;
Phonetic Anagrams; Backward Speech
Day 3: Word-Fluency 2; TBR; Story Two
Day 4: Auditory Slurvians; Word Association

All tests for which the subject's performance was cued by auditory signal were prerecorded on high-fidelity, reel-to-reel tape at 7.5 inches per second. The recordings were made by a male speaker who had had professional training, and employment, as a radio announcer. The tests recorded were: Word Association, Phonetic Anagrams, Backward Speech, and Auditory Slurvs. The latter three tests had time limits for each item; the time limits and announcement of the number of each item were incorporated into the recording. Presentation of the items in the Word Association recording was controlled by the experimenter.

For those measures requiring that the subject write, his final product was inspected for legibility immediately after completion.

Procedures for the Individual Tests

Description of the individual procedure for the several different measures, will follow the same order of presentation as in the earlier section of this chapter in which these measures and the rationale for their use were presented. In the following descriptions the nature of the instructions for each test will be indicated only to the extent necessary to convey the essence of the procedure.

PMA Vocabulary

Administration of this test was straightforward and routine; the subject was given a pencil, a copy of the test booklet that had been turned to the proper page, and an answer sheet. He was then given the instructions according to the manual.

The score on this test consisted of the number of correct items, scored according to the test manual.

WAIS Vocabulary

Administration of this subtest of WAIS involved some modification of standard format in that it was presented as a written task (instead of orally as prescribed in the WAIS Manual). The items (words) making up this test were typed on two sheets of paper on which each word was set in a block of space that allowed sufficient room for the subject to write his definition. The instructions given were consistent with those printed in the WAIS Manual. Subjects were then allowed to complete the test without further instruction. The standard reply to any question was to "Just tell as well as you can, in your own words, what each word means." As in the WAIS format, there was no time limit.

The primary data gained from this measure was the overall vocabulary score, obtained in careful reference to the WAIS Manual. (Scoring was done by the author, who had had extensive experience administering the test in the standard fashion.) In addition to the formal score for this measure, two derived values were recorded: total number of words and the number of different words used. Special note was also made of the use of synonyms.

Word-Fluency

This test was given twice, simply for purposes of obtaining a scoring base of greater breadth. In each administration the task was carefully explained, with appropriate demonstration, practice, and citation of constraints.

The basic score on this test was the number of acceptable words produced, the score typically obtained for this test. Another score, developed by the author, is the extent of "Alliterative Assonance," represented in the number of items involved in "runs" of assonance. An assonant "run" is the number of immediately sequential words that contain the same vowel (phone, not letter) as the (first) syllable[11] nucleus in that run. For example, "sit, sick, sift," and so on; but also counting words beginning with the same /s/ cluster and sequential vowel, for example, "spook, spool, spoon," and so on.

Story One

A microphone was placed unobtrusively to the left and front of the subject, with the tape recorder positioned out of his view. He was given the task instructions and handed the picture card, at which time a timer was started and allowed to run until his story was finished. This procedure yielded three time measures: the overall time elapsed; the amount of time actually spent telling the story; and the difference between the two, identified as "formulation time," the span of time presumably required to formulate a schema for the story.

It was important that this task yield data based on a genuinely spontaneous expression, in which the subjects were free to speak as they would, including the amount of time spent talking. Therefore they were simply given the pertinent instructions and allowed to proceed independently. When a subject indicated he had finished he was not encouraged to talk more in order to attain a certain minimum size of sample.[12]

The recordings were transcribed by a skilled stenographer who typed each story verbatim, including anything identifiable as a meaningful word. These transcriptions were reviewed by the author, first to check their accuracy to that point and then to insert the remaining audible features, such as filled pauses, word fragments, and isolated sounds. The transcriptions were then reviewed a final time to locate and record perceptible silent intervals of 1 second or longer.

The primary scores for this test were the total number of words and the number of different words used. Words repeated immediately (i.e., in word repetitions or phrase repetitions) were counted only once. Other measures derived from these protocols were: the amount of time presumably used to formulate a story, overall word rate as represented in actual story time, certain data on grammatical and phonetic structure, and extent of nonfluencies and stutters.

Story Two

The subject was provided a pad of lined paper and a container holding four sharpened wooden pencils from which the erasers had been removed. Subjects were asked to cross out errors they made, thereby identifying the errors they recognized. The subject was given the task instructions, then handed the picture card, whereupon the timer was started and allowed to run until his story was finished. A notation was made of the elapsed time at the moment the subject began to write, so that three time measures, comparable to those for Story One, were also recorded for this measure.

The primary scores for this test were the total number of words and number of different words used. Other measures obtained were: the amount of time presumably used in story formulation, and in actual production; also, the kinds and number of errors made during production.

Word Association

This measure was administered as a written test, for several reasons. Writing could be expected to "equalize" the performance demands for the two groups; it also provided a permanent record of the associations; and, with the instrumentation used, yielded a precise record of response times.

A special pad was used to record each subject's performance. The pad consisted of a sheet of plain, legal-size paper, covered by carbon paper and topped with a sheet of aluminum foil. This pad was overlaid with a specially made stencil and clamped to a masonite board of accommodating size. The stencil was made of heavy duty stencil grade paper in which were cut 100 rectangular openings, arranged in a 10 by 10 pattern, spaced evenly, with the long dimension of the openings aligned with the long dimension of the pad. The rectangular slots, each ample for the purpose, provided spaces in which the subject could write his associations on the aluminum foil exposed through each slot.

The subject wrote with a ballpoint pen, the upper end of which was wired to one lead of an electronic timer, from which another lead was connected to the aluminum foil. The timer was activated by a voice relay; it was started as each word of the Kent-Rosanoff list, on the prerecorded tape, was spoken; it was stopped when the stylus made contact with the aluminum foil as the subject wrote his answer. An override switch could interrupt the sequence at any point; it was used to reset the timer after the elapsed time for each item had been recorded, by the experimenter, on a separate record form. The switch that reset the timer also started the tape again, and the process repeated.

Prior to actual administration of the Word Association test the subject's reaction time to an auditory stimulus was determined by having him touch the stylus to the foil as soon as he heard a tone, also prerecorded on the tape. An average value for five trails was later subtracted from each of his word association reaction times, the resulting values being accepted as the actual associative reaction times. Also, immediately prior to the test proper, five trial words were presented to ensure that the subject heard each word clearly and well.

In view of the beliefs that stuttering reflects emotional disturbance it seemed plausible to expect that word association might be sensitive to emotional influence. Some suggestion of such an effect was contained in a study reported by Travis (1928). He found that stutterers, in contrast to normal speakers, produced fewer words during a chain association task when performing in the presence of other persons. Assuming that the threat of electric shock would be emotionally disruptive, and that the effect would be relfected in lengthened response time, the following procedure was implemented.

Half of the subjects in each group heard the Kent and Rosanoff list in its original form; the remaining subjects heard the last 50 words of the list first. For all subjects the test was interrupted at the midpoint, at which time the subject was advised that, at varying intervals during the remainder of the test, he would receive five shocks calcuated to be annoying but not necessarily painful. Since individuals vary in their tolerance of electric shock an apparatus was constructed that permitted calibration of the amount of charge actually delivered. After strapping the electrodes to the inner surface of the wrist just below the heel of the hand not used for writing, a "tolerance level" was established by administering three or four shocks of increasing intensity. Once the subject indicated that his tolerance level had been reached the testing was resumed. Immediately, and unknown to the subject, the charge setting was increased by approximately 10% beyond the tolerance level established, the object being to ensure that the shock was uncomfortable. In view of the observation that each subject almost always gave unmistakable evidence of sensing the shock, and from their subsequent verbal report, it can be considered that the shocks were, at least momentarily, unsettling.

The shocks were delivered after words number 53, 61, 67, 80, and 90. The intent of this spacing was that the subject should experience the shock soon after resuming the test, but that the irregular and then longer intervals might create a negative (and therefore presumably interfering) state of anticipation. The subjects were questioned immediately afterward about their reactions in this regard. All reported that they did not like being shocked, but claimed that they took the shocks as they came and concentrated on listening for the next word. Roughly 30% of both groups reported noting how many shocks they had received, and therefore how many were still to come; the others lost count.

The associations were "scored" according to three classifications: "Common," "Nonspecific," or "Different." An association was identified as Common if it were listed among the most common associations in the norms published by Russell and Jenkins (1954).[13] This reference was chosen because the data were obtained from a large subject population of an age and educational level comparable to the subject groups in this study. Actually, the common associations reported in this source are very much the same as those listed in other studies of word association that have used the Kent and Rosanoff list (cf. Palermo & Jenkins, 1964; Postman & Keppel, 1970).

The Nonspecific and Different categories were intended to reflect "unusual" associations. Both of these categories can be scored more objectively than the category of Individual responses, which was used in previous research. The Nonspecific category, adopted from Kent and Rosanoff, refers to "words which are so widely applicable as to serve as more or less appropriate reactions to almost any of our stimulus words" (Kent & Rosanoff, 1910, p. 319). Although noting that such words are ordinary enough, Kent and Rosanoff considered them to be "inferior" to the common (specific) associations, and that their very generality or indefiniteness implied "some pathological significance." An association was classified as "Different" if it were heterogeneous with the stimulus word, that is, of a different grammatical class. Typically, associated words are homogeneous with the stimulus word (Deese, 1962; Ervin, 1961).

A secondary measure was average reaction time, for the total test, the two halves separately, and the items immediately following delivery of a shock. Special note was made of the class of associations to the words following the shocks. A separate count was made of the number of synonyms and antonyms used.

Visual Slurvs

All items of the two forms of the Slurvians test, and the four demonstration-example items, were printed in 2-inch block letters on strips of poster board. The four demonstration items were used with both forms of the test and shown to the subject in the course of giving the instructions. The items of the form being used in the visual presentation wre placed, sequentially, on an easel situated approximately 6 feet in front of the subject. The exposure time of each item, 30 seconds, was controlled by the experimenter.

The score on both versions of this test was the number of items correct. Solution of parts of items was not credited.

Auditory Slurvs, Backward Speech, Phonetic Anagrams

The items used in each of these tests, and the format of delivery, were prerecorded on tape. Demonstration-example material was also prerecorded for each of these measures and was employed in conjunction with the instructions pertinent to each measure. Scores on these measures were the total number of correct items.

Test of Behavioral Rigidity

This measure was administered according to the sequence and instructions contained in the TBR Manual.[14] Raw scores obtained from subjects' performance are converted into "Rigidity Quotients" having a mean of 100 and a standard deviation of 15. Separate scores are computed for each of the three subtests (Motor-Cognitive, Psychomotor Speed, and Personality-Perceptual), and an overall Composite rigidity score summarizes total performance. Scoring was done according to the manual.

Footnotes

[1]Primary Mental Abilities (1949). Published by Science Research Associates, Chicago, IL.

[2]In contrast to free association, the type expressed in the usual word association test, and to continuous or "chain" association tasks.

[3]Data I have gathered periodically over more recent times have continued to confirm these findings. Further, other research contains corroborative evidence (see Chapter 8).

[4]Originally published in 1910, the list was later printed as a formal test by the Stoelting Company and has subsequently appeared in many sources.

[5]The list by Rapaport et al. contains many words reflecting psychodynamic, including psychoanalytic, concepts.

[6]A wide range of other research in the psychology of stuttering also does not support the assumption of an emotional basis for the disorder. See Wingate (1976, chap. 2).

[7]This group included two "recovered" stutterers.

[8]The difficult items were too difficult for everyone. Similarly, all subjects in the present research failed to solve some of the Slurvians.

[9]It is worth noting that certain differences between the sexes in King's results were sufficient to contraindicate combining the sexes in making the comparisons between the stutterers and normal speakers.

[10]In some cases the interval was slightly longer, but never longer than two weeks.

[11]Although most words were of one syllable, a word of more than one syllable qualified if the first vowel met the criterion.

[12]For instance, in Johnson's (1961a) collection of spontaneous speech samples, subjects were prompted to continue speaking until they had produced samples of a minimum size comparable across subjects.

[13]The number of words in the "most common" category varied among the stimulus words, ranging between one and four, and was determined by the proportional occurences of these words to the total number recorded.

[14]The interested reader should consult the TBR Manual.

8
Results and Discussion

The principle objective of this research was to investigate certain dimensions of language function in stuttering and to identify probable interrelationships among them. A second, related, objective was to obtain data on normal nonfluency and stuttering, and the relationship of these two phenomena to certain structural aspects of the language. Results bearing primarily on the principal objective of the research will be presented in the first section of the chapter. The data most pertinent to issues of fluency will be presented in the second section.

Linguistic Dimensions

Direct Comparisons on Pertinent Variables

The pertinent data are presented in Table 8.1, arranged vertically in the sequence in which they will be reviewed. The left half of the table lists the dimensions that constitute the core of the analysis. As noted in Chapter 7, some of the measures afforded an opportunity to extract other data that would be pertinent, in varying measure, to certain aspects of the investigation. These data are listed at the bottom of Table 8.1 as "secondary measures." They will be incorporated into the review of results where it seems most appropriate.

The performance of the stutterers differed substantially from that of the normal subjects on most of the principal dimensions of comparison, and on certain of the derived measures. Table 8.1 shows the extent of these differences on the variables for which such comparisons are pertinent.

WAIS Vocabulary

It was surprising to find the extent of difference between the two groups on WAIS vocabulary scores. As revealed in the Tables 8.2 and 8.3, the correlations between PMA vocabulary and WAIS vocabulary scores are high

TABLE 8.1. Comparison of subject groups on the various language test variables: main variables

	Stutterers		Normals		
	$\bar{X}$	σ	$\bar{X}$	σ	P
WAIS-score	13.1	2.3	14.9	2.6	.02
W-Fl-score	36.9	17.1	53.6	14.8	.002
Word association					
Common	41.0	10.0	44.0	10.0	.41
Nonspecific	2.6	2.1	1.4	1.0	.08
Different	25.0	8.1	18.0	6.5	.004
TBR					
Composite	101.0	9.3	112.0	14.0	.006
Motor-Cognitive	96.0	15.1	107.0	12.6	.02
Psych. speed	98.0	25.8	111.0	12.4	.06
Pers.-Percptl.	101.0	18.2	107.0	16.3	.30
Sound mindedness					
Visual Slurvians	7.0	3.4	10.3	2.5	.001
Auditory Slurvians	4.9	2.7	8.3	2.4	.0004
Phonetic anagrams	5.2	3.2	8.8	4.3	.005
Backward speech	9.7	6.2	14.7	5.3	.01
Story One					
Number of words	249.1	144.8	209.6	147.5	.40
Number different words	156.1	76.5	102.3	51.1	.01
Story Two					
Number of words	203.4	124.0	224.3	111.0	.58
Number different words	108.8	50.7	121.3	50.8	.45
	Secondary measures				
WAIS					
Number of words	251.0	126.0	215.6	86.6	.30
Number different words	155.3	63.3	134.8	34.4	.21
Number synonyms	9.5	—	9.0	—	—
Word association					
Number synonyms	2.0	—	2.0	—	—
Number antonyms	13.2	8.0	16.8	6.8	.02
Number of errors, Story Two	21.0	9.2	15.0	12.5	.08

for both groups. Though the correlation values for the two groups are comparable, the one for the normal speakers is higher. This difference may express the fact that the stutterers clearly did not do as well as the normal speakers on the WAIS vocabulary, the expressive vocabulary measure. The difference cannot be attributed to problems of oral expression because the subjects' definitions of the words were written. The difference also cannot be accounted for in terms of the effort made to give an adequate definition because, individually as well as on the average, the stutterers used more words in giving their definitions than did the normal speakers. Although this difference between the two groups was not statistically significant, it was sizable enough to carry two implications. One has already been mentioned: namely, that achievement on this measure is not due to the number of words used. The second implication is that, since stutterers used more words but received lower scores, their word usage evidently was less efficient than that of the normal speakers.

It is of some interest that the stutterers also used fewer synonyms as definitions than did the normal speakers. The difference is not statistically significant, but sufficient to contradict the claim that stutterers learn synonyms for many words as a way of avoiding stuttering (see, for example, Bender, 1939, p. 244; Van Riper, 1971, p. 168).

Word-Fluency

In contrast to the results for the WAIS vocabulary, the difference in scores between the two groups on the word-fluency test was not surprising. The significantly better performance of normal speakers on this measure was anticipated, in view of the previous findings (Wingate, 1968) that normal speakers were clearly superior to stutterers on this measure. The present evidence, confirming previous findings, is also corroborated substantially by results obtained in certain other studies (Okasha, Bishry, Kamel, & Hassan, 1974; Weuffen, 1961) in which a measure of word-fluency was incorporated in the procedure.

It is pertinent to mention here that this recurring evidence that stutterers do not do well with a word-fluency task contributes a great deal to a psycholinguistic conceptualization of the nature of stuttering, which will be discussed at length in Chapter 9. In fact, the evidence centering in word-fluency performance is pivotal in a theoretical construction that nicely interweaves other salient features of the disorder with pertinent findings from research in normal speech.

It is of some interest that both groups showed significant improvement in their second performance on the word-fluency task. This finding suggests that although word-fluency capability is evidently a kind of special skill (see Chapter 9), it is evidently subject to improvement with practice. Nonetheless, the stutterers' mean score on the second adminstration still did not equal the average score of the normal speakers on the first administration.

The superior achievement of the normal speakers on this measure was not due to the normal speakers listing more "simple" or "easy" words. Although, on the average, the normal speakers gave slightly more words that are listed in both the "A" and "AA" categories of the Thorndike and Lorge (1944) compilation, the difference was not significant. Interestingly, the stutterers listed more polysyllabic words but, again, the difference was not significant.

An unplanned, but useful, by-product of the word-fluency task with stutterers derives from the fact that the focal constraint required in this test was that the words to be listed begin with the letter "s." Now, since both "speech" and "stutter" begin with "s," this task afforded a kind of specialized projective measure. If, as is so widely believed, stutterers are typically preoccupied with speech, or with the fact that they stutter, one could expect that the words "stutter" and "speech" (or a variant) should surface quickly in stutterers' lists of words beginning with "s." Certainly, if the belief is credible, one should expect to find that these words would occur more frequently to stutterers than to normal speakers. However, the protocols do not provide any support for this expectation. The word stutter was listed infrequently by both stutterers and normal speakers. Speech occurred slightly more often among normal speakers, but still infrequently.[1]

Note that the difference between the two groups on the measure of Alliterative Assonance is at a level of statistical significance comparable to that for word-fluency (*p.* = .001). The two measures are clearly correlated, as one could expect since the former is part of the latter. Still, Alliterative Assonance represents an aspect of word-fluency performance that is of special interest, because such productions are marked by the combination of initial consonantism *and* succeeding vowel; the syllable nucleus is made part of the associative base.

Word Association

The results relative to the Word Association test show values for "Common," "Nonspecific," and "Different" associations.[2] The comparison for the Common responses is included here, even though showing no difference, because this is one dimension of word association analysis typically reported in the relevant literature. Several other comparisons made between the two groups in the present research also showed no differences. These comparisons included: (1) reaction time for the entire list, for each half of the list separately, and for words following the shocks; and (2) the nature of the associations to words following the shocks. The very comparable values of the two groups on these latter comparisons thus suggest that the stutterers do not differ from the normals in the readiness with which they make some kind of verbal association. The significance of the shocks remains unclear.

On the other hand, there is evidence that in certain qualitative aspects the nature of stutterers' word associations depart from that found typically among normal speakers. Note that the stutterers tended to give fewer common associations. Although this particular trend was not statistically significant, notable differences in stutterers' associations were revealed in the other two categories, both of which represent the inverse of Common associations. The stutterers gave substantially more Nonspecific associations than did the normal subjects ($p = .08$), and they differed very significantly from the normal speakers in the extent to which they gave Different (heterogeneous) associations ($p = 004$).[3]

The results of the word association test in this study are consistent with previous findings in indicating that, while stutterers' performance on a measure of this type is not, in general, remarkably different from that of normal speakers, there is among stutterers a clear tendency for verbal associations to depart in subtle ways from the verbal associative trends shown by normal speakers. Recall that in reviewing the findings of previous studies of word association in stutterers (Chapter 7) the following trend was noted. In studies using the Kent and Rosanoff list, which contains many common words, stutterers do not differ significantly from normals in length of time to produce associative words; however, more of their associations are uncommon ones. In comparison, when presented with special lists, composed of predominantly uncommon words, stutterers do differ from normals in terms of the length of time to give associations.[4] It seems that these two findings, each suggesting a subtle deviance in verbal associative function among stutterers, are interrelated in respect to the dimension of word frequency.

Test of Behavioral Rigidity

The dimensions of the TBR that assess flexibility involving language-related cognitive skills show the normal speakers to be clearly superior to the stutterers. On the Composite Rigidity score, which reflects overall flexibility and speed in performance, the difference between the two groups is highly significant. Taken alone, the Motor-Cognitive score, which most directly reflects this flexibility per se, also shows a significant difference between the two groups. The Psychomotor Speed score, of itself, barely fails a standard significance level. The Personality-Perceptual scores, in contrast, reveal the two groups to not be notably different on this dimension of the test, which is designed to assess flexibility (or rigidity) in traits of personality.

The TBR results are consistent with those obtained in the previous use of this measure (Wingate, 1966a) in which 12 young adult male stutterers evidence significantly less flexibility than did matched normal speakers on the Motor-Cognitive subtest. These findings add to certain other evidence, reported earlier, that a "perseverative tendency" in stutterers is most apparent in tasks that involve a rapid and contiguous change of set. In the relevant tasks of the TBR, and in the task that N.D. Solomon (1951) found to show a significant difference, the "rapid and contiguous change" involves language-related functions.

Tests of "Sound Mindedness"

It seems appropriate to consider the results for the Phonetic Anagrams test, the Backward Speech test, and the two forms of the Slurvian test under one heading because these measures evidently share a common focus. As discussed previously, the overall commonality in these four tests most likely reflects some kind of skill in dealing flexibly with phonetic patterns. Clearly, the Phonetic Anagrams and Backward Speech tests are addressed to the level of phonemes and the phonetic structure of words. Evidently the Slurvians also involve some amount of capability for phonetic "manipulation." However, success with Slurvians seems to also require a facility with larger language structures—phonetic patterns of word groups and related prosodic aspects of spoken language.

The results obtained reveal that the normal speakers were clearly superior to the stutterers on all four of these measures. It bears mention that the most dramatic difference between the two groups occurred with the Auditory Slurvians. As noted earlier this test is particularly demanding when administered in the format of presentation used in this research.

The striking differences between the stutterers and normal speakers on these measures of sound mindedness, results corroborated by other research, strongly suggest that stutterers lack the level of skills, found in normal speakers, to deal with a wide range of structural features and patterns of the language.

Story-Telling

The two main variables of interest in these data, from a language standpoint, were the total number of words and the number of different words used in each task. The first to be considered is the data from Story Two, as it was intended to be the comparative reference base.

The Story Two data for the two subject groups are similar for both total number of words and number of different words used. It should be noted that the stutterers actually wrote less than did the normal speakers; they used fewer words, and fewer different words—in fact, approximately 10% less of both.[5] This difference was not found to be statistically significant, so the two groups may be considered to be comparable in respect to extent and diversity of word usage in this task of written expression. An essential equivalence of the two groups on this measure is reflected in Figure 8.1, in which a single curve expresses the relationship between number of different words and total words used by each of the subjects in both groups.

The data for Story One, however, yield a different picture. In this oral story-telling the stutterers used *more* words than did the normal speakers,[6] in fact 19% more total words. Although a test of this difference between the two groups did not indicate statistical significance, it is pertinent to men-

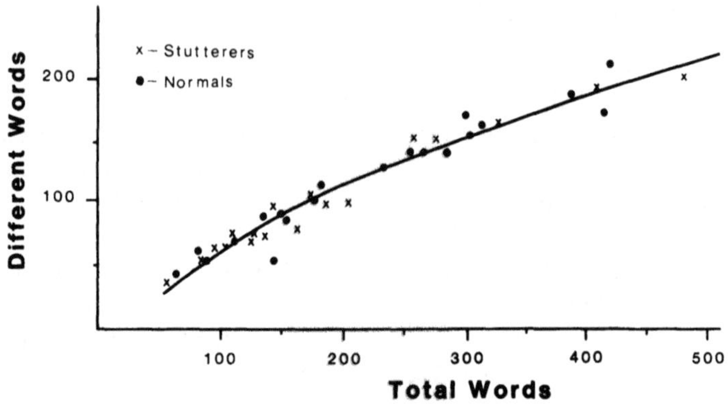

FIGURE 8.1. Relationship of the number of different words to total number of words used by stutterers and normal speakers in *writing* a story (Story Two).

tion that, except for one instance (the longest story of all) stutterers' stories were consistently longer than those of the normal speakers. It is in terms of the number of *different* words used that a difference between the two groups is very clear. The stutterers used 53% more different words than did the normal speakers, a difference that statistical test indicates is highly significant.

Figure 8.2 represents the relationship between the total number of words and number of different words used by individuals of the two groups in telling Story One. Here the data for the individuals of each group are expressed by different curves. The paramount distinction be-

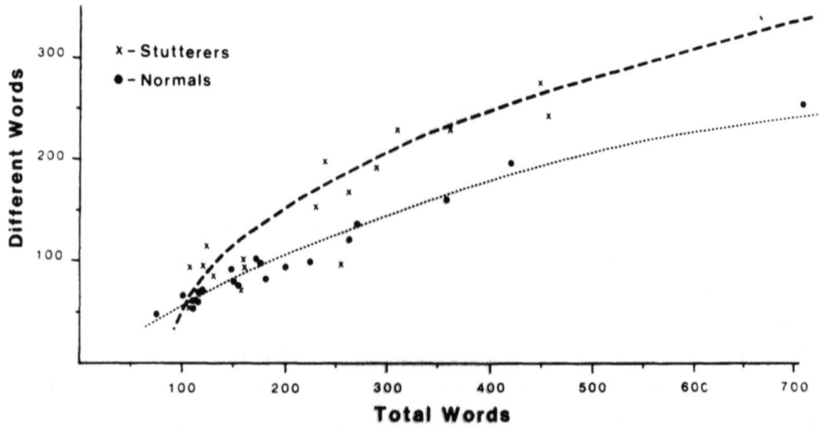

FIGURE 8.2. Relationship of the number of different words to total number of words used by stutterers and normal speakers when *telling* a story (Story One).

tween the two curves is, clearly, the significantly greater number of different words used by stutterers in telling Story One.

As noted earlier in this chapter the formula derived by Sankoff and Lessard (1975) expresses the relationship between the number of different words and the total words in a corpus based on large samples of spontaneous speech. The Sankoff-Lessard formula was used to assess the extent to which the data reflected in the curves of Figures 8.1 and 8.2 conform to what might be considered a normative reference. Using the formula, a series of D scores was computed to correspond to 20-word intervals over the range of total words (T) used in Stories One and Two by each group. It was then tested for statistical difference between the distributions of these formula-derived D values and the corresponding actual D values (number of different words) in each data set. The data represented by both of the curves in Figure 8.1, and the data for the normal speakers' curve in Figure 8.2, did not differ from the formula-derived values. However, the data represented in the stutterers' curve in Figure 8.2 did differ significantly from the reference data. This result augments the evidence, derived from direct comparison of the two groups, that the stutterers' diversity of word usage in narration is deviant.

Figure 8.3 is a composite in which the curves for all the story-telling data may be compared to a reference curve computed from the Sankoff-Lessard formula. The latter has the clear character of a mathematically derived curve of uniform shape. Because it is based on large samples it may be somewhat flatter than one might expect to find for samples of the size constituting the present research. Nonetheless, it has acceptable

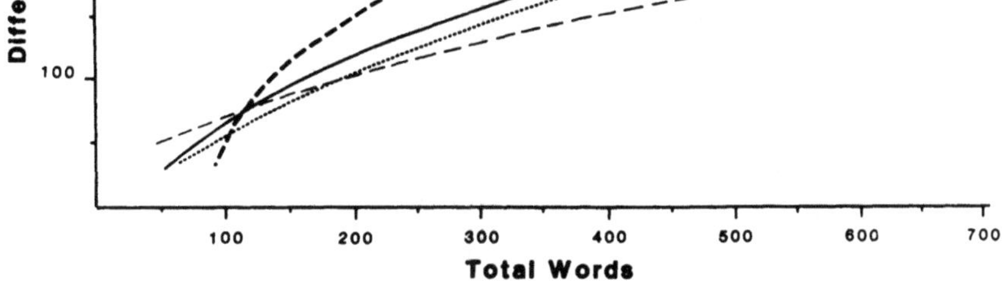

FIGURE 8.3. Word usage curves for oral and written stories of the two subject groups relative to a reference curve based on a large normative sample.

reference value for the data of this study and illustrates graphically the extent of deviance in the stutterers' Story One data.

There is another reason to characterize the stutterers' word diversity in oral expression as remarkably excessive, and as deviant from normal expectation. It has been known for some time that written material contains a wider range of words than does spoken discourse (see, for example, French et al., 1930). Research undertaken specifically to compare written and spoken samples, from normal speakers, is particularly relevant. This work (Drieman, 1962; Fraisse & Breyton, 1959; Horowitz & Newman, 1964; Moscovici & Humbert, 1960)[7] routinely has found that written samples contain considerably fewer total words but, at the same time, relatively more different words than oral samples produced by the same individuals. The reasons regularly given to account for these contrasts are those that should be evident to reflection on the likely differences between the two activities. For instance, in contrast to speaking: writing is more effortful; it is a skill that clearly is taught; it employs an entirely different motor system than speaking; and it is learned only after lengthy and laborious instruction and practice. Also, writing takes more time, in the course of which one has more opportunity to plan, to prepare, to reflect, to be more deliberate in proceeding, and so forth.[8] The curves in Figure 8.3 show that the stutterers and normal speakers differ markedly relative to the standard pattern found in comparing written and spoken expression. The normal speaking subjects in this study conformed to the pattern found in previous research with normal speakers:[9] their written stories are shorter, and have a higher diversity of word usage, than their spoken stories. In contrast, the stutterers, though also producing shorter written than spoken stories (the typical pattern), evidenced markedly greater diversity of word usage in their *spoken* stories, which is clearly the opposite of the usual pattern.

The greater number of different words occurring consistently in the stutterers' spoken stories is a distinctive and unique finding. It reflects a clearly atypical aspect of oral verbal expression, yet one that does not seem to be evident to a less detailed form of analysis. Using transcriptions of the 40 stories, from which all indications of stuttering had been removed, were submitted, in random sequence, to five speech pathology graduate students for appraisal of the extent to which "the story gives the impression of being coherent, sequential, and continous in development, generally organized in presentation." The resultant ratings, made in reference to a five-point scale, were very similar for the two groups of stories in terms of range, distribution, and central tendency. Evidently there were no discernible differences at this level. Two of my colleagues, who had had substantial experience with the Thematic Apperception Test (TAT), were asked to rate the stories, using a five-point scale, relative to "the amount of redundancy or extent of detail superfluous to the theme."

These ratings reflected a difference between the two groups which, though failing the standard level of statistical significance, indicated more superfluity in stutterers' stories.

Also two structural comparisons were made between the stories of the two groups: (1) the relative proportions of content and function words, and (2) the distribution of word lengths in both of these grammatical categories. The findings are presented in Table 8.2. The relative proportions of content and function words are identical for the two groups, for both the spoken and written stories. The content/function proportions for the spoken stories are consistent with the values reported by other sources that have analyzed spontaneous speech samples (Blankenship & Kay, 1964; Howes & Geschwind, 1969). Note that the proportion of content words is considerably higher in the written stories: this finding is consistent with previous content/function analysis of written material (e.g., Miller, Newman, & Friedman, 1958) and, as well, with the frequent evidence, cited previously, of greater word diversity in written, vis-á-vis spoken, material.

The data reflecting word-length usage reveals that the stutterers used considerably more short words than did the normal speakers. This dif ference, evident but not statistically significant for the written stories, is highly significant for the spoken stories, where it shows up in both content and function word categories. This highly significant difference between the two groups relative to the distributions of word length was something of a surprise. Diversity of word usage usually is assumed to reflect "vocabulary richness," which seems to imply something more than a larger stock of one-syllable words. Further, in this particular case vocabulary richness is contradicted by the fact that these subjects failed to give evidence of it in their WAIS vocabulary definitions. Also, any attempt to explain the evident diversity of word usage in terms of the claim regard-

TABLE 8.2. Content/function word proportions relative to word length distributions in Story One and Story Two

	Content words					Function words		
	Percent of total corpus	Word lengths in syllables				Percent of total corpus	Word lengths in syllables	
Task		1	2	3	4		1	2
Story One								
Stutterers	53	64	30	6	0	47	97	3
Normals	53	58	29	9	4	47	95	5
Story Two								
Stutterers	57	61	25	10	4	43	96	4
Normals	57	58	26	10	6	43	96	4

ing stutterers' presumed use of synonyms[10] is contradicted by the fact that, for both the WAIS vocabulary and the word association tests, the stutterers' use of synonyms was no different than that of the normal speakers. Diversity in word usage is also not to be explained in terms of literal redundancy, that is, repetition of words and phrases, because such occurrences do not contribute to number of *different* words.

It is possible, however, that diversity might be inflated by a kind of redundancy taking the form of unnecessary elaboration or recycling on a theme. This consideration raises the issue of circumlocution, often said to characterize stutterers' speech. Typically, circumlocution is explained as resulting from the stutterers' efforts to avoid "difficult words." The findings yielded in this research suggest that such circumlocution as occurs in the speech of stutterers is more likely to reflect certain limitations in the ability to generate verbal utterances.

Table 8.2 does not show another significant difference between the two groups on Story One, namely story time. The groups did not differ on "formulation" or "preparation" time for either Story One or Story Two, but the stutterers' time spent in telling Story One was significantly longer than the time used by the normal speakers. In some small measure this difference was due to the longer stories told by the stutterers, but the principal reason for the lengthier story time of the stutterers was the time consumed by instances of stutter and other disfluencies. This highly significant difference will be discussed in the section on "Disfluencies."

Among the several dimensions of verbal function, just considered, that compare the stutterers' and normal speakers' story-telling the differences are clearly related to the mode of expression. The findings indicate that in the speaking task the stutterers were remarkably less focused and less efficient in their verbal formulation and expression than were the normal speakers. Referring to the typical differences between written and oral expression mentioned earlier, one is inclined to think particularly of the differences attendant on the amount of time available, wherein writing affords ample time to reflect, deliberate, reconsider, recast, and so forth. In other words, time pressure on verbal formulation would seem to be a critical factor. But there are also other relevant matters to consider. Recall the differences between the two groups on the WAIS vocabulary. In that task too the mode of expression was writing, which should have afforded the same advantages to expression that are afforded in writing a story. The fact that the stutterers clearly did not benefit from such advantages when writing definitions seems related to the nature of the task. There are some important differences between writing a story and writing word definitions. In the latter activity, one's orientation to the task is determined externally, and many constraints immediately become operative, constraints expressed particularly in respect to word choices and word arrangements. In the definition task the stutterers revealed inferior linguistic function in two ways: (1) they used more words, and more different words, in their efforts to succeed in the task; but (2) their achievements were still inferior to those of the normal speakers. Since their recognition vocabulary scores indicate a level of word knowledge equivalent to the normal speakers, it seems that their effort with WAIS definitions gives additional evidence of ineffectiveness in verbal formulation and expression, an ineffectiveness that is not to be explained simply in terms of time-related pressure attendant on speaking.[11]

It may be instructive to present here an overall quantitative comparison between the two groups on the three tasks that involved connected expression: the WAIS definitions, Stories One and Two. Table 8.3 shows, for each of the three measures, the number of words and number of different words used, and a ratio expressing this relationship. Note that the ratios for the two groups are identical for the written story (Story Two). In giving WAIS definitions, both groups show a higher ratio than in the written story. Giving definitions constitutes a series of brief tasks in which the task focus emphasizes content, so one might expect some increase in the ratio of number different words to total number of words, as is found. However, the ratio is considerably higher for the stutterers. In writing definitions, the stutterers used 21% more words overall, and 15% more different words, than did the normal speakers.

One should expect, in reference to normative data presented earlier in this chapter that, of these three measures, the spontaneous speech samples obtained as Story One would yield the lowest ratio of different-to-total-words. The normal speaker's samples conform to this expectation, but the ratio for the stutterers' samples remains high.

TABLE 8.3. Comparison of extents of word usage in the three tasks involving spontaneous expression

Task	Stutterers	Normal
Story Two		
Number of words	203	224
Number of different words	109	121
ratio	.57	.57
WAIS Vocabulary		
Number of words	251	215
Number of different words	155	135
ratio	.67	.61
Story One		
Number of words	249	210
Number of different words	156	102
ratio	.63	.49

Intercorrelations

For clarity of reference all correlations between +.20 and −.20 have been omitted in the correlation matrices presented in Tables 8.4 and 8.5.[12] Most of the values entered in the tables are significant beyond the .10 level. The levels of significance, from .10 to .001 and greater, are indicated in footnotes of the tables. Generally, level of significance is related directly to correlation value. Some correlation values that did not attain the .10 level of significance were retained in the tables primarily to indicate patterns of similarity and difference among the correlations for each subject group.

There are several high, and highly significant, correlations found to be common to each subject group. As expected, the two measures of Vocabulary are highly related, although more so for the normal speakers—an evident reflection of the stutterers' poorer performance with the WAIS. The high positive correlations between Number of Words and Number of Different Words in Story One, and the high negative correlations between Common and Different word associations, could also be expected. Interestingly, both of these correlations are higher for the normal speakers. Both subject groups also show high positive correlations between the two versions of the Slurvians test, and between the Phonetic Anagrams and Backward Speech tests, indicating that each of these pairs of tasks tap common sources and that the functions involved operate similarly among individuals of the two subject groups.

In contrast, there are two highly significant correlations that are dramatically different for the two subject groups. Among the stutterers there is a very substantial negative correlation between the Word-Fluency measure and the Number of Different Words in Story One, whereas for the normal speakers there is no relationship (r = .02) between these two variables. The other correlation that is dramatically different between the two subject groups is the high positive correlation between Alliterative Assonance and Auditory Slurvians evidenced by the normal speakers, which contrasts with the low negative correlation between these variables evidenced in the stutterers' data. This difference between the two groups actually extends to all correlations between the two measures of word-fluency and the two Slurvian measures. In fact, there is a notably different pattern between the two subject groups for correlations between the two word-fluency measures and most of the other variables.

In regard to the other correlations it seems most parsimonious to consider evident patterns rather than to compare even the more notable individual pairs. A pattern common to both groups is that of moderate correlations between both Vocabulary measures and the measures of word manipulation skills: the Slurvians, Phonetic Anagrams, and Backward Speech. A major difference in pattern is that, overall, there were more correlations among the stutterers' data than among the normal speakers; which rather suggests that among the stutterers the functions tapped by

TABLE 8.4. Normal speakers: intercorrelations among the variables measured[a]

Variable	WAIS	WF1	Allit.	Words WAIS	Words Story One	D/Wrd. Story One	Words Story Two	W-A Com	W-A Dif	TBR MC	TBR PS	TBR CR	Vis. Slurv.	Aud. Slurv.	Anagr.	Bk-Sp
PMA	.87			.42						−.25	.53	.24	.34	.21	.30	.41
WAIS		.20		.44						−.21	.50	.39	.42	.21	.55	.60
WF1			.54	.23				.28	−.36		.33	.26	.30	.49	.30	.27
Allit								.27	−.27		.29	.22	.49	.77		
Words, WAIS							.26			−.29						
Words, Story One						.98		−.37	.23							
Dif. wrds, Story One								−.36	.28							−.20
Words, Story Two									−.28	−.29		−.22				
W-A. Com									−.81		.25	.33	.45	.29		
W-A. Dif											−.36	−.45	−.42	−.21	−.20	−.29
TBR, MC											−.21					
TBR, PS												.80	.54	.50	.61	.65
TBR, CR													.45	.32	.60	.65
Vis. Slurv.														.73	.49	.56
Aud. Slurv.															.32	.33
Anagr.																.83

[a]Correlation values less than ±.20 excluded.
[b]Correlation values of: ±.70 and above have a minimum significance level of .0001
±.61 and above have a minimum significance level of .002
±.54 and above have a minimum significance level of .01
±.42 and above have a minimum significance level of .05
±.39 and above have a minimum significance level of .10.

TABLE 8.5. Stutterers: intercorrelations among the variables measured[a]

Variable	WAIS	WF1	Allit.	Words WAIS	Words Story One	D/Word Story One	Words Story Two	W-A Com	W-A Dif.	TBR MC	TBR PS	TBR CR	Vis. Slurv.	Aud. Slurv.	Anagr.	Bk-Sp	Stutt. Rating
PMA	.81			.29		.20					.36	.22	.39	.48	.50	.55	
WAIS				.34			.24					.38	.32	.31	.52	.48	
WF1			.65	−.46	−.55	−.69	−.32	.55	−.41	.51	.39	.54	−.25		.46	.33	
Allit				−.33	−.42	−.44		.33	−.33	.37		.47	−.40	−.21	.30		
Words, WAIS					.40	.43	.49	−.23	.48		−.20						
Words, Story One						.94	.42	−.29	.25	−.56		−.33			−.20		
Dif. words, Story One							.49	−.44	.32	−.54		−.37			−.20		
Words, Story Two										−.29		−.43					
W-A, Com.									−.72	.41	.25	.59		.22	.25		−.25
W-A, Dif.										−.22		−.33	−.20	−.29	−.46	−.29	
TBR, MC												.49			.22		
TBR, PS												.32	−.24				
TBR, CR															.36	.23	
Vis. Slurv.														.68	.39	.45	
Aud. Slurv.															.48	.59	
Anagr.																.89	.20
Bk-Sp																	

[a]Correlation values less than ±.20 excluded.

[b]Correlation values of: ±.68 and above have a minimum significance value of .0001
±.59 and above have a minimum significance value of .002
±.52 and above have a minimum significance value of .01
±.44 and above have a minimum significance value of .05
±.37 and above have a minimum significance value of .10

the various measures represent a more common substance than is the case for the normal speakers. Another notable difference centers on correlations involving Composite Rigidity, the overall flexibility score of the TBR. The stutterers' matrix shows negative correlations between this flexibility score and the several measures reflecting amount of words used. In contrast, the normal speakers' matrix shows, quite differently, high positive correlations of the flexibility measure with variables reflecting facility with words and their structure.

Factor Analyses

Substantial overall differences between the stutterers' and the normal speakers' functioning with these various linguistic measures are well reflected in the results of factor analyses of the data. Separate analyses were made of the data from each subject group. The results, obtained from Varimax orthogonal rotation, are presented in Table 8.6.

The analysis for the normal speakers' data yielded four factors that account for 70% of the variance. The four factors can be indentified readily in reference to the variables loading them, and constitute a logical and sequentially coherent structure. The first factor, having the heaviest loading, is based on six variables as listed in Table 8.6. It is readily identifiable as a word knowledge factor. The central dimension of this factor reflects the type of word knowledge traditionally expressed in the term vocabulary. In addition, the composition of Factor I includes dimensions of word knowledge that reflect: (1) facility in identifying the phonetic structure of words and (2) a certainty, quickness, and flexibility in expressing their semantic value.

The second factor, based on five variables, is clearly identifiable as representing word access, the facility with which words that are appropriate for a particular context are "brought up" from the lexicon.

The third and fourth factors reflect word usage. Factor III represents word use in oral expression, and Factor IV represents word use in written expression. It is of considerable interest that oral usage is the heavier contribution to the factorial structure.

Corresponding analysis of the stutterers' data reveals a factor structure that is different from that of the normal speakers. The composition of Factor I has certain similarities to Factor I for the normal speakers, but it is not as easily rationalized. For instance, although vocabulary is a dimension of the stutterers' Factor I it is not as clearly a major element as in the normal speakers' first factor. Also representation of Slurvian skill in this factor is not as sensible as is the appearance of this variable among those that constitute Factor II in the normal speakers' data.

The stutterers' Factor II is identical to the normal speakers' Factor III, representing word usage in oral expression. The stutterers' Factor III is

TABLE 8.6. Composition of factor loadings for stutterers and normal speakers

Stutterers			Normals		
Factor		Cumulative percent of variance	Factor		Cumulative percent of variance
Variable	Contribution		Variable	Contribution	
Factor I		27	Factor I		30
Aud. Slurv.	.85		WAIS	.85	
Bk. Sp.	.81		Bk Sp	.82	
Vis. Slurv.	.80		Anagr	.80	
Anagr.	.77		TBR-PS	.76	
SRA	.64		SRA	.73	
WAIS	.56		TBR-CR	.65	
Factor II		47	Factor II		47
Words in Story One	.94		W-A Com.	.79	
Different words in Story One	.85		Allit.	.70	
			A. Slurv.	.69	
			Vis. Slurv.	.63	
			WF1	.56	
Factor III		58	Factor III		59
WF1	.71		Words in Story One	.90	
Allit	.68		Different words in Story One	.88	
TBR-PS	.62				
TBR-CR	.62				
Factor IV		67	Factor IV		70
W-A Diff.	.71		Words in Story Two	.75	
			Different words in Story Two	.61	

identifiable as a word access factor. However, it shows only a partial resemblance to the normal speakers' word access factor. Note that the sequence of these two factors is inverted in the analysis of the stutterers' data.

If it is assumed that word access represents the ready availability of words specifically pertinent to an utterance being generated, the foregoing result of the factor analysis is consistent with other evidence, presented earlier in this chapter, which suggests that limitations in word access function is a substantial dimension of the excessive and inefficient word usage that characterize the stutterers' oral expression.

Factor IV from the stutterers' data might be looked on simply as anomalous, except that its presence in the factor structure is consistent with the description presented in the foregoing paragraph.

Overall, the analysis of the stutterers' data does not show the coherence in factor composition nor the logical sequence in factor structure that is clearly evident in the analysis of the normal speakers' data.

Disfluency Dimensions

The disfluency analyses to be presented here were derived from the spontaneous speech samples obtained as Story One. The first level of analysis is a review of the kinds and extent of disfluencies evidenced by the two subject groups. The relevant data, presented in Table 8.7, are arranged in the same categories used in Tables 2.4 through 2.10, which reviewed the findings of other studies that had compiled comparative data on disfluencies in stutterers and normal speakers. The Type N category refers to the kinds of disfluencies typically considered to be normal. The Type S category refers to the two disfluency types that are the characteristic markers of stuttering. The Indeterminate category includes those types that, on occasion, may be associated with a stutter event even though in most instances the incident is likely to be normal in character. The only notable difference in the categories of Table 8.7 vis-á-vis the tables of Chapter 2 is that, unlike previous research reports. Filled Pauses ("uh" and the like) are not included within the class of Interjections.

TABLE 8.7. Average disfluencies per 100 words in Story One[a]

	Type of disfluency				
			Indeterminate		
Subject group	Type N[b]	Type S[c]	Single syllable word[d]	Inter-jection	Filled pauses
Stutterers	5.8	12.3	3.2	2.1	7.3
Normals	1.0	0.3	1.1	0.7	3.1

[a]The classifications of disfluency types correspond to those used in Chapter 2.
[b]Revisions, phrase repetitions, polysyllabic word repetitions, incomplete words.
[c]Sound and syllable repetitions, prolongations.
[d]Includes instances of one and more-than-one repetition per repetition instance.

Inspection of Table 8.7 reveals findings clearly similar to those presented in the relevant tables of Chapter 2. As could be expected, the greatest difference between the two groups is in regard to the Type S category, the stutters. The miniscule amount found among normal speech samples are benign; they are stutters only in the descriptive sense, as reported in a few of the "hesitation phenomena" studies reviewed in Chapter 2. The data from the present study thus show what the research comparing the speech of normal speakers and stutterers has always shown: that stutters characterize the speech of individuals identified as stutterers.

The data presented in Table 8.7 also corroborate other comparative data on another important dimension—namely, that the speech of stutterers contains more disfluencies of *all* kinds. As noted in Chapter 2, this important contrast has been overlooked in previous research; largely, it seems, because of theoretical predilections. This finding contradicts the claim that stutters develop in reaction to normal disfluency. If this claim were true, one should find the speech of stutterers to contain only, or mostly, stutters—and no, or only a few, normal disfluencies. Research has consistently revealed a very different picture.

Beyond refuting the "reaction" conjecture, there is a more valuable and enduring significance to the recurring evidence that stuttered speech contains more disfluencies of all kinds than does normal speech. It indicates that the speech (oral language) production process of stutterers breaks down at several levels. At certain levels the breakdown in continuity resembles—and in many instances may well be the same as—similar occurrences in the speech of normal speakers: for instance, some of the filled, and unfilled, pauses, or repetitions of a word, or of longer verbal units. At these levels the break in continuity might well be conceived as occuring relative to units that are "lexically intact," or "lexically complete." But the breakdowns intrinsic to a stutter event are in language units *below* the level of the word; they reflect "lexical fracture." As suggested in the discussion developed in Chapter 6, this fracture occurs along the "fault line," at the juncture of initial consonantism and syllable nucleus—a feature illuminated by the syllable structure hypothesis.

Linguistic Features of the Stutters

For several reasons[13] only two structural dimensions of the words involved in stutters will be considered: grammatical class and initial phone.

Figure 8.4 displays the frequencies of stutter occurrence involving words of the various grammatical classes. The letter codes on the abscissa represent the first distinctive letter in each class name, thus: *N*oun, *V*erb, ad*J*ective, adver*B*, pr*O*noun, au*X*iliary, ∞ (infinitive), *C*onjunction, *P*reposition and a*R*ticle. This curve of stutter distribution reflects the same

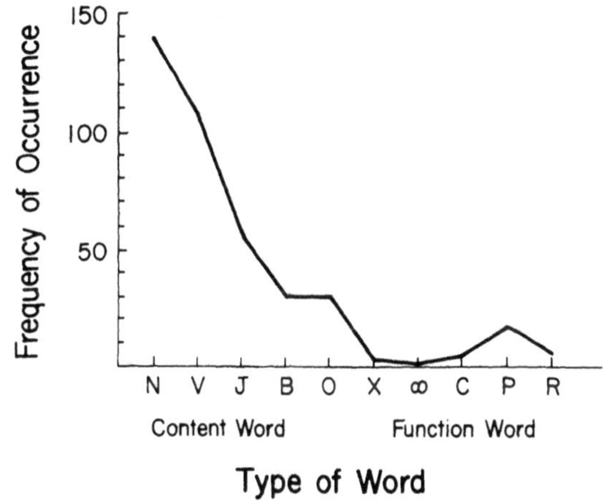

FIGURE 8.4. Frequency of stuttering associated with words of various grammatical classes. (*N*oun, *V*erb, ad*J*ective, adver*B*, pr*O*noun, au*X*iliary, ∞ (infinitive), *C*onjunction, *P*reposition, and a*R*ticle.)

finding reported so regularly in previous work, that *content* words are stuttered significantly more often than *function* words. As previous research has also indicated, there is evidently little reason to make much point of the absolute rank order of word classes stuttered, even within the content category (see Table 4.1). Again, as found repeatedly in previous work, the pattern of significantly more stuttering on content words was found to be consistent among the individual subjects.

In regard to a phonetic factor, stuttering occurred significantly more often with initial consonants than with initial vowels. The pertinent data have been entered in Table 5.17. Again, consistent with the findings of previous research, the ratio of stuttering on initial consonants is approximately double the ratio of consonant-initial occurrence in the corpus even though, in this corpus, the latter ratio is unusually high.

The frequency of stuttering on individual phones was also found to be very similar to that reported in previous research. The frequency of stuttering on the various phones was computed relative to the frequency with which the phones occurred initially within the corpus. The rank order of occurrence of initial phones correlated significantly ($r = .62$) with normative data of initial frequency, although not as highly as is found for larger samples. Nonetheless, the most frequently occurring initial consonants were /s, h, w, and t/, a typical finding. These four phones were also, proportionately, the least frequently stuttered. The phone /hw/ occurred infrequently, and was involved in only one stutter. These findings are thus consistent with the data previously reported regarding "the easy" consonants, and with the analysis of these data that is developed in Chapter 5.

Linguistic Aspects of a Normal Nonfluency

I have made the point in previous publications (Wingate, 1964, 1976) that single-syllable word repetitions are a somewhat unique class of nonfluency. Because of their monosyllabic character they can resemble the syllabic iterations that are one of the characteristic markers of a stutter event and may, therefore, be mistaken as stutters. However, like other normal nonfluencies they are not themselves stutters even though they may at times be associated with a stutter event.

Figure 8.5 shows, for both the stutterers and normal speakers, the frequencies with which single-syllable words of the various grammatical classes occurred as whole-word repetitions. There are two important points to be made regarding these curves. First, except for the section representing content words, the curves have a generally similar form that indicates a tendency for repetition of pronouns, conjunctions, and articles. This finding is consistent with the evidence reviewed earlier (Chapter 4) that words of these grammatical classes frequently occur, and often are repeated, in phrase-initial position. Notably, the stutterers evidenced significantly more repetition of both pronouns and conjunctions, and more word repetition overall. Second, comparison of both of these distributions with the curve for distribution of stutters (Figure 8.4) shows them to be clearly different. This difference supports the analysis developed in Chapter 4 that the repetition of single-syllable words is a normal type of nonfluency, which must be excluded from tallies of "stutterings."

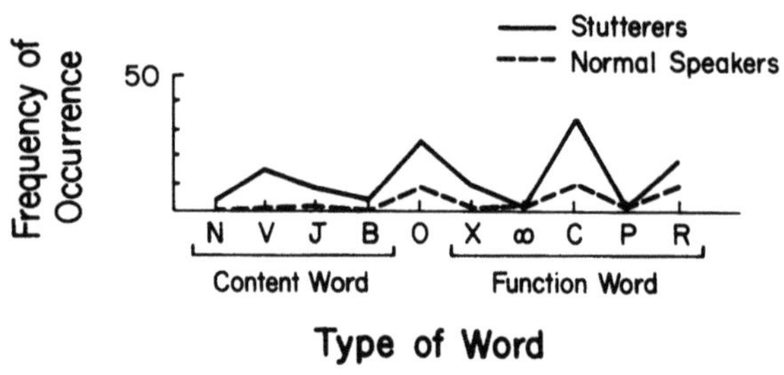

FIGURE 8.5. Frequency with which single-syllable words of the various grammatical classes occurred as whole-word repetitions in the spontaneous speech of the two subject groups. (*N*oun, *V*erb, ad*J*ective, adver*B*, pr*O*noun, au*X*iliary, ∞ (infinitive), *C*onjunction, *P*reposition, and a*R*ticle.)

Sequelae to Nonfluencies

Certain dimensions of the "hesitation phenomena" research have shown that events subsequent to the nonfluencies of normal speech contribute substantially to understanding the nature of nonfluencies. The significance of events that occur subsequent to a nonfluency is that they afford grounds for rationalizing the occurrence of the nonfluency. In this section the relevant data regarding events sequential to the several types of nonfluency recorded in the present study will be presented.

The curves in Figure 8.6 display the distribution of events immediately sequential to four nonfluency types. (The data for a fifth type of nonfluency, filled pause, will be presented separately.) The categories of sequential events include, in addition to grammatical classes: filled pause /ə /, true interjections (I), and isolated phones (Ph). It is of some interest that, except for a few notable differences, the distribution curves for the two groups are similar in form, although the stutterers' speech contains more nonfluencies of all kinds—in several cases with significant departure from the normal samples. One notable exception to similarity in form is evident in the second display, wherein adverbs are shown to occur with dramatic frequency as sequelae to monosyllabic word repetitions. One should relate this finding to the evidence (see Figure 8.5) that, among stutterers, verbs were a prominent type of monosyllabic word repetition. Curiously, the stutterer samples showed fewer instances, than did the normal samples, of adverbs occurring as sequelae to silent pauses of one second, whereas verbs were frequent sequelae to these brief pauses. At this time one can only speculate as to why the verb–adverb sequence was evidently a special nonfluency locus for the stutterers. Two other notable exceptions to similarity in form of the curves are the indications of the (statistically significant) differences between the two groups in the occurrence of filled pause /ə/ and isolated phones (Ph) following silent pauses (of any length). The isolated phones clearly suggest a word that was only started; that is, that they are word-initial phones. They occurred rarely among the normal speakers but frequently among the stutterers, in whose samples they are suspect of incipient stutters. The occurrence of filled pause sequential to silent pause suggests that whatever was to follow next in the speech sequence was not readily "available." A separate analysis of events involving pauses is particularly illuminating.

Pause

As noted in Chapter 2, consideration of pause has been omitted in the research of stuttering, a particularly significant omission in view of the fact that research concerned with the nonfluencies of normal speech has found pause to be a major nonfluency type that is important to the understanding of language processes.

The research on normal nonfluency identifies two types of pause, Filled Pause ("uh" or some variant) and Silent Pause (of indefinite lengths). Broadly speaking, much of the pause research has yielded evidence that

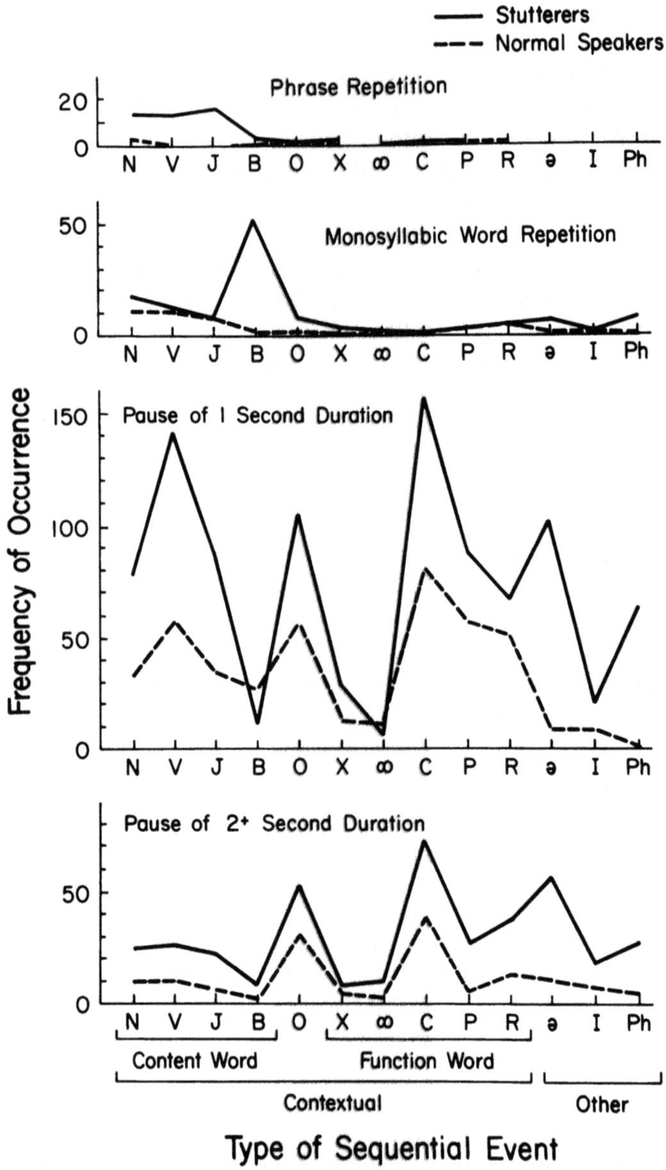

FIGURE 8.6. Frequency with which words of the various grammatical classes and certain other events occurred immediately sequential to four types of nonfluency. The "Other" categories that now appear on the abscissa are: /ə/ or filled pause; "I" for interjection; and "Ph" indicating an isolated phone.

pauses, of both kinds, reflect delays incident to utterance planning: the choice of words and the organization of longer speech units (phrases, sentences). Although there is some reason to believe that the two forms of pause may function somewhat differently, such possible differences have not yet been reliably identified. Curiously, the literature on pause has given little consideration to the fact that there is an obvious difference in the substance of the pause types: one of them, the filled pause, is vocalized; the other is not.

This notable difference between the two pause types can be characterized, at least, as activity versus inactivity. Now, it seems justifiable to assume that this activity, reflected in the filled pause, is initiated at some conscious or preconscious level of speaker intention, and represents an adjustment incident to maintaining utterance continuation—time to retrieve or choose a word, organize a phrase, and so forth. This supposition carries the implication that certain features of forward planning are in process before, as well as during, the occurrence of a filled pause. In contrast, silent pausing does not carry these implications. A silent pause seems more likely to indicate a locus where an expressive choice or decision is not adequately anticipated, or only vaguely grasped, or where choices are amorphous, faint, or some similar problem. Silent pauses, then, might well reflect a more fundamental discontinuity in the speech planning or speech activation process than do filled pauses. This matter remains to be studied in the pause research. However, certain findings in the present research, to be considered shortly, bear pointedly on this difference.

Before presenting the analyses of pause data contained in the present research it is pertinent to note first that, as with the other forms of disfluency the stuttered speech samples contained more of both kinds of pause than did the samples from the normal speakers.

The analysis of pause data from this study[14] centers on filled pauses and their loci. Filled pauses were chosen as the focus because of: (1) their substance, as discussed previously, and (2) the fact that this pause type has received some previous consideration in comparisons of stuttered and normal speech (and, moreover, is claimed to have the same properties in normal and stuttered speech). The essential objective, of course in reference to the findings from pause research is to identify pause sequelae.[15] As it turned out, the analysis also yielded two categories of antecedents to filled pause, along with evidence that they are related to the type of filled pause sequelae.

Categories for identifiying "type" of filled pause emerged as the analysis proceeded. At one time, five different categories were in use, but eventually it became evident that the following three categories were adequate. Filled pauses were found to occur either: (1) *as word addition*—instances in which a filled pause follows a word quickly (in open juncture); (2) *after a silent pause*—instances in which a filled pause occurs after a silent pause of one second or longer; and (3) *in repetition*—instances in which a filled pause is repeated, either alone or with other sounds, syllables, or word iterations.

Instances of the first two types of filled pause were found in both the normal and stuttered speech samples. Significantly, instances of the third category occurred only in (a majority of) the stutterer records.

The immediate sequelae of each filled pause were identified as either: (1) a word or (2) a silent pause. Part-word items (sounds or syllables) were not considered as separate events if they were the initial parts of the forthcoming word, and no effort was made to distinguish such words from words not characterized in this way. In effect, no effort was made to distinguish words that might have been stuttered from those that were not.

Figure 8.7 presents a graphic comparison of the normal and stuttered speech samples relative to the event immediately sequential to filled pauses. The upper figure reflects data for the first filled pause category, "as word addition." Here the two curves are much the same across all classes of sequential event. The lower figure is based on the second category,

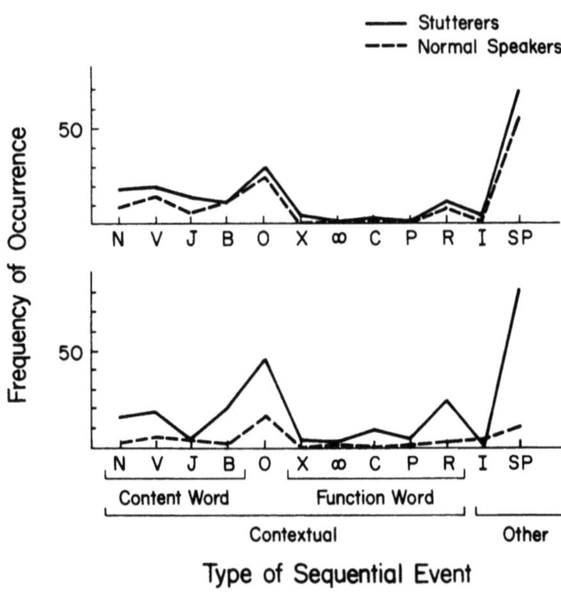

FIGURE 8.7. Frequency with which words of the various grammatical classes and certain other events occurred immediately sequential to a filled pause. The "Other" events are: *I*nterjection, and *S*ilent *P*ause. The upper curve displays data for the category of "filled pause as word addition;" the lower curve represents data for the category of "filled pause after silent pause."

"after a silent pause." In this display the curves show notable differences, occasioned by certain kinds of sequelae; in particular the striking difference in amount of silent pause. The latter finding indicates that, in respect to pausing, the stuttered speech samples are characterized by a filled pause bracketed by silent pauses.

A statistical analysis of these data is presented in Table 8.8 wherein the types of sequelae have been collapsed into categories of "word" and "silent pause" and all values are expressed in terms of incidence per 100 words. Values for filled pauses occurring "in repetition" (stuttered samples only) are included. To retain simplicity in table structure, relevant significance values for these comparisons are presented in Table 8.9.

The two speech samples are similar only in respect to the values representing the frequency with which a silent pause was sequential to a filled pause occurring "as word addition." Otherwise the findings differ markedly. As reflected in Figure 8.7, a filled pause bounded by silent pauses is practically unique to the stuttered speech samples. The two sets of data also differ significantly in regard to the occurrence of words as sequelae to filled pause. In the normal speech samples a word occurs more often as the sequel to a filled pause expressed "as word addition" than "after a silent pause." The pattern is just the opposite for the stutterer samples. Note that a word is almost always the sequela to a filled pause expressed "in repetition."

In general, these comparisons indicate that, in the normal speech samples, filled pauses are much more likely to occur as word additions than following a silent pause, and more likely to be followed by a word than by a silent pause. Also, when a filled pause occurs after a silent pause, it is much more likely to be followed by a word than by another silent pause; in fact, the latter event is rare. Quite differently, in stuttered speech filled pauses occur more frequently after a silent pause than as a word addition, and very often they are followed by another silent pause.

TABLE 8.8. Sequelae to filled pauses occurring in three loci in stuttered versus normal speech samples[a]

Sample source	Locus of filled pauses	Sequel to filled pauses locus		
		Word	Silent pause	Total
Normals	As word addition	2.55	1.61	4.17
	Silent pause	1.49	0.34	1.83
Stutterers	As word addition	1.27	1.29	2.96
	Silent pause	2.72	1.14	3.96
	In repetition	1.67	.12	1.79

[a]Data expressed in terms of incidence per 100 words.

TABLE 8.9. Significance levels[a] of differences between comparison values in Table 8.8

	Normal versus stuttered samples			Word versus silent pause		
	Word	Silent pause	Total	Normal	Stutterer	Total
As addition	0.09	ns	ns	ns	ns	0.07
After silent pause	0.04	0.05	0.003	0.0005	0.02	ns

[a]By appropriate t-test (for related or unrelated measures).

At one level of analysis, the overall pattern differences between the two samples can be described in terms of the cooccurrence of filled pauses and silent pauses. In stuttered speech, the filled pauses are bounded by a silent pause at one or both ends for 80% of their occurrences; however, the same circumstance obtains for only 57% of the filled pauses in the normal speech samples. These data indicate a difference in pause structure between the two samples, evidence that is elaborated by noting other relevant differences.

In the normal speech samples, filled pauses occurred most often (70%) as additions to a word, and in a majority of instances (61%) these filled pauses were followed immediately by another word. The remaing 30% of the filled pauses in the normal speech samples occurred sequentially to a silent pause; in 81% of these instances the filled pause was also followed immediately by a word.

The stuttered speech samples show a very different pattern. In almost the inverse of the normal samples, filled pauses in stuttered speech occurred more often (57%) after a silent pause; also, a smaller percentage (69%) of these instances were followed by a word. When filled pauses occurred as additions, they were more often followed immediately by a silent pause (57%) than by a word (in contrast to 39% in the normal speech samples).

Two studies of pause in normal speech bear pointedly on these differences in pattern and provide a frame of reference for interpreting their significance. Boomer (1965), reporting results obtained from 16 subjects speaking extemporaneously for 3 minutes, found that only 28% of filled pauses were preceded by a silent pause. Brotherton (1976), using data gathered from fewer subjects (10) but longer samples (10 minutes), reported that only 38% of filled pauses were preceded by a silent pause. The values for silent pause/filled pause sequence in these two studies are very comparable to the relevant proportion for the normal speech samples of the present study, which is 30%. However, the relevant proportion for the stuttered speech samples, 57%, departs considerably from these values.

The predominant pattern in the normal samples—filled pause as addition, followed by a word—suggests the following sequence: awareness of imminent decision arises during ongoing production, time to make the decision is "arranged" coincidental with a lexical unit and its termination, during the course of which the decision is resolved and production continues. About half as often, additional time is needed to resolve the decision (the pattern of "silent pause following filled pause-as-addition"). However, when a filled pause was preceded by a silent pause, more time was rarely needed.

The predominant pattern in the stuttered samples was one in which a silent pause preceded a filled pause. The nature of a silent pause is not clear, particularly in this sequence, but at least it does not suggest intention. In fact, the opposite seems more likely; namely that, at the point of discontinuity in verbal expression, what should come next was, at best, only nascent in the speaker's mind. This supposition is supported by evidence that often additional time apparently was needed to continue the verbal sequence (a silent pause also *followed* the filled pause). Moreover, in those considerably less frequent instances when a filled pause occurred "as addition" the immediate sequela was more often a silent pause than a word. Again, evidently more time was needed to resolve whatever decision was imminent.

In respect to patterns of pausing on which the two subject groups can be compared directly, it seems clear that the stuttered speech samples give evidence of less effective word retrieval and generally less efficient utterance planning. This evidence is enlarged by considering the category "in repetition." The filled pauses of this category are unique in several ways. First, they characterize the stuttered samples. They are also unique in terms of locus, that is, they occur with other filled pauses or other vocalized elements of speech (sounds, syllables, words) that are also iterated. Such occurrences, heard under ordinary circumstances, are distinctive and reliably identified as markers of stutter events. Typically, they are judged to reflect difficulty in saying what comes next. Very often such occurrences are construed as difficulty "with" a word, on the assumption that the stutterer "knows the word but can't say it." (It is noteworthy that in these samples a word was the immediate sequela to practically all such filled pauses.) However, the nature of the stutterers' presumed difficulty "with" a word is not clear. Certainly the difficulty in such instances is not with motor execution; it must be at some higher level, such as the level of phonological representation or beyond. This matter will be discussed further Chapter 9.

Footnotes

[1]On the first and second word-fluency administrations respectively: "stutter" appeared in the lists of seven and four stutterers; three and five normals. "Speech" occurred in the lists of one and two stutterers; six and three normals.

[2]The "Common" were those listed among the most common by Russell and Jen-

kins (1954); the "Different" words were those classifiable as "heterogenous;" see Chapter 7.
[3]Homogenous associations are more typical in the general population (see, for example, Deese [1962]; Ervin [1961]).
[4]If broadly based normative association data were available for such lists, stutterers would give more uncommon associations to words in these lists, too.
[5]One should have expected the opposite here too if it is true, as is often claimed, that stutterers have a need to express themselves that is suppressed by a reluctance to talk.
[6]This is not a simple average value. Except for one pair, every stutterer used more total words, and more different words, than his comparison normal speaker.
[7]Mann (1944) reported the same finding in comparing her large (2,800-word) written samples to the comparably large (3,000-word) oral samples obtained by H. Fairbanks. The finding held for comparisons of both normal college-student subjects and hospitalized schizophrenics, although different subjects participated in the two studies.
[8]An incidental contribution of this research, of considerable significance, is that similar findings have been found in at least three languages so far: English, French, and Dutch.
[9]And the schizophrenic subjects in the Mann (1944) and H. Fairbanks (1944) studies.
[10]The claim that stutterers know many synonyms as a means of avoiding stuttering. Moreover, none of the stutterer subjects in this study made this claim. (In my experience stutterers rarely do.)
[11]It is appropriate to note at this point that, overall, the stutterers also produced more written errors (corrected and uncorrected combined), and that the difference approached statistical significance ($p = .08$).
[12]The complete correlation matrices are included in the Appendix as Tables 8.4A and 8.5A.
[13]Grammatical class (principally the content/function word distinction) has shown the most stable relationship to stutter occurrence. As discussed in Chapter 5, grammatical class overlaps the other language factors. Special attention is directed to initial phone because of its focal and consistent concurrence with stutter events.
[14]This part of the research was published as a separate article (Wingate, 1984b).
[15]This information also has value relative to the sequelae of other kinds of disfluencies, identified in this chapter. Incidently, the "marker" concept of stuttering, presented in several places earlier in the book, also directs attention to sequelae.

Part IV: A New Departure

This final section, consisting of a single chapter, extends the analyses developed in the chapters of Part II, which culminated in a concept of stuttering as a disorder that is credibly and economically characterized in psycholinguistic terms. This final chapter enlarges the base of that concept through incorporating several other dimensions of evidence into the analysis. The results of the research reported in Part III provide a substantial part of that enlargement. In addition, other especially relevant dimensions of evidence are contained in findings from certain other literature on stuttering, studies of verbal function in normals, and clinical and research reports from the field of neurolinguistics.

Interrelating these several dimensions of evidence leads to deductions that constitute a new departure in understanding the nature of stuttering. Overall, the analyses supporting this new departure also generate inferences applicable to conceptualizing the functional structure and organization of normal oral language.

9
Outlines of a Language Dysfunction

A hair, perhaps, divides the False and True; Yes; and a single Alif were the clue—
Could you but find it.

Quatrain 50
The Rubaiyat

The results of the research reported in Part III constitute evidence that substantiates the implications, contained in certain earlier sources, that stuttering is a disorder of oral language expression. More specifically, in corroboration of certain previous work (e.g., Wingate, 1966b, 1967a, 1967b, 1968, 1971, 1979a), these findings also constitute evidence that stuttering is a defect in the language production system, a defect that extends beyond the level of motor execution. Stuttering may give the appearance of being a peripheral disorder, and from time to time it has been described as a problem involving one or another of the peripheral systems (breathing, phonation, articulation), or some incoordination among the three. Such accounts are limited to superficial aspects of the disorder. There is ample evidence to indicate that the defect is not simply one of motor control or coordination, but that it involves more central functions of the language production system.

The evidence of disturbance in the language production system of stutterers emerges clearly in all levels and dimensions of the analyses reported in Chapter 8, from the significant differences revealed in comparisons on individual variables to the clear contrast in factor composition and structure yielded by the factor analysis. The findings of this research provide a focus and a framework for interrelating the many dimensions of information about stuttering and normal speech that were presented in the earlier chapters and, as well, other relevant dimensions not yet considered. The objective of this chapter is to attempt an integration of several major lines of evidence, with the anticipation that such integration will constitute the basis for an eventual neurolinguistic explanation of stuttering and, as well, contribute to the understanding of normal language production processes.

In developing the psycholinguistic integration that is the objective of this chapter the reference foci will be the two stutter-related linguistic features that have recurred consistently in the analyses developed in the earlier chapters: *word-initial position* and *linguistic stress.*

Word-Initial Position

Data and implications relevant to word (syllable)-initial position, the universal feature of stuttering, come into prominence very early in an assay of the findings. Among the variables that significantly differentiated between the normal speakers and the stutterers one variable, *word-fluency*, stands out as central to understanding stuttering as a defect in the language production system.[1] Actually, the term word-fluency is not the most suitable referent for the mental function represented by this factor. In selecting a name for the word-fluency factor Thurstone (1938) had in mind that the task obviously reflects the readiness with which an individual can produce a series of words. Note that the idea of "readiness" in word production is the essence of dictionary definitions of "fluency," although with the important distinction that ordinary use of fluency implies the production of words in meaningful connected sequence. Had the word-fluency factor been discovered in more recent times it might well have been given a name that is more appropriate; most suitably, *Lexical Access.*

"Lexical access" aptly describes the function demanded by the word-fluency task; namely, word search and retrieval. Moreover, the search and retrieval function must operate under the constraint of a salient structural feature of the items sought—the word-initial phone. The special pertinence of the word-fluency test is that the activity involved in this task is directly comparable to a process by which we evidently access words in ordinary connected utterance. In both the word-fluency task and the process of "bringing up" words in the course of speaking one finds an important common dimension: the use of a word-initial segment as the cue for word search and retrieval. The important role of initial segments was demonstrated in the research reported by Brown and McNeill (1966) and Shattuck-Hufnagel (1981), who worked with normal speakers. Similar supporting evidence is to be found in studies done with aphasics (Barton, 1971; Goodglass, Kaplan, Weintraub, & Ackerman, 1976; Goodglass & Stuss, 1979; Pease & Goodglass, 1978). Evidently other structural aspects of words may also be used in word retrieval, such as number of syllables and stress pattern. However, consistent with common experience as well as with research findings, word-initial sound/letter is a major key in lexical access. There are, of course, certain differences between word-access function in the word-fluency test and in spontaneous speech. In the word-fluency task the words do not express a message; they are not organized into a larger structure; they are all content words, all of which have the same initial sound; and they are produced at a much slower rate than are words in connected speech. At the same time, in both of these word-access processes the initial letter/phone is "in place" and the task is to generate the remainder of the word.[2]

The significant difference between normal speakers and stutterers on the word-fluency task indicates that stutterers are much less capable than are normal speakers in a language function critical to maintaining ongoing speech: the quick retrieval of appropriate words.

This finding assumes particular significance in the effort to understand stuttering when such evidence is aligned with a description of the essence of a stutter event. In several places earlier in the book, particularly in Chapter 6, it has been emphasized that the cardinal (although badly neglected) universal characteristic of stuttering is the feature of word-initial position. In the occurrence of a stuttered word, performance of the initial phone persists—either in oscillation, in steady state, or some combination of the two.[3] The point has been made that these phenomena simply *mark* a stutter event, that contrary to appearance and common belief the stutter does not occur *on* the initial phone; and that the difficulty is not with the initial phone, which actually *is* being produced—in fact, it is being produced excessively. The aberration consists in the fact that the speech production sequence has been interrupted at that point; it is not moving on to the rest of the word. Here too, as in word-access function, the initial phone is "in place" and the remainder of the word remains to be filled in. However, in stutter events the speaker is unable to generate the rest of the word. Apparently something has gone wrong at a critical stage in the process of lexical retrieval.

The inference that stuttering reflects some disturbance in lexical access appears to contradict what seems evident to direct observation of instances of stutter occurrence. It appears, and it is generally assumed, that the stutterer knows the word he is apparently attempting to say, that he has the entire word "in mind." In fact, stutterers frequently complain that they know what they want to say but can't say it. However, the appearance of the stutter event and the introspective testimony regarding it may be misleading. At what level, or to what extent, or in what detail does the stutterer "know" the word that clearly is not forthcoming? The suspicion that he does *not* know the word in the completeness he claims, and for which he is regularly given credit, is enlarged by the frequent observation that typically he can say the word immediately after it is said for him. He is, then, able to copy a model of what he could not produce himself. Such occurrences indicate that his difficulty is not simply one of motor execution, as is regularly assumed, but that it involves some level of representation of the word pattern. It is pertinent to note here how well this finding articulates with the evidence that stuttering is influenced favorably by word familiarity: familiarity as represented in word frequency and related dimensions (see pertinent sections of Chapters 4 and 5) and as reflected in the influence of practice (Wingate, 1986a, 1986b).

One of the long-term and persisting problems in the literature of stuttering is the way in which words are conceived to be the source of difficulty. It is assumed that certain properties of words (their initial phone, meaning, previous associations, etc.) have somehow acquired the capacity to *elicit* stuttering. A concurrent assumption is that words are stored as whole and invariable entities, and retrieved in this form. The former assumption is contradicted by work that is not of particular concern here;[4] the latter assumption is contradicted by findings from various sources in psycholinguistics, particularly the literature dealing with speech errors (see Cutler, 1982; Fromkin, 1973b; Hill, 1973). Writers in the field of stuttering have shown little awareness of evidence that word form is not the same at all stages between the level of ideation and the final acoustic product. Evidently, as indicated by findings in psycholinguistic research, the representations of a word at these two ultimate levels differ considerably; in fact, there is reason to envision differences between phonological and phonetic representations of a word. Thus, while it may be that a stutterer can be said to "know" the stuttered word in its abstract, ideational, or even phonological representation, the critical factors in speaking[5] are the complete phonetic representation of the word (including its suprasegmental features) and its availability, intact, at the precise time required in the utterance sequence.

The stutter event signals a breakdown in the speech production process at a point I called "the fault line" (Chapter 6), a term intended to carry the implication of a defect that extends beyond what is directly observable. Significantly, the locus of the fault line corresponds to the boundary between the two syllable constituents identified in the syllable-structure hypothesis: the boundary between *onset* and *rime*. In a stutter event the syllable onset is produced, but the rime is missing. Note that the same description applies to lexical access function as reflected in the word-fluency measure, in which the initial phone is "in place."

There is a clear isomorphism to the three major features of the preceding discussion: (1) the process of lexical access, (2) the stutter event, and (3) the syllable-structure hypothesis. This isomorphism constitutes a foundation not only for understanding the true nature of stuttering but, as well, for suggesting the contribution that psycholinguistic analysis of stuttering can make to the investigation and eventual understanding of normal language processes.

It is relevant to note here that Telser (1971) reported finding evidence of word-finding difficulty in young stutterers. Contradictory results were reported by Boysen and Cullinan (1971), who found no difference in their study of children similar in age to those in the Telser study. Such equivocal results present no essential difficulty for the discussion developed here. Several different word-finding tasks have been used in language research, especially in aphasia, of which the object-naming or picture-naming task, used by Telser and by Boysen and Cullinan, is the most common. Such tasks are referred to in the psycholinguistic literature as measures of "naming on confrontation," which is recognized as involving functions different from the process of lexical retrievel in spontaneous speech (Barton, Maruszewski, & Urrea, 1969; Davis, 1983; Geschwind, 1967).

At this point it is pertinent to mention that the word association test, too, is a kind of word-finding task, with a unique range of constraints for accessing the lexical pool. Stutterers and normal speakers do not differ as dramatically on this measure as they do on word-fluency, yet the evident differences are notable. There are two dimensions along which findings regarding word-association are relevant to a psycholinguistic analysis of stuttering. First, word association has been shown to express the frequency with which words occur in general use. Howes (1957b, 1964)[6] demonstrated some time ago that the average probability that a given word will occur as a response in word-association is the same as the probability with which that word occurs in general usage. This finding indicates that although each stimulus word evidently induces a specific pattern within the lexicon, the underlying word-frequency distribution remains influential. Of course, individual differences qualify this general correspondence. Still, as a general finding it is relevant to the evidence that stutters are related to word frequency and that word association function among stutterers shows departures from the normal pattern. Second, word associations are properly understood as a reflection of linguistic competence. The original explanation of word associations, accepted for many years, was that they are based on simple recall and represent "associative bonds." In contrast to this account, it has been recognized for some time that word associations reflect a system of category structure in vocabulary and are generated by various rules (Brown & Berko, 1960; Clark, 1970; Deese, 1965; McNeill, 1966). Word association function tells something about the ability to understand and produce language.

Note that there is evidence of a link between word association function and lexical access as reflected in the word-fluency task. Anderson (1965) had normal speakers give word associations to individual letters. Most of the words given as associations to a letter were words that began with that letter; further, the number of associations given to a letter was related to the frequency with which that letter occurs in word-initial position.

More on Word-Fluency

Throughout the years it has been well documented, from both clinical report and pertinent research, that stuttering "runs in families." Although the pattern of stuttering inheritance[7] does not follow classic Mendelian "laws," modern methods of analysis (Kidd, 1980, 1983, 1984; Kidd, Heimbuch, & Records, 1981) provide models of genetic transmission that give a satisfactory fit to the data.

In view of the grounds for suspecting a genetic basis for stuttering, and the consistent finding that stutterers evidence limitations in the word-fluency task, it is of particular interest to find strong evidence that the word-fluency factor is, as Vandenberg (1967) put it, "under genetic control." Vandenberg summarized the findings from four separate twin studies[8] that had used Thurstone's *Test of Primary Mental Abilities* in studying dimensions of mental function. These four studies, which involved in toto 152 pairs of dizygotic twins and 192 pairs of monozygotic twins, yielded data that consistently revealed highly significant evidence of a hereditary component in two of the six factors: the verbal factor and the word-fluency factor. Vandenberg noted that these two factors are independent in the general population, but suggested that their remarkably consistent concurrence in the four independent studies might indicate that the two factors share, or reflect, some common genetic base.

There are certain other findings regarding word-fluency that are more immediately pertinent to the topic of cerebral asymmetry, laterality, and language function. A number of studies concerned with functions of the frontal lobes, particularly the prefrontal areas, have included the word-fluency measure among psychological tests employed.

In view of the divergent opinions and claims regarding frontal lobe functions Milner (1964) reported the results of selected psychological tests administered to patients undergoing brain surgery for relief from focal seizures. She found that defects after frontal lobectomy "are indeed elusive," as evidenced in the fact that patients having frontal lobe lesions show much less impairment on many verbal and nonverbal tests than do patients with lesions in posterior loci. However, certain tasks turned out to be discriminative. Milner found the standard Thurstone word-fluency measure to be the one test that was selectively affected by left frontal lesions. Typically, a left frontal lobectomy (which leaves Broca's area intact) did not result in any lasting dysphasia, and the patient's scores on most verbal tests returned rapidly to normal preoperative level. However, the word-fluency achievement of these patients suffered, and it was significantly lower than that of patients who had had right frontal, or left temporal, excisions. Milner cited an earlier report by Rylander (1948) who has also observed that patients' achievement on a word-fluency test was impaired by radical bilateral lobotomy. Several years later Milner (1967) reported that reexamination of the patients in her study showed that the word-fluency deficiency had persisted.

Later Benton (1968) used a series of psychological tests with 25 patients who had either left, right, or bilateral frontal lobe lesions. He found that, in contrast to patients with right lesions only, the achievement of patients with left frontal or bilateral frontal lesions were decidedly inferior on the word-fluency test he used, which was an oral counterpart of the standard Thurstone measure.[9]

Wertz and Lemme (1974) reported that the word-fluency performance of 131 patients with left hemisphere damage was only a little more than a third as good as that of 40 patients with right hemisphere damage. They also compared the word-fluency achievement of 63 patients, who had left-hemisphere damage, to normal individuals matched with the patients for age, sex, and education. The patients' scores were less than one fifth that achieved by the normal individuals.

Perret (1974) reported the results of several psychological tests administered to 118 patients whose lesions were distributed almost equally in frontal, temporal, and posterior sites. His findings corroborated previous results indicating word-fluency deficit in patients with left frontal lesions. Perret related these findings to a symptom frequently found in frontal lobe patients, namely, difficulty in "shifting," or dealing readily with change in circumstance; in other words, perseverative tendencies.

Clinically based reports yield findings regarding word-fluency that are similar to the investigative reports. Zangwill (1975) reported two cases in which Broca's area was either excised or undercut who, several weeks postoperatively, had no residual dysphasia evident to standard neurological examination but who evidenced loss in word-fluency ability. Clinical reports that give a descriptive characterization of the speech of patients with prefrontal injury are particularly pertinent to the discussion being developed here, inasmuch as they constitute of kind of link between three related areas: word-fluency test findings, actual word-finding in ongoing speech, and disturbance of fluency. Zangwill (1966) summarized the observations made by Feuchtwanger (1923) and Kleist (1928) regarding the verbal deficits of patients with left prefrontal lesions. These patients showed: (1) a certain loss of spontaneity of speech, in the absence of articulatory disorder, (2) difficulty in evoking appropriate words or phrases, and (3) in some cases definite impairment of verbal thought processes. Zangwill reported noting similar characteristics in a number of patients he had observed who had left frontal lesions. The conversational speech of these patients appeared normal, with no articulatory defect and no sign of naming disorder, but the patients complained of real difficulty evoking appropriate words and phrases.

Luria (1966) reported that patients with a lesion in superior aspects of the left prefrontal cortex frequently find it difficult to produce connected speech, "pronunciation and sometimes the finding of each word requires a special impulse" (p. 206). Later, Luria (1970, pp. 176–185) expanded this topic, giving case examples in which particulars of the description are very reminiscent of certain aspects of stuttering. He characterized these symptoms as reflecting a disturbance in "inner speech," as conceived by Vigotsky; that is, disturbance of "the abbreviated schema of speech which precedes the speech act itself," in other words, disturbance in the processes of utterance organization and planning.

Reports containing similar findings continue to appear (see, for instance, Jonas, 1981; Kaczmarek, 1984). Zangwill (1978) noted that the range of evidence previously reviewed indicates that the left prefrontal cortex is involved in the generation of propositional utterance. In particular, it participates in some important way in the production of fluent, well-organized speech.

It is pertinent to include in this section some mention of the many reports on forms of expressive aphasia (e.g., Head, 1963; Luria, 1970; Weisenberg & McBride, 1964) or cases of brain injury with and without aphasia (Rosenbek, Messert, Collins, & Wertz, 1978) that describe speech symptoms identifiable as stutters. Recently Brown and Cullinan (1981) reported findings that bear specifically on the interrelationship between stuttering, disfluency, brain damage, and difficulty in word access. Brown and Cullinan found, in a group of anomic aphasics, that amount of overall disfluency and extent of word-retrieval difficulty were directly related and, further, that as these two variables increased the proportion of disfluencies identifiable as stutters also increased.

Linguistic Stress

In a fashion complementary to word-initial position, linguistic stress, too, is interrelated with stuttering, lexical access, and syllable structure. The nexus of this interrelation is the syllable nucleus: (1) the syllable nucleus is the segment through which linguistic stress is expressed; (2) it is also the major dimension in the rime constituent of syllable structure (and, *pari passu,* the salient aspect of the syllable/word "remainder" in lexical access); and (3) it is the phone next in sequence beyond the fault line, which corresponds to the locus of a stutter event.[10]

(No attempt is made to review the considerable amount of research that has been addressed to the study of linguistic stress. The several studies to be cited are included as representative indices of the complexity of the topic).

Since the work of Tiffin and Steer (1937) it has been known that stressed syllables typically are characterized by some combination of changes in intensity, duration, and pitch. Subsequent work (e.g., Cutler & Foss, 1977;

Fonagy, 1966; Fry, 1955; Ladefoged, 1963; Lieberman, 1960) has yielded findings that have illuminated the variation among these changes as they occur in any particular stressed syllable; the trading relationships among these variables; and, as well, other variables such as vowel color. Other research has demonstrated, for example, the influence of stress on length of utterance as a function of induced variations in vowel length (Ladefoged, 1968), effect of stress on the length of abutting consonants and the variation in this influence as a function of word length (Klatt, 1974), relationships of stress and rate (Gay, 1978). It is especially appropriate to note that linguistic stress is related inversely to word frequency (Berry, 1953; Howes, 1957a; Lieberman, 1963; Savin, 1963), and to recall that stressed words more often have a consonant as initial phone (Berry, 1953; Denes, 1963). Of special relevance is the evidence reported by Allen (1972) that the stress pattern in English centers on a ballistic release of the initial consonant into the stressed vowel, with the release involving respiratory, laryngeal, and articulatory activity.

Briefly summarized, the results of research in this area continue to expand the statement made by Chomsky and Halle (1968, p. 59) that "one of the most complex aspects of the phonetics of English is its intricate system of stress contours, both within the word and within the phrase." The complexities of linguistic stress involve semantic and syntactic dimensions as well. In fact, there is mounting evidence that the prosodic aspects of language play a pivotal and determining role in utterance planning.

The literature of stuttering contains another conceptual limitation that is closely related to the problem mentioned in the preceding section, (the problem that words are considered to be the source of difficulty). The second limitation is posed by the assumption[11] that speech is organized and produced in a manner that is mirrored in how we perceive the acoustic signal. Speech is conceived as being arranged and run off in the way we seem to hear it, as a series of words in temporally ordered sequence. This happens to be the same way that words appear on the printed page and, very likely, familiarity with the printed page has influenced and supported the conception. Stated briefly, this conception presupposes a left-to-right model of speech production, in which words are the planning units and are entered into the sequence as needed. Although this model has a clear commonsense appeal it cannot explain a great deal of what has been discovered in the study of oral language—and in other intricate and complicated human activities. In his seminal article regarding the matter of "serial order in behavior" Lashley (1951) explained that many complicated activities, like playing the piano, but especially speech, must be organized through the operation of some high-level planning system. In respect to speech, such a system determines the order of sounds within words and words within sentences. The substance of Lashley's explanation is contained in descriptions of the speech process which recognize that a speaker organizes what he says as he proceeds; that when he begins to talk he has an idea of what he is going to say but does not have all the words selected, and certainly does not have them arranged in the final sequence.

Such description, which has appeared more frequently since the time of Lashley's classic paper, was also voiced by certain other authors in the same era (see Miller, 1951). The central idea is one of a system that, in the process of transducing thoughts into the eventual acoustic signal, organizes neural representations into "structures" capable of being rendered into final acoustic form. Several levels of organization are envisioned, the two most general being concerned with the lexical dimension (which subsumes the phonetic and the morphologic aspects) on one hand, and the suprasegmental dimension on the other. The distinction between these two dimensions is not simply conceptual; there are many lines of evidence that contribute to identifying them as functionally separate in the generation of the final output. In fact the evidence from these sources indicates that the suprasegmental dimension has prior entry into the formulation of the linguistic sequence (Boomer & Laver, 1968; Butterworth & Goldman-Eisler, 1979; Fromkin, 1973a; Martin, 1972). Moreover, there is, further, other reason to believe that the prosodic system is central to the organizing process. J.G. Martin (1972) emphasized that phoneme (and syllable) durations in words are context dependent; they vary from one time to another as a function of their role in an utterance. Therefore, neither the phones, nor the words of which they are a part, can be stored as stable entities. Their configuration must be determined at the time of utterance production. In Martin's analysis stressed syllables are focal in the organization of an utterance; the prosodic pattern is fundamental, though accommodating the lexical elements with their phonetic constituents. Support for the sort of analysis proposed by Martin comes from the rather extensive research on speech errors. One of the most common findings is that errors of stress assignment are rare; instead, stress similarities are the foci for the phonetic errors. A corollary of this distinction is that errors involving vowels, the syllable nuclei, are much less frequent than those that involve consonants. In Shattuck-Hufnagel's (1983, 1987) production planning concept, derived from the error literature, the production unit is established on a suprasegmental framework.

Propositionality

As noted in Chapter 1, (Orton 1927) surmised that stuttering reflects a problem in language formulation, that it is associated with "the plane of the speech effort" or, in other words, the level of propositionality. Reference was also made in subsequent chapters to certain findings in stuttering research that provided support for Orton's inference. Before proceeding to expand the scope of such evidence, material relative to the propositional nature of ordinary speech will be presented as a frame of reference.

Propositionality in Normal Speech

The essence of propositional utterances is that they are novel, designed uniquely for a particular communicative circumstance, and generated at the time of expression. Put in somewhat different terms, propositionality implies planning, and the ability to implement and execute the plans. Propositional utterances are internally coherent, appropriate in reference, relevant to the situation, and have a communicative value that is intended by the speaker and so perceived by the listener.

Traditionally, propositional speech is contrasted with "automatic" speech which, typical of dysphasia, is describable as the opposite of propositional speech. Most often the differentiation ends with the designation of these two classes. Little effort has been made to differentiate and characterize other kinds of utterance that can be "scaled" in reference to the categorical distinction between propositional versus automatic speech.[12] Cursing is one of such other kinds of utterance. In the speech of normal individuals, curses consist of words or brief word strings that, even as isolated utterances, are selected by the speaker, used appropriately in the overall context, and relevant to the situation. They are certainly not "automatic" in the normal speaker, as evidenced by the fact that curses of different "quality" can be, and often are, employed as befitting one situation or another. However, curses have no linguistic communicative value, either intended or perceived. They are best considered to be fixed, highly routinized verbal elements having a heavy emotional loading but no propositional value. However, although not propositional, curses are not produced "automatically" in the expressions of a normal speaker.

Another "midground" kind of utterance is represented in the typically brief expression referred to in certain linguistic sources as "phatic communication." Phatic utterances, such as the quickly rendered, "How are you?" and the like, also are not properly identified as either automatic or truly propositional. Unlike truly automatic utterances of dysphasics, phatic expressions are relevant to the situation, appropriate in content, and have communicative value. Clearly they are intended, selected, and fit into the proper communicative slot. At the same time they have minimal propositional value; they are best described as highly overlearned, routinized semantic strings. Lengthier rote memory verbalizations, such as recitative readings in religious ceremony, the pledge of allegiance, and other memorized oaths are similar in nature to phatic communication. All of these expressions lack a truly propositional character, they are not novel, unique to a particular circumstance, intended as communication, nor specially generated at the time. But they are also not automatic.

The preceding discussion suggests that there are various levels of propositional speech; that differing degrees of organizational and planning demands are occasioned by different circumstances, conditions, and ideational content. There is evidence for other levels of propositionality too, higher on the "scale." For instance, consider the difference in the manner and content of what one says to a small child as compared to any level of conversation with an adult. Relevant research (Sachs, Brown & Salerno, 1976; Snow, 1972) confirms what one could expect—adults adjust their language to the child's linguistic level. In speaking to children adults use simpler sentences, repeat themselves, and speak more slowly. Different levels of propositionality are also induced by other circumstances, in the speech of children as well as of adults. For example, work reported by Goldman-Eisler (1968), with adult subjects, yielded evidence that explaining the meaning of cartoons requires more reflective formulation and more planning, than giving descriptions of them. Similar results were reported by Levin, Silverman, and Ford (1967), whose subjects were young children.

Reading aloud represents a special type of speaking performance. The task facing the oral reader of ordinary prose is not a simple one, but it is a task more of discovery than of creation. One could expect oral reading and spontaneous speech to be qualitatively different, which is the issue central to Abercrombie's objection to the linguistic study of what he called "spoken prose" (Abercrombie, 1963; see discussion in Chapter 2). There are several ways in which one might describe differences between oral reading and spontaneous speech. A fundamental difference, and one that is specific to our immediate interest, is that in ordinary prose the message is already formulated; most of the organization and planning, at least of the kind demanded in spontaneous speaking, has already been done.

Evidently there has been little comparative study of the oral reading and spontaneous speech of normal speakers. There are two studies, done many years apart, that were addressed specifically to such comparison. One study, by Snidecor (1943, 1944), was mounted from an interest in certain acoustic parameters of speech. The other study, by Henderson, Goldman-Eisler and Skarbek (1965), emerged from the research interest in hesitation phenomena. The results of these two studies concur in indicating a notable difference between the two speech modes. Snidecor found, among superior speakers, that spontaneous speech was slower and contained more pauses, and also that pauses occurred at different loci than those observed during oral reading. Henderson et al. also found that spontaneous speech is slower, contains more pause, and that the pattern of pausing is different than in oral reading.

Comparable findings have emerged in the course of certain other research that has had different objectives. Ptacek and Sanders (1966), investigating voice characteristics associated with age, obtained samples of both oral reading and spontaneous speech. They found spontaneous speech to be 20 to 30% slower than oral reading. Lass and Noll (1970), interested in differences in speech rate between cleft palate and normal persons, found that the impromptu speaking of both groups was slower, with more pause time, than when they read aloud. In Johnson's major study comparing normal speakers and stutterers (Johnson, 1961a) the spontaneous speech rate of both groups was approximately 25% slower than their oral reading rate. Johnson did not include pause in this study; however, both groups evidenced substantially less other disfluency during oral reading than in spontaneous speech.

As discussed by Henderson and colleagues (1965) and later by Goldman-Eisler in relation to her other research on speech fluency (Goldman-Eisler, 1968), the substantial differences found consistently in this research (comparing oral reading with speaking) reflect the demands that arise in the process of generating spontaneous speech.[13] The differences in speaking performance between oral reading and spontaneous speech are not unlike those between description and explanation. The task of oral reading does not place as extensive demands on the language system as are posed in generating speech. In fact, Clark (1971) made the point that someone who has a good idea of what he is going to say by virtue of being "primed" with focal words talks more like a reader than a spontaneous speaker. On a hypothetical scale of propositionality, oral reading is not of the same rank level as spontaneous speech.

Propositional Influence in Stuttering

There are several sources of data, both experimental and observational, that bear directly on the matter of propositional influence on stuttering.

Observation

It has been noted repeatedly for many years that stutterers' apparent fluency varies with the circumstances of speaking. Such circumstances are sufficiently noteworthy that many of them appear in lists of "facts" about stuttering.[14] It is widely reported that stutterers do not stutter when they exclaim in surprise, joy, pain, fear, and so forth, nor when they curse. They are said to seldom stutter in making offhand remarks or in using simple, brief utterances—that is, phatic expressions. They do not stutter when speaking recitatively, for instance in responsive speaking in church or saying standard prayers, or when speaking to pets. Stutterers have no trouble speaking a role in a play, and stutter very little when talking to small children. They tend to have somewhat less trouble when engaged in "small talk," but have their greatest difficulty when intending to tell something "important."

The reader may already have recognized that the circumstances associated with increasing levels of stuttering, reviewed in the previous paragraph, parallel exactly the levels of propositionality in spontaneous utterance that were discussed in the preceding section. This concurrence, which indicates that stuttering is some function of propositional level, is also found in data derived from the oral reading of stutterers.

Pertinent Research

Another frequently reported observation is that stutterers are more fluent when reading aloud than when speaking spontaneously.[15] This observation is corroborated by research addressed to the topic. The stutterer subjects in Johnson's (1961a) major study had substantially fewer stutters (*and* other disfluencies) when reading aloud than when speaking. Cohen's (1952) subjects stuttered significantly more during impromptu speaking than when reading aloud. Sitzman's (1968) subjects stuttered significantly less when they read aloud the written transcripts of their own spontaneous speech that had been recorded previously. This extensive evidence that less stuttering occurs during oral reading than in spontaneous speech concurs with the analysis presented earlier that reading aloud is not of the same level of propositionality as ordinary speaking.

In addition to the findings presented in the preceding paragraph, there also is clear-cut evidence that the amount of stuttering is related directly to the level of propositionality of the material being read. Several studies, reviewed earlier (Chapter 4), yielded evidence that the amount of stuttering directly reflects the level to which the reading material approximates ordinary prose (Conway & Quarrington, 1963; Eisenson & Horowitz, 1945; Van Riper & Hull, 1955), and is least frequent of all when reading words presented as a list (Brown, 1938a). (It is of considerable interest that Brenner, Feldstein, and Jaffe (1965) found that normal speakers evidenced *more* disfluency in reading material having a low approximation to English than when reading ordinary prose—the opposite of what has found for stuttering.)

The substance of the discussion to this point is represented in outline form in Table 9.1. The arrangement of the table contents is intended to interrelate, in their approximate relationships, the essential points developed in the foregoing discussion.

A Third Dimension

For many years unusual movements of the eyes have been observed to be linked with stutters during both oral reading and spontaneous speech (see Brutten, Bakker, Janssen, & van der Meulen, 1984; Craven, 1972; Jasper

TABLE 9.1. Probability of stutter occurrence at varying "levels" of utterance

Probability	Spontaneous speech	Oral reading
100%	Important explanations, etc.	
	Ordinary conversation	
	"Small talk"	
		Ordinary prose
	Talking to small children	nth order approximation
	Talking to pets	2nd order approximation
	Recitative speaking	Word list
	"Asides"	
	Phatic statements	
	Curses	
0%	Exclamations	

and Murray, 1932; Kopp, 1963; Moser, 1935, 1938; Murray, 1931). A variety of actions have been reported, the more notable of which include aimless vertical or horizontal eye movements, extended fixation of gaze, variations in pupillary size, and binocular incoordination.[16] The authors of the earlier studies just mentioned interpreted their findings in neurological terms; Jasper and Murray, for example, considered their results to indicate "a relative decrease in the control of cortical over subcortical centers." Authors of the more recent investigations (Brutten et al., 1984; Craven, 1972), reflecting the long-standing influence of Johnson's "evaluation" notion, have attempted an explanation in terms of "expectancy." One investigator (Kopp, 1963), noting that ocular anomalies were minimal during the stutterers' viewing of nonlinguistic material, suggested that these unusual actions were "associated with both language and speech."

The research findings regarding ocular pecularities during speech in stutterers are paralleled by long-term clinical observations of, and concern with, stutterers' eye movements. One finds frequent mention in the clinical literature that stutterers do not maintain adequate "eye contact" with their auditors (see, for instance, Fiedler & Standop, 1983, p. 5; Luper & Mulder, 1964, p. 164; Sheehan, 1970, p. 289; Van Riper, 1971, p. 28). The extent to which inadequate eye contact is "a problem" among stutterers is well represented in the fact that "Maintaining Eye Contact" is prescribed as Rule 6 in *Self-Therapy for the Stutterer.*[17] Clinical concern with eye contact is based on the assumption that the stutterer looks away from his auditor because he feels ashamed or embarrassed or as an effort to "deny his stuttering." Typically, the clinical prescription to the stutterer is that he should not "avoid" eye contact but should instead "look the world squarely in the eye" (*Self-Therapy for the Stutterer*, p. 98).

In the past 25 years several loosely related lines of research have explored human ocular phenomena, particularly gaze, as they relate to certain other actions, functions, and characteristics of the individual. One dimension of particular interest is the work of Gur (1975) and Kinsbourne (1972) who found evidence that direction of gaze is related to laterality. Certain other work, addressed to very specific acts, has also yielded results that are of particular relevance to the present discussion. For instance, Condon and Ogston (1971) found that eye blinks are closely associated with word boundaries, especially the word-initial boundary.

A major portion of the interest in gaze has been in respect to its role in social interaction, especially in conversation (see Argyle, Ingham, Alkema, & McCallin, 1973). Out of this research has come evidence that gaze is intimately linked to formulative dimensions of language function (see Beattie, 1978; Day, 1964; Duke, 1968; Kendon, 1967). The evidence from this work, as concluded by Beattie (1978, p. 48), is that "gaze is organized in a coordinated system with the plans underlying speech, and the speech flow itself." Butterworth and Goldman-Eisler (1979) discuss how averting one's gaze is a form of speaker adjustment that supports utterance planning, and that maintaining gaze interferes with utterance formulation.

The assumption that stutterers break eye contact due to feelings of shame and embarrassment has evidently been maintained in ignorance of the findings that indicate the role of gaze in utterance planning. The evidence just reviewed, regarding the considerable extent to which gaze aversion is "a problem" in stutterers, would seem to be explained more appropriately as revealing the degree to which utterance planning is a significant problem in stuttering, a problem reflected in the surface observation of "inadquate eye contact."

The Laterality Connection

A link between laterality and stuttering was suggested early in this century by several reports that described a concurrence of left-handedness and speech defect, especially stuttering, in certain children (e.g., Ballard, 1912; Claiborne, 1917; Grossman, 1910; Nice, 1915; Whipple, 1911). Often a report carried the implication, or claim, of a cause–effect relationship by describing the appearance and/or disappearance of stuttering on change of handedness. Investigation of this apparent relationship was pursued well into the 1930s (e.g., Bryngelson, 1939; Bryngelson & Rutherford, 1937; Daniels, 1940; Johnson, 1937; Johnson & Duke, 1935; Van Dusen, 1939), with both clinical reports and research yielding evidence that was supportive in some instances, but either equivocal or contradictory in others. At least by the early 1930s it was recognized (see Jasper, 1932) that there is no simple relationship between stuttering and handedness, and that laterality is a complex matter. In a review and discussion of some 20 publications dealing with the subject Travis and Johnson (1934), while expressing reservations about a direct link between stuttering and handedness, found reason to support the conception of stuttering as a disorder that has a significant relationship to the functional organization of the central nervous system. This conception, the "cerebral dominance theory of stuttering," generally has been attributed to Travis and Orton.[18] The crux of this position is that those neurologic functions necessary to produce the final output, identifiable as normal speech, must operate under a "dominant gradient of control," which was conceived as a hierarchy of neurophysiological centers. Laterality participated in this gradient concept as a representation of the evidence, from the field of neurology, of a dominant or "leading" cerebral hemisphere. According to the concept, at least the ultimate level of control in the gradient was lateralized.

The flurry of interest in the cerebral dominance explanation of stuttering gradually dissipated, partly because of equivocal or actually contradictory findings, but also because of the burgeoning preoccupation with psychological explanations of stuttering that began in the 1940s. Over the intervening years many persons in the field have considered the laterality matter in stuttering to be a dead issue. However, the evidence implicating laterality in stuttering evidently has been sufficiently persuasive that the topic has continued to reappear in relevant literature (see, for instance, Records, Heimbuch, & Kidd, 1977; Rosenfield, 1980). In fact, the essence of Travis' original position was republished just a few years ago (Travis, 1978a) at which time Travis (1978b) also revealed that over the intervening 40 years, he has continued to believe that the dominance concept has validity. Recently the development of more sophisticated means of assessing laterality and dominance have supported a resurgence in the investigation of laterality in stuttering (e.g., Cross, 1987; Johannsen & Victor, 1986; Luessenhop, Boggs, Laborowit & Walle, 1973; Pinsky & McAdam, 1980; Sussman & MacNeilage, 1975; Wood, Stump, McKeehan, Sheldon, & Proctor, 1980).

When considered in regard to what is known about human laterality, especially as it pertains to language function, the laterality connection in stuttering takes on a substance that deserves consideration. The literature on the subject of human laterality is extensive and complex, and the interested reader is referred to several recent sources that deal adequately with the subject.[19] Only a brief and rather general reference will be made to those aspects of this literature that pertain to major issues that are necessary to address here, where stuttering is the primary focus.

Sidedness (or lateral "preference"), which is observable in actions that involve only one side of the body, has long been used to infer "dominance," in which it is assumed that one cerebral hemisphere takes the lead in actions involving both sides of the body. It is of considerable relevance to our considerations that an intererst in language function has, from the beginning, made a major contribution to the recognition and exploration of dominance. It has been known since the latter half of the 19th century that speech, an obviously bilateral activity, is seriously disturbed by insult to cortical tissue of one hemisphere, in most cases the hemisphere that also is linked to the individual's sidedness. This seemingly straightforward relationship has needed considerable qualification and adjustment over the years that it has been investigated. For instance, it has become clear that sidedness is not as simple a concept, nor as validly measured, as was once thought. "Dominance," too, is thereby compromised. At the same time, the past several decades have seen the accretion of evidence that, in certain major respects, the human brain is structurally and functionally asymmetric and, also, that this asymmetry is somewhat independent of sidedness, which is itself a complex matter.

Throughout this whole endeavor of investigating laterality, and language, and the interrelationships between them, a major complication in both developing questions and deriving answers is posed by those persons who give evidence of being left-handed (-sided). Historically left-handedness has been considered an anomaly, on actuarial grounds if no other. In an organism bilaterally structured there are two alternatives for lateral preference, and if sidedness is simply an expression of probabilities one would find approximately 50% of each in the population. But only about 6% of the population is left-sided. The ancient view of sinistrality as anomalous is therefore justified. In fact, the basis for this view has been expanded through the extensive investigation of laterality conducted in approximately the past 20 years. Left-sidedness is not simply the alternative (reversed) state of central nervous system structure or organization; rather, it seems to represent varying degrees of departure from right-sidedness. In fact, there is growing support for the position maintained by Annett (1978) that there are, properly, only two classes of laterality: *right-sidedness* and *nonright-sidedness,* with the latter class including various degrees of left-sidedness and ambilaterality. Annett also makes the point, now quite well established, that language lateralization is more stable and consistent in those individuals who are right-sided than in those who are nonright-sided.

There is extensive clinical and research evidence that the two cerebral hemispheres "have major responsibility" for different functions. These findings have led to comparisons of hemispheric functions in which an effort is made to establish categories of operation that characterize the functioning of each hemisphere and distinguish it from the other. Beaton (1985, chaps. 4 and 14) discusses these efforts—and their limitations. Interestingly, the limitations to which Beaton draws attention arise largely from the evidence of varying degrees of overlap in hemispheric function that surfaces along with those findings that suggest the hemispheric differences. Still, certain general characterizations of hemispheric function can be stated. The one that is most pertinent to the present discussion has to do with the lateralization of language.

There is extensive, consistent evidence that, in most individuals, the left hemisphere is crucial to language perception and production. This evidence articulates with indications that left hemispheric "structures" are designed more for certain types of function, such as seriation, that are evidently generic to a process such as spoken language, with its sequences of segments, morphemes, and syllables. At the same time, the view that language "resides" in the left hemisphere is no longer tenable; other areas of the brain are also involved, not only in the final product but most likely in certain organizational stages as well.

The extent of right hemispheric contribution to language function remains uncertain but evidence is gradually accumulating that the right hemisphere does participate in language—in fact, that its contribution involves a fundamental dimension of spoken language, namely, its prosody. Recognition that the right hemisphere evidently contributes at least substantially to the prosodic dimension of language has come about gradually within the past 30 years, beginning with work that revealed a right hemispheric advantage for the perception of music (Curry, 1967; Kimura, 1964; Milner, 1962; Shankweiler, 1966). An adequate review, tracing the development of this topic, is beyond the scope of the present discussion. However, it is pertinent to set forth a brief summary of the major points to be found in this literature.

First, there is a growing realization that it is not enough to distinguish language from speech and thought, that "language" includes several general types of function, such as gestural, prosodic, semantic, and syntactic divisions, and that they show varying patterns of lateralization (see Benson, 1986).

Second, prosody is receiving more attention as an important aspect of spoken language, with a growing recognition that it contains dimensions more linguistically significant than simply contributing "emotional coloring" to verbal expression. For most of this century, following Hughlings Jackson's identification of propositional speech and its association with the "leading" hemisphere, it has been widely accepted that the contribution of the right hemisphere is essentially to provide the emotional element of speech; what has been generally considered to be intrinsic to the "automatic" aspects of speech. Too little attention has been paid to the fact that the prosodic dimension of language is not so simply construed, that, among other features, it has clear semantic properties as well as those associated with affective expression. In fact, prosodic variation can easily produce considerable change in the meaning of a lexical string. For instance, prosodic variation can yield five different meanings of the four-syllable utterance, "He's got a knife." Four different meanings are signaled by stressing one or another of the four syllables, a fifth meaning is achieved by placing especially strong stress on the last syllable, a modification traditionally coded in standard orthography by placing an exclamation mark after the last word. Another illustration of the semantic value of prosody is found in the not infrequent use of intonation to completely invert the meaning carried by the lexical units, a form of sarcasm. For example, the intonation pattern underlying the utterance, "Isn't that nice?" might either directly support the meaning of the lexical string or directly contradict it.[20]

Some years ago Monrad-Krohn (1947, 1963) identified and discussed four classes of prosody, of which only two—*emotional* prosody and *inarticulate* prosody—fit the nonpropositional role ascribed to the affective component of prosody. The other two classes, *intrinsic* prosody (the standard melodic pattern of a language) and *intellectual* prosody (represented in the examples given previously) are an integral part of the meaning of an utterance; they clearly have propositional value. In the course of producing ordinary spoken language, these prosodic aspects must be an integral part of utterance planning. It is particularly germane to recall here the evidence, discussed earlier (Chapter 8), that stress pattern is entered early into the planning of an utterance.

There are now many sources in both clinically based and experimental literature that give evidence that the prosodic dimension of language is largely a right hemispheric function (Behrens, 1985; Blumstein & Cooper, 1974; Blumstein & Goodglass, 1972; Boller & Green, 1972; Ross, 1981; Ross & Mesulam, 1979; Shapiro & Danly, 1985; Weintraub, Mesulam, & Kramer, 1981). Such findings, particularly those relating to intrinsic and intellectual prosody, suggest that propositionality is not exclusively a left-hemispheric function. This implication, incidently, is corroborated by reports that some left-hemispherectomy patients are able to generate some limited spontaneous speech (Butler & Norrsell, 1968; Gott, 1973; Levy, Nebes, & Sperry, 1971; Smith, 1966; Zangwill, 1967).

There is another well-documented observation that relates pointedly to the evidence that music, melody, and prosody are "specialties" of right-hemispheric function. Reference to the reports of patients who, though unable to speak because of either localized or extensive left-hemispheric damage, are still able to sing, producing "well-articulated and linguistically accurate words" in doing so (Bogen, 1969; Gott, 1973; Smith, 1966; Yamadori, Osumi, Masuhara, & Okubo, 1977).[21] However, such performances are generally recognized to be nonpropositional; also, certain reports (e.g., Bogen & Gordon, 1971; Gordon & Bogen, 1974) seem to claim that singing and speaking are very dissimilar processes. On the other hand, notable success in working with aphasics has been achieved using Melodic Intonation Therapy (Sparks, Helm, & Albert, 1974). The core of this therapy method is to have the patient concentrate on the prosodic pattern of sentences; the appropriate intonation is imitated, emphasized by accompanying hand movements, and supported by unison speaking with the therapist. Sparks et al. also cited other sources (Gerstman, 1964; Ustvedt, 1937) that reported the successful use of comparable methods. Along similar lines, Luria (1972) has described the considerable improvement in verbal facility achieved by an aphasic patient after he developed a form of expression described as "a kind of prose which was close to poetry," a manner of speaking that effected "a dominance of prosodic organization."

These findings have direct relevance to stuttering. A most compelling correspondence is that one of the relatively few "universal" facts about stuttering (Wingate, 1983) is that stutterers do not stutter when they sing. In apparently similar vein, stuttering is substantially reduced, if not eliminated, when the stutterer speaks to rhythm or in chorus with another speaker. These effects have seemed to me to be different expressions of the influence of prosody, and certain other speaking conditions that have a demonstrated ameliorative effect on stuttering can be explained along the same lines (Wingate, 1969a, 1970b).[22] Further, these observations regarding speaking conditions that ameliorate stuttering, coupled with the consistent evidence for the concurrence of linguistic stress and stuttering, strongly suggest that the prosodic factors have a significant role in the disorder (Wingate, 1976, 1977c, 1979a, 1979b, 1981, 1984a, 1984b, 1984c).

The "laterality connection" in stuttering, then, rather than being explained as incomplete cerebral dominance, seems better conceived as an inadequate integration of those aspects of the functional "specialties" of the two hemispheres that are specifically requisite for language production (without necessarily abandoning the assumption that one hemisphere "leads" in the sense of orchestrating). Moreover, it is necessary to take account of evidence that the generation, organization, and production of language is not exclusively (perhaps not even predominantly) a cortical-level process. Recognition that subcortical structures participate in the production (and perception) of spoken language is a third major development in the relatively recent literature concerned with the neurology of language. The bulk of this literature deals with evidence that structures in the limbic system, particularly certain thalamic nuclei, are integral to language processes (see Crosson, 1985; Mateer & Ojemann, 1983; Robinson, 1976; and especially Lamendella, 1977).

The findings contained in the literature on subcortical participation in language are, like other content mentioned earlier, not amenable to an adequate brief summary because of their extent, detail, and in many instances, uncertain nature. Also the relevance of much of this information is not, at least now, directly appreciable in respect to an analysis of stuttering. At the same time, certain matters deserve mention.

It has been known for some time that midbrain structures are the source of the ebb and flow of activation and suppression of cortical area function, and that their processes underly both affective and volitional activity. The literature just mentioned extends this level of knowledge to the "activities" of language; for instance, there is the recurring evidence of a close relationship between the affective functions of limbic structures and the prosodic dimensions of language. This literature also provides indication, from several directions, that lateralization of language functions extends to subcortical structures; that naming activity and articulatory adequacy have at least partially separable sites or systems; that certain pathways seem particularly involved in conveying phonological information. A most dramatic indication of the role of subcortical structures is reflected in the finding that electrical stimulation of certain thalamic nuclei has elicited words and phrases (Schaltenbrand, 1965; Schaltenbrand, Spuer, Wahren, & Rummler, 1971). This result contrasts markedly with that obtained from stimulation of cortical tissue, which has yielded only voicing.[23] Lamendella (1977) noted that this finding might indicate, not that the thalamic nuclei generate words, but that some dimensions of the cortical speech system are being accessed by thalamic projections. At the same time, Robinson (1972, 1976) gives examples of what he calls, credibly, "limbic speech." Both authors would undoubtedly deny propositional capacity to limbic structures alone. At any rate, Schaltenbrand's finding illustrates the important role of limbic structures.

There is other evidence of significant thalamic participation in speech mechanisms. Aphasia, especially anomia, and other significant disturbances in speech have been reported to result from: thalamic hemorrhages (Cappa & Vignolo, 1979; Ciemins, 1970; Fisher, 1961; McFarling, Rothi, & Heilman, 1982; Penfield & Roberts, 1959); thalamic tumors (Botez, 1962; Cheek & Taveras, 1966; Smyth & Stern, 1938); electrical stimulation of the thalamus (Ojemann, Fedio, & Van Buren, 1968); and thalamotomy (Allen, Turner, & Gadea-Ciria, 1966; Almgren, Andersson, & Kullberg, 1969; Bell, 1968; Ojemann, Hoyenga, & Ward, 1971; Samra et al., 1969; Selby, 1967; Vilkki & Laitinen, 1974, 1976). The extent to which various thalamic structures are involved remains unclear, but there is considerable evidence that the left ventrolateral nucleus participates actively in speech production. In fact, certain authors (Botez & Barbeau, 1971; Ojemann & Ward, 1971) conceive of the lateral thalamus as an integrating center through which cortical speech areas are related to verbal memory processes and to the subcortical respiratory substrate for speech.

Two dimensions of this research on thalamic function deserve special mention and are of particular relevance to the analysis of stuttering developed in this book. Almgren and co-workers (1969, 1972), Ojemann and Ward (1971), and Riklan and Levita (1970) report evidence that perseverative tendencies in dealing with verbal material result from lesions in the left ventrolateral nucleus. Botez and Barbeau (1971) and Vilkki and

Laitinen (1974, 1976) found diminished scores on the Thurstone form of word-fluency test to be associated with lesions in the left ventrolateral nucleus. These findings have direct significance for understanding the speech production system as a functional circuitry that interrelates several levels of the central nervous system that span phylogentically old and new structures. The reader should recall that relevant research in stuttering (see Chapters 7 and 8) yields similar evidence regarding verbal-specific perseveration and word-fluency limitations in stutterers. Stuttering and stutter-like symptoms are mentioned in certain of these reports regarding the effects of thalamic lesions (see especially Markham & Rand, 1963; Riklan & Levita, 1970).

It seems pertinent to mention at this point the concept of a "starting mechanism of speech," or *elementary system* proposed by Botez (1960). This mechanism is conceived to be based in phylogenetically older levels of the central nervous system, although extending to the supplementary motor area of the cortex. It is said to be concerned with the initiation of speech and the maintenance of speech volume, fluency,[24] articulation, and motor patterning of words in connected speech. The idea of such a mechanism was developed to explain clinically observed symptomatology in which patients evidenced mutism without akinesia.[25] The concept lacks many refinements, especially from a linguistic standpoint, but the notion has a certain pertinence for stuttering relative to the inital-position variable and to the matters of accessory features and emotional influences on speech.

Of related interest here is the evidence that facial movements and voicing, in both their affective and volitional expressions, are activated by related neurologic systems. One of the most notable findings reported by Schaltenbrand (1965; Schaltenbrand et al., 1971) was that the words and phrases elicited by thalamic stimulation were almost always accompanied by a grasping movement of the contralateral hand and a turning of the eyes toward the contralateral side. The interrelationship of vocalization and facial (and certain other body) movements is best appreciated through reference to the phylogenetic development of vocalization (see, for example, Lieberman, 1984; MacLean, 1978; Myers, 1978; Robinson, 1972). Its relevance for stuttering emerges in regard to the occurrence of certain *accessory* features of stuttering. Such features consist mainly of extraneous movements that accompany stutter events, but are not clearly related to the speech act. For many years they were called "secondary mannerisms," a designation which carries the assumption that these acts are acquired in reaction to the stutter or in struggling with it. The term accessory is preferable, for several reasons (see Wingate, 1964, 1976, pp. 48–49); in fact, the designation accessory and its subcategories,[26] was devised largely in consideration of the kind of neurologic phenomena mentioned here, namely that many of these features, particularly those involving motions of the face, suggest involuntary movement resembling "overflow" motor activity as seen in cerebral palsy.

Consideration of the phylogenetic development of speech leads to reflections on the essence of the speech code and its primary elements. Vocalization is a communicative function that humans share with other mammalian life forms, and even though there are certain substantial differences between human and nonhuman neural systems for vocalization both systems involve phylogenetically old structures. There is little, if any, doubt that vocalization is the primordial dimension of distance communication among humans, and that the evolution of this function over millions of years has progressed through many modifications and refinements in variety and degree of controls. Evidently this modification has come about through progressive changes in structure and function of the oral apparatus (see Lieberman, 1975, 1984), along with changes occurring in the expanding central nervous system tissue. An apparently concurrent change was the shift from a continous, or *graded*, signaling system to one that is predominantly discrete, or *categorical*, in nature (see Marler, 1975). The system is described here as "predominantly" categorical because speech incorporates both discrete and continous dimensions. The continuous, or graded, component of the system is expressed in the suprasegmental dimension of speech. The discrete, or categorical, dimension of the system is represented in the segmental aspects of speech, the phonemes.[27]

This conception of oral language is somewhat confounded by the fact that certain of the segmental items—vowels—are of the same substance as the suprasegmental dimension, namely, vocal resonance. Moreover, it is the resonance of the vowels that serves as the vehicle for prosodic expression.

Vowels are the simplest (least extreme) modifications of vocalization, as well as being the oldest. They constitute the body of the speech stream, as recurring pulses of resonance that are the foundation of the syllabic structure of language—although it is the consonants that create the units of this structure. Dudley (1940), later Ohman (1966), and most recently Fowler (1980) have described speech in essentially these terms, as a sequence of vowels produced by smooth, relatively slow movements of tongue and lips that modulate the vocal stream.[28] The consonants interrupt this vowel stream in brief, partial or complete, closures of the vocal tract; closures effected by ballistic type movements that are more rapid and precise than the movements producing vowels. Consonants are thus boundary phenomena, occurring as the limits of vowel pulses, setting the syllable boundaries.

A possible additional complication in this conception of oral language is the fact that certain of the non-vowel segmental items, the voiced consonants, include a resonance component. However, few of these segments participate in the suprasegmental dimension of speech, and then only rarely. Obviously, the remaining segment type, the voiceless consonants, do not.

Clearly, the classes segmental and suprasegmental are not isomorphic with, respectively, categorical and graded. This lack of correspondence is due primarily to the considerable suprasegmental involvement of vowels. The segmental features of speech merit further consideration.

Consonant and Vowel Again

The designations "consonant" and "vowel" represent one of those highly useful dichotomies whose boundaries are not at all as clear as usage of terms implies. Both of these classes continue to elude clear definition (Studdert-Kennedy, 1975; Zipf, 1935).[29] The lack of a clear distinction between consonant and vowel is exemplified most simply in the fact that certain consonants are identified as "semi-vowels." A more formal representation of this circumstance is found in the "sonority hierarchy" (Hooper, 1976; Malmberg, 1963) in which the segmental phonemes are arranged on a continuum. Vowel forms, placed at one end of the continuum, and voiceless stops at the other, represent the extremes of the sonority ranking.

The fact that the constituents of what are generally considered to be two separate classes of phonemes fit into a single continuum seems to reflect a central reality for understanding the nature of speech. The crux of the matter is that the sonority hierarchy describes the range over which vocalization is modified by differing, and varying, "articulatory" actions. It therefore represents the segmental domain of speech not only in its present-day form, but also in reference to its phylogenetic background, its origin and development out of vocalization, as described in the previous section.

At the same time, in spite of the underlying continuity, a difference between the segment classes of consonant and vowel has a clear psychological reality, and a functional reality.[30] Also the two classes have separable physical (acoustic) identities, and evidently some physiological individuality (see earlier discussion, Chapter 6). Consonant and vowel are fundamental to the description and analysis of speech and language from the time of its onset in the individual, near the the 12th month of life. Moreover, the *anlage* of consonant and vowel are discernible in the very early oral activity of infants. Stark (1980) and Oller (1980) described two sound-making systems of infants evident in the first few months of life, a "consonantal" system and a "vocalic" system, that are independent of adult forms even though certain dimensions of them will, relatively soon, merge into true phonemes. Once actual vowels and consonants have become evident in the early stages of speech development, vowels appear earlier and stabilize much more readily than do consonants, a difference that is noted throughout early childhood. It is of great interest that this difference in developmental progression can be seen to parallel the phylogenetic progression of speech sound making. That is, the phonemes that are most readily acquired by the child are the ones that are closest to vocalization, that involve the least modification of vocalization, and that appeared earlier in the evolutionary progression toward speech (see, for instance, Lieberman, 1972, 1975, 1984).

Another parallel between speech development in the individual and in phylogeny, which is intrinsically related to the one based in consonants and vowels, is that communication through vocalization predates actual speech. The infant's communicative use of prosody appears long[31] before its intentional use of phonemes, especially those phonemes appearing as sequences that constitute early words. Crystal (1973, 1976) noted the agreement among most observers that language-specific intonational patterning emerges between 6 and 7 months of age. It is clearly evident by the time the average infant is 9 months old. As Crystal put it, intonation is "the earliest kind of linguistic structuring in the vocalization of the child." Wode (1980) makes the point, too often overlooked, that the basic properties of the prosodic system are already quite well established in the holophrastic and two-word stages of language development. Further, the prosodic variation evident at these levels obviously is used in a linguistically contrastive fashion.[32]

There is one further comparison between consonant and vowel that is particularly relevant to the present analysis: the evidence that they differ in respect to lateralization. Shankweiler (1971) reported the results of several studies of dichotic listening, using both synthetic and actual speech, in which the results concurred in indicating that the perception of stop consonants is highly dependent on the function of the (dominant) left hemisphere but that, in contrast, vowels may or may not be processed by the dominant hemisphere. The lateralization effect was not tied to any particular acoustic feature, but evidently reflected some dimension more central to what characterizes consonant or vowel. The evidence indicated that vowels are processed "neither like music," acknowledged as a right hemisphere function, "nor like what is most characteristic of speech," traditionally viewed as a left hemispheric function. By "most characteristic of speech" Shankweiler meant "those phonetic properties of speech that are a consequence of encoding." Very similar conclusions are presented in a landmark paper by Liberman (1970) in which he discussed the similarities of speech and language as code. In reference to the consonant-vowel contrast in lateralization, Liberman remarked that stop consonants seem to be "more deeply linguistic, more different from nonspeech, than the vowels." Although these findings are based on studies of speech perception, it seems highly defensible to consider them relevant to speech production as well. As Liberman noted, it is very unlikely that man has two separate mechanisms, one for producing speech and one for perceiving it, but rather a more unitary device that functions similarly in all its operations.

The idea of consonants being more "encoded," and more "linguistic," than vowels is consistent with certain of the various generalized descriptive characterizations of left hemisphere versus right hemisphere specializations, such as: that left hemispheric function is more serial, analytic, focal, and temporal, and that right hemispheric function is more holistic, diffuse, and atemporal. However, as emphasized in earlier discussion, proper recognition of the prosodic dimension of language substantially qualifies attribution of "language function" solely to the left hemisphere. Actually, the idea that consonants are more encoded, or linguistic, than vowels aligns more neatly with the distinction between "discrete" and "graded," as discussed earlier in this section. It may still be proper to conceive of the left hemisphere as "leading," but more in the sense of a focus for organization, for imbricating the relevant functions of each hemisphere that contribute the discrete and graded aspects to the final product.

In view of the substantial relevant evidence that has now accrued, it seems reasonable to conceive of the long evolutionary history of speech as originating in a kind of vocalization similar to that found in other hominid life, gradually shading into the form manifested in intonation, then being further modified into the shapes we now call vowels, and culminating in the sounds produced by the more extreme sort of gestures that we identify as consonants. It seems likely that this progression, almost certainly an expression of enlarging and refining brain structures, would be closely linked to developments in lateral specialization of function. One could then surmise, in reference to pertinent findings presented previously, and consistent with the hypothesized evolutionary progression, that the phylogenetically earlier levels in the system (those having a graded character) are more bilaterally represented in the brain, and that lateralization characterizes the later dimensions of the system. It follows that the consonantal-type gestures are the ones likely to be strongly lateralized.

In this conception the lateralization of consonantal forms will be understood to be one aspect of a generalized evolutionary development of sidedness, intimately linked to the refinement in motor control associated with sidedness and to the type of specializations in function that evidently have come to characterize the left hemisphere (such as seriation, sequencing, timing, etc.). It is then comprehensible that the focus for the generation and organization of speech should have become established in this matrix, wherein the division of the vowel stream into syllables, which is accomplished through consonantal gestures, creates the essential structure of language.

These considerations have direct relevance to stuttering, and to certain psycholinguistic concepts given special attention in this book, particularly the syllable-structure hypothesis. It seems to me that consonant and vowel, discrete and graded, prosody, laterality, and lexical access form a kind of matrix that has explanatory linkage with the syllable-structure hypothesis and the fault line concept of stuttering presented in Chapter 6. Exploring that linkage constitutes another "new departure" in the study of language organization and speech production.

Synopsis

The data and analyses presented in this chapter represent an extension, and a denouement, of the content developed in preceding chapters. As in the earlier chapters, the findings that emerge here are not only directly pertinent to understanding stuttering but contribute, as well, to a conception of normal expressive language processes. Much of the material presented in this chapter is, again, highly consistent with certain psycholinguistic concepts given special attention here, particularly the syllable-structure hypothesis, originated by Hockett (1967) and elaborated in the work of Shattuck-Hufnagel (1983, 1987). In fact, the final psycholinguistic analysis developed in this chapter arrives essentially at an enlargement of the syllable-structure hypothesis, through the inference that the syllable constituents may be differentially lateralized. In this enlarged image of the syllable-structure hypothesis one finds a clear correspondence between the discernible structure of stutters and the structure of the basic linguistic unit, the syllable.

As for stuttering per se, the converging lines of evidence indicate that the disorder reflects a special kind of neurologic dysfunction involving, at least as the principal focus, neuronal systems of the left prefrontal cortex and related subcortical structures. At the same time, neural activity on the other side of the central nervous system evidently is part of the problem. There are many parallels between stuttering and aphasia, ordinarily not clearly evident, that become discernible once the parameters of comparison are brought into focus. At the same time there are notable differences between the two disorders, of which the most striking concerns etiology; while it seems clear that both disorders can be induced by cortical damage,[33] there is substantial evidence that much, perhaps most, stuttering is genetic in origin.

The actual occurrence of stutter events remains to be explained in terms of a lack of proper synchrony of linguistic elements. Reference is made here, not to motor acts, but to synchrony in terms of utterance planning and assembly. Stutter events clearly represent a lack of synchrony in word assembly, which itself implies functions above the level of motor execution. Moreover, as presented in this and earlier chapters (2, 4, 7, and 8), evidence from several dimensions of inquiry in stuttering indicate some anomaly in expressive language function beyond the level of the word, its retrieval, and its assembly. Stuttering is not simply a problem of words per se, but of words as the pivotal elements in a system that can transduce ideas and thoughts into an audible code—speech. When functioning properly, as it does in the normal speaker, the system produces and transmits the code with a form and degree of continuity identifiable as having a normal flow. In stutterers the system is not functioning properly.

Footnotes

[1]Recall that the significant difference found in this research is supported by results obtained in previous research using a word-fluency measure (Okasha et al., 1974; Weuffen, 1961; Wingate, 1968).

[2]I recognize that the central representation of a phoneme may be more abstracted than its representation at the surface (production), but this possible distinction does not seem of particular significance here.

[3]The marker sometimes includes a phonatory aspect that resembles the "neutral vowel," but which is more properly identified as an abortive vocal gesture.

[4]The interested reader is referred to Wingate (1966c, 1966d, 1986a, 1986b.)

[5]This description also applies to reading aloud.

[6]Howes' results are supported by findings like those reported by Beattie and Butterworth (1979), Freedman and Loftus (1971),and Saporta (1955).

[7]Meaning *genetic* transmission. The "social heredity" hypothesis (Gray, 1940), which expresses the explanatory notions of Wendell Johnson, purports to explain the inheritance of stuttering as a psychological phenomenon. Although still accepted by certain sources as credible (Bloodstein, 1981; Taylor, 1976), the "social heredity" account is thoroughly untenable (see Wingate, 1986c).

[8]Blewett (1954), Thurstone, Thurstone, and Strandskov (1955), and Vandenberg (1962, 1964).

[9]Both Milner and Benton found certain other, nonlanguage related, differences associated with lesions of the right hemisphere. They are not directly pertinent to the present discussion.

[10]As noted earlier, to speak accurately of stuttering in regard to specific phones would require denoting the *vowel* as the "difficult" phone, rather than the immediately preceding consonant.

[11]This assumption is not limited to the field of stuttering.

[12]Generally speaking, I maintain a serious reservation about the use of the term "automatic" in reference to *any* aspect of speech production in the normal speaker. The word may be used properly to refer to certain aphasic utterances and to ictal utterances. However, especially at the present state of knowledge I believe that assumptions about "automaticity" in normal speech processes are unwarranted. A special term is needed to refer to certain highly routinized verbal acts that seem to occur indepedent of intent.

[13]Keep in mind that pause is not the only kind of "hesitation phenomena" to be found more frequently in spontaneous speech than in oral reading. The recurring

reference to pause in this discussion simply reflects the fact that attention to other hesitation phenomena was not included in most of these studies.

[14]See, for instance Bloodstein (1949), and the "facts" references cited earlier.

[15]One may find an occasional report of a stutterer who stutters more when reading aloud, in which case the inversion of the general rule seems due to marked pressures felt by the individual. Such cases are evidently few in number.

[16]The latter is tantamount to a temporary strabismus. It is of interest here that the infamous Dieffenbach surgery for stuttering, done in the middle of the 19th century (see Wingate, 1976, p. 285), was based indirectly on his observation of some concurrence between stuttering and strabismus.

[17]This publication of the Speech Foundation of America, now in its fourth edition, is prepared by professionals in the field who are considered to be leading clinicians.

[18]Travis (1933a) credited M.W. Sachs and Orton with having developed this position.

[19]Some recent good reviews and summaries of the topic are presented in: Beaton (1985); Bryden (1982); Corballis (1983); Geschwind and Galaburda (1984).

[20]Or, also, indicate indifference or only superficial interest.

[21]Bogen (1969) notes that this observation was recorded as early as 1745.

[22]This account does not ignore the importance of timing.

[23]Stimulation at both levels has produced speech arrest.

[24]Note that here, as in the aphasia literature generally, "fluency" is used to mean word retrieval; in essence, the inverse of anomia.

[25]Cases in which facial and vocal activity are absent or markedly diminished although general motor activity is relatively unaffected.

[26]Extraneous movements of the facial area are identified as *speech-related* features and certain *ancillary* features.

[27]The categorical nature of speech segments is discussed in pertinent literature on categorical perception. See, for instance, Blumstein (1987, pp. 260–264; Foss and Hakes, (1978, pp. 79–88). Of particular relevance to the ensuing discussion are findings like those reported by Fry, Abramson, Eimas, and Liberman (1962) and Liberman, Harris, Kinney, and Lane (1961) that consonants are identified more categorically while vowels are identified on a more graded basis.

[28]Research reported by MacNeilage and Scholes (1964) is especially pertinent to this description: they found that electrical activity of tongue muscle during vowel articulation shows "a complex pattern of finely graded changes." (See also Perkell (1969), and previous discussion, chapter 6.)

[29]Studdert-Kennedy quotes Sweet as having made the same point in his *Handbook of Phonetics* (1877).

[30]There are several ways to document this reality. The most impressive comes from the research on speech errors: errors involve either consonants or vowels, but not interchanges between the two classes.

[31]In the temporal compression of infant development, two or three months is, maturationally, a very long time.

[32]Wherein prosodic pattern changes the meaning of even brief utterances.

[33]Many sources of evidence presumptive of organic etiology in stuttering were not included in the material considered in this book.

Appendix

Table 8.4A. Normal speakers: intercorrelations among the variables measured[a]

Variable	WAIS	WF1	Allit.	Words WAIS	Words Story One	D/Wrd. Story One	Words Story Two	W-A Com	W-A Dif	TBR MC	TBR PS	TBR CR	Vis. Slurv.	Aud. Slurv.	Anagr.	Bk-Sp
PMA	.87	.12	.18	.42	.11	.11	.17	−.07	−.06	−.25	.53	.24	.34	.21	.30	.41
WAIS		.20	.12	.44	.14	.17	.13	0.0	−.13	−.21	.50	.39	.42	.21	.55	.60
WF1			.54	.23	.07	.02	−.18	.28	−.36	−.10	.33	.26	.30	.49	.30	.27
Allit				.12	−.05	−.05	.10	.27	−.27	.15	.29	.22	.49	.77	.16	.18
Words, WAIS					.03	.06	.26	−.07	−.17	−.29	.12	.16	.09	.13	.12	.09
Words, Story One						.98	.08	−.37	.23	.04	.13	−.01	−.11	.18	0.0	−.13
Dif Wrds, Story Two							.09	−.36	.28	.09	.05	−.04	−.14	.15	−.04	−.20
Words, Story Two								.08	−.28	−.29	−.11	−.22	−.11	−.01	−.18	−.16
W-A, Com									−.81	−.09	.25	.33	.45	.29	.03	.16
W-A. Dif										.15	−.36	−.45	−.42	−.21	−.20	−.29
TBR, MC											−.21	.02	−.11	−.04	0.0	−.05
TBR, PS												.80	.54	.50	.61	.65
TBR, CR													.45	.32	.60	.65
Vis Slurv														.73	.49	.56
Aud Slurv															.32	.33
Anagr																.83

[a]All values included.

[b]Correlation values of: ±.70 and above have a minimum significance level of .0001
±.61 and above have a minimum significance level of .002
±.54 and above have a minimum significance level of .01
±.42 and above have a minimum significance level of .05
±.39 and above have a minimum significance level of .10.

TABLE 8.5A. Stutterers: intercorrelations among the variables measured[a]

Variable	WAIS	WF1	Allit.	Words WAIS	Words Story One	D/Wrd Story One	Words Story Two	W-A Com	W-A Dif.	TBR MC	TBR PS	TBR CR	Vis. Slurv.	Aud. Slurv.	Anagr.	Bk-Sp	Stutt. Rating
PMA	.81	.01	−.06	.29	.13	.20	.15	−.09	.13	.06	.36	.22	.39	.48	.50	.55	−.01
WAIS		−.03	.16	.34	.05	.19	.24	−.10	.06	.15	.16	.38	.32	.31	.52	.48	.16
WF1			.65	−.46	−.55	−.69	−.32	.55	−.41	.51	.39	.54	−.25	−.16	.46	.33	−.10
Allit				−.33	−.42	−.44	.04	.33	−.33	.37	.12	.47	−.40	−.21	.30	.16	−.01
Words, WAIS					.40	.43	.49	−.23	.48	−.17	−.20	−.04	.05	.07	−.11	−.06	.13
Words, Story One						.94	.42	−.29	.25	−.56	.12	−.33	−.06	.01	−.20	−.10	.10
Dif Wrds, Story One							.49	−.44	.32	−.54	−.02	−.37	.08	.09	−.20	−.09	.14
Words, Story Two								−.17	.17	−.29	−.14	−.43	−.19	.09	.02	.06	.16
W-A, Com									−.72	.41	.25	.59	.03	.22	.25	.10	−.25
W-A, Dif										−.22	−.15	−.33	−.20	−.29	−.46	−.29	0.0
TBR, MC											.08	.49	.03	.05	.22	−.04	.14
TBR, PS												.32	−.24	−.06	.19	.14	.07
TBR, CR													.11	.01	.36	.23	−.19
Vis Slurv														.68	.39	.45	.10
Aud Slurv															.48	.59	.06
Anagr																.89	.20
Bk-Sp																	.02

[a]All values included.

[b]Correlation values of: ±.68 and above have a minimum significance value of .0001
±.59 and above have a minimum significance value of .002
±.52 and above have a minimum significance value of .01
±.44 and above have a minimum significance value of .05
±.37 and above have a minimum significance value of .10.

References

Abercrombie, D. (1963). Conversation and spoken prose. *English Language Teaching, 18*, 10–16.

Aborn, M., Rubenstein, H., & Sterling, T.D. (1959). Sources of contextual constraint upon words in sentences. *Journal of Experimental Psychology, 57*, 171–180.

Adams, M.R. (1982). Fluency, nonfluency, and stuttering in children. *Journal of Fluency Disorders, 7*, 171–185.

Adams, M.R., & Dietze, D. (1965). A comparison of the reaction times of stutterers and nonstutterers to items on a word association test. *Journal of Speech and Hearing Research, 8*, 195–203.

Adams, S. (1932). A study of the growth of language between two and four years. *Journal of Juvenile Research, 16*, 269–277.

Allen, C.M., Turner, J.W., & Gadea-Ciria, M. (1966). Investigation into speech disturbances following stereotaxic surgery for Parkinsonism. *British Journal of Disorders of Communication, 1*, 55–59.

Allen, G.D. (1972). The location of rhythmic stress beats in English: An experimental study, I. *Language and Speech, 15*, 72–100.

Almgren, P.-E., Andersson, A.L., & Kullberg, G. (1969). Differences in verbally expressed cognition following left and right ventrolateral thalamotomy. *Scandinavian Journal of Psychology, 10*, 243–249.

Almgren, P.-E., Andersson, A.L., & Kullberg, G. (1972). Long-term effects on verbally expressed cognition following left and right ventrolateral thalamotomy. *Confinia Neurologica, 34*, 162–168.

Anderson, N.S. (1965). Word associations to individual letters. *Journal of Verbal Learning and Verbal Behavior, 4*, 541–545.

Andrews, G., Craig, A., Feyer, A., Hoddinott, S., Howie, P., & Neilson, M. (1983). Stuttering: A review of research findings and theories circa 1982. *Journal of Speech and Hearing Disorders, 48*, 226–246.

Andrews, G., & Harris, M. (1964). *The syndrome of stuttering.* London: Heineman.

Annett, M. (1978). Genetic and non-genetic influence on handedness. *Behavioral Genetics, 8*, 227–249.

Argyle, M., Ingham, R., Alkema, F., & McCallin, M. (1973). The different functions of gaze. *Semiotica, 7*, 19–32.

Arnold, G. (1966). Stuttering and language development: The written language of stutterers. *Asha, 8*, 365 (Abstr.).

Ballard, P.B. (1912). Sinistrality and speech. *Journal of Experimental Pedagogy, 1*, 298–310.

Barton, M.I. (1971). Recall of generic properties of words in aphasic patients. *Cortex, 7*, 73–82.

Barton, M.I., Maruszewski, M., & Urrea, D. (1969). Variation of stimulus context and its effect on word-finding ability in aphasics. *Cortex, 5*, 351–365.

Beaton, A. (1985). *Left side, right side: A review of laterality research.* London: Batsford Academic and Educational Publishers.

Beattie, G. (1978). Sequential temporal patterns of speech and gaze in dialogue. *Semiotica, 23*, 29–52.

Beattie, G.W., & Butterworth, B.L. (1979). Contextual probability and word frequency as determinants of pauses and errors in spontaneous speech. *Language and Speech, 22*, 201–211.

Behrens, S.J. (1985). The perception of stress and lateralization of prosody. *Brain and Language, 26*, 332–348.

Bell, D.S. (1968). Speech functions of the thalamus inferred from the effects of thalamotomy. *Brain, 91*, 619–638.

Bender, J.F. (1939). *The personality structure of stuttering.* New York: McGraw-Hill.

Bender, J.F. (1943). The prophylaxis of stuttering. *Nervous Child, 2*, 181–198.

Benson, D.F. (1986). Aphasia and the lateralization of language. *Cortex, 22*, 71–86.

Benton, A.L. (1968). Differential behavioral effects in frontal lobe disease. *Neuropsychologia, 6*, 53–60.

Berger, K. (1967). The most common words used in conversation. *Journal of Communication Disorders, 1*, 201–214.

Bergmann, G. (1986). Studies in stuttering as a prosodic disturbance. *Journal of Speech and Hearing Research, 29*, 290–300.

Bernstein, N.E. (1981). Are there constraints on childhood disfluency? *Journal of Fluency Disorders, 6*, 341–350.

Berry, J. (1953). Some statistical aspects of conversational speech. In W. Jackson, (Ed.), *Communication theory* (pp. 391-399). London: Butterworth Scientific Publications.

Berry, M.F. (1938). A study of the medical history of stuttering children. *Speech Monographs, 5*, 97–114.

Bever, T.G., Fodor, J.A., & Weksel, W. (1965). Is linguistics empirical? *Psychological Review, 72*, 467–482.

Beveridge, W.I.B. (1957). *The art of scientific investigation.* New York: Random House.

Bjerkan, B. (1980). Word fragmentations and repetitions in the spontaneous speech of 2-to-6-year old children. *Journal of Fluency Disorders, 5*, 137–148.

Blankenship, J. (1964). "Stuttering" in normal speech. *Journal of Speech and Hearing Research, 7*, 95–96.

Blankenship, J., & Kay, C. (1964). Hesitation phenomena in English speech: A study in distribution. *Word, 20*, 360–373.

Blewett, D.B. (1954). An experimental study of the inheritance of intelligence. *Journal of Mental Science, 100*, 922–933.

Blood, G.W., & Seider, R. (1981). The concomitant problems of young stutterers. *Journal of Speech and Hearing Disorders, 46*, 31–33.

Bloodstein, O. (1949). Conditions under which stuttering is reduced or absent: A review of the literature. *Journal of Speech and Hearing Disorders, 14*, 295-302.

Bloodstein, O. (1958). Stuttering as an anticipatory struggle reaction. In J. Eisenson, (Ed.), *Stuttering: A symposium* (pp. 3-69). New York: Harper & Row.

Bloodstein, O. (1960). The development of stuttering: I. Changes in nine basic features. *Journal of Speech and Hearing Disorders, 25*, 219-237.

Bloodstein, O. (1969). *A handbook on stuttering.* Chicago: The National Easter Seal Society.

Bloodstein, O. (1974). The rules of early stuttering. *Journal of Speech and Hearing Disorders, 39*, 379-394.

Bloodstein, O. (1975). Stuttering as tension and fragmentation. In J. Eisenson (Ed.), *Stuttering: A second symposium* (pp. 3-95). New York: Harper & Row.

Bloodstein, O. (1981). *A handbook on stuttering* (3rd ed.). Chicago: National Easter Seal Society.

Bloodstein, O., & Gantwerk, B.F. (1967). Grammatical function in relation to stuttering in young children. *Journal of Speech and Hearing Research, 10*, 786-789.

Bloodstein, O., & Grossman, M. (1981). Early stutterings: Some aspects of their form and distribution. *Journal of Speech and Hearing Research, 24*, 298-302.

Bluemel, C.S. (1913). *Stammering and cognate defects of speech.* New York: Stechert.

Bluemel. C.S. (1957). *The riddle of stuttering.* Danville, IL: Interstate Press.

Blumstein, S.E. (1973). *A phonological investigation of aphasic speech.* The Hague: Mouton.

Blumstein, S.E. (1987). Speech perception and modularity: Evidence from aphasia. In E. Keller & M. Gopnik (Eds.), *Motor and sensory processes of language.* Hillsdale, NJ: Erlbaum.

Blumstein, S., & Cooper, W. (1974). Hemispheric processing of intonation contours. *Cortex, 10,* 146-158.

Blumstein, S., & Goodglass, H. (1972). The perception of stress as a semantic cue in aphasia. *Journal of Speech and Hearing Research, 15,* 800-806.

Bogen, J.E. (1969). The other side of the brain. II. An appositional mind. *Bulletin of the Los Angeles Neurological Societies, 34,* 73-105.

Bogen, J.E., & Gordon, H.W. (1971). Musical tests for functional localization with intracarotid amobarbitol. *Nature, 230,* 524-525.

Boller, F., & Green, F. (1972). Comprehension in severe aphasics. *Cortex, 8,* 382-394.

Boomer, D.S. (1965). Hesitation and grammatical encoding. *Language and Speech, 8,* 148-158.

Boomer, D.S., & Dittman, A.T. (1962). Hesitation pauses and juncture pauses in speech. *Langage and Speech, 5,* 215-220

Boomer, D.S., & Laver, J.D.M. (1968). Slips of the tongue. *British Journal of Disorders of Communication, 2,* 1-12.

Borghi, R. (1955). *A study of the reaction time of stutterers and non-stutterers to verbal stimuli.* Masters thesis, University of Redlands, Redlands, CA.

Botez, M.I. (1960). Clinical contribution to the study of tumoral frontal syndrome. *Psychologie Neurologique, 140,* 347-368.

Botez, M.I. (1962). Aphasia and correlated syndromes in intracranial expanding processes. *Editura Academici R.S.R.,* Bucharest. (Rumanian text, English summary.)

Botez, M.I., & Barbeau, A. (1971). Role of subcortical structures, and particularly the thalamus, in the mechanisms of speech and language. *International Journal of Neurology, 8,* 300–320.

Boysen, A.E., & Cullinan, W.L. (1971). Object-naming latency in stuttering and non-stuttering children. *Journal of Speech and Hearing Research, 14,* 728–738.

Branscom, M.E. (1942). *The construction and statistical evaluation of a speech fluency test for young children.* Masters thesis, University of Iowa, Iowa City.

Branscom, M.E., Hughes, J., & Oxtoby, E.T. (1955). Studies of nonfluency in the speech of preschool children. In W. Johnson (Ed.), *Stuttering in children and adults.* Minneapolis: University of Minnesota Press.

Brenner, M.S., Feldstein, S., & Jaffe, J. (1965). The contributions of statistical uncertainty and task anxiety to speech disruption. *Journal of Verbal Learning and Verbal Behavior, 4,* 300–305.

Brotherton, P.L. (1976). Aspects of the relationship between speech production, hesitation behavior, and social class. Doctoral dissertation, University of Melbourne, Melbourne, Australia.

Brown, C.S., & Cullinan, W.L. (1981). Word-retrieval difficulty and disfluent speech in adult anomic speakers. *Journal of Speech and Hearing Research, 24,* 358–365.

Brown, R. (1973). *A first language: The early stages.* Cambridge, MA: Harvard University Press.

Brown, R., & Berko, J. (1960). Word association and the acquisition of grammar. *Child Development, 31,* 1–14.

Brown, R., & McNeill, D. (1966). The "tip of the tongue" phenomenon. *Journal of Verbal Learning and Verbal Behavior, 5,* 325–327.

Brown, S.F. (1935). *An investigation of the relative frequency of stuttering on various speech sounds during oral reading.* Masters thesis, University of Iowa, Iowa City.

Brown, S.F. (1937a). *A quantitative investigation of certain phonetic, grammatical and semantic factors influencing the incidence of stuttering.* Doctoral dissertation, University of Iowa, Iowa City.

Brown, S.F. (1937b). The influence of grammatical function on the incidence of stuttering. *Journal of Speech Disorders, 2,* 207–215.

Brown, S.F. (1938a). A further study of stuttering in relation to various speech sounds. *Quarterly Journal of Speech, 24,* 390–397.

Brown, S.F. (1938b). Stuttering with relation to word accent and word position. *Journal of Abnormal and Social Psychology, 33,* 112–120.

Brown, S.F. (1938c). The theoretical importance of certain factors influencing the incidence of stuttering. *Journal of Speech Disorders, 3,* 223–230.

Brown, S.F. (1943). An analysis of certain data concerning loci of "stutterings" from the viewpoint of general semantics. *Papers from the Second American Congress of General Semantics, 2,* 194–199.

Brown, S.F. (1945). The loci of stutterings in the speech sequence. *Journal of Speech Disorders, 10,* 181–192.

Brown, S.F., & Moren, A. (1942). The frequency of stuttering with relation to word length during oral reading. *Journal of Speech Disorders, 7,* 153–159.

Bruner, J.S., & O'Dowd, D. (1958). A note on the informativeness of parts of words. *Language and Speech, 1,* 98–101.

Brutten, G.J. (1975). Stuttering: Topography, assessment and behavior change. In J. Eisenson (Ed.), *Stuttering: A second symposium* (pp. 201-262). New York: Harper & Row.

Brutten, G.J., Bakker, K., Janssen, P., & van der Meulen, S. (1984). Eye movements of stuttering and non-stuttering children during silent reading. *Journal of Speech and Hearing Research, 27,* 562-566.

Bryden, M.P. (1982). *Laterality: Functional asymmetry of the intact brain.* New York: Academic Press.

Bryngelson, B. (1939). A study of laterality of stutterers and normal speakers. *Journal of Speech and Hearing Disorders, 4,* 231-233.

Bryngelson, B., & Rutherford, B. (1937). A comparative study of laterality of stutterers and non-stutterers. *Journal of Speech Disorders, 2,* 15-16.

Bushnell, P.P. (1930). An analytic contrast of oral with written English. *Columbia University Teachers College Contributions to Education,* (451).

Butler, S., & Norrsell, U. (1968). Vocalization possibly initiated by the minor hemisphere. *Nature, 220,* 793-794.

Butterworth, B., & Goldman-Eisler, F. (1979). Recent studies on cognitive rhythm. In A.W. Siegman & S. Feldstein (Eds.), *Of speech and time* (pp. 211-224). Hillsdale, NJ: Erlbaum.

Cappa, S.F., & Vignolo, L.A. (1979). "Transcortical" features of aphasia following left thalamic hemorrhage. *Cortex, 15,* 121-130.

Carroll, J.B. (1938). Diversity of vocabulary and the harmonic series law of word-frequency distribution. *Psychological Record, 2,* 379-386.

Carroll, J.B. (1964). *Language and thought.* Englewood Cliffs, NJ: Prentice-Hall.

Carterette, E.C., & Jones, M.H. (1974). *Informal speech.* Berkeley, CA: University of California Press.

Chaney, C.F. (1969). Loci of disfluencies in the speech of non-stutterers. *Journal of Speech and Hearing Research, 12,* 667-668.

Cheek, W.R., & Taveras, J.M. (1966). Thalamic tumors. *Journal of Neurosurgery, 24,* 505-513.

Chomsky, N. (1965). *Aspects of the theory of syntax.* Cambridge, MA: MIT Press.

Chomsky, N., & Halle, M. (1968). *The sound pattern of English.* New York: Harper & Row.

Chotlos, J.W. (1944). Studies in language behavior: IV. A statistical and comparative analysis of individual written samples. *Psychological Monographs, 56,* 77-111.

Ciemins, V.A. (1970). Localized thalamic hemorrhage. *Neurology, Minneapolis, 20,* 776-782.

Claiborne, J.H. (1917). Stuttering relieved by reversal of manual dexterity. *New York Medical Journal, 105,* 577-581, 619-621.

Clark, H.H. (1970). Word associations and linguistic theory. In J. Lyons (Ed.), *New horizons in linguistics* (pp. 271-286). Baltimore, MD: Penguin Press.

Clark, H.H. (1971). The importance of linguistics for the study of speech hesitations. In D.L. Horton & J.J. Jenkins, (Eds.), *The perception of language* (pp. 69-78). Columbus, OH: Merrill.

Clark, H.H., & Haviland, S.E. (1974). Psychological processes as linguistic explanation. In D. Cohen (Ed.), *Explaining linguistic phenomena* (pp. 91-124). Washington, DC: Hemisphere.

Claxton, G.I. (1974). Initial consonant groups function as units in word production. *Language and Speech, 17,* 271–277.

Cohen, E. (1952). A comparison of oral reading and spontaneous speech of stutterers with special reference to the adaptation and consistency effects. Doctoral dissertation, University of Iowa, Iowa City.

Cole, R.A. (1973). Listening for mispronunciations: A measure of what we hear during speech. *Perception and Psychophysics, 13,* 153–156.

Condon, W.S., & Ogston, W.D. (1971). Speech and body motion synchrony of the speaker-hearer. In D.L. Horton & J.J. Jenkins (Eds.), *The perception of language* (pp. 150–173). Columbus, OH: Merrill.

Conture, E.G., Schwartz, H.D., & Brewer, D.W. (1985). Laryngeal behavior during stuttering. *Journal of Speech and Hearing Research, 28,* 233–240.

Conway, J., & Quarrington, B. (1963). Positional effects in the stuttering of contextually organized verbal material. *Journal of Abnormal and Social Psychology, 67,* 299–303.

Cooper, E.B. (1977). Case-selection procedures for school-aged disfluent children. *Language, Speech and Hearing Services in Schools, 8,* 264–269.

Cooper, E.B., Cady, B.B., & Robbins, C.J. (1970). The effect of the verbal stimulus words wrong, right and tree on the disfluency rates of stutterers and nonstutterers. *Journal of Speech and Hearing Research, 13,* 239–244.

Corballis, M.C. (1983). *Human laterality.* New York: Academic Press.

Craven, D.C. (1972). An investigation of pupillary response preceding expectancy and stuttering. Doctoral dissertation, University of Southern California, Los Angeles.

Cross, D.E. (1987). Comparison of reaction time and accuracy measures of laterality for stutterers and normal speakers. *Journal of Fluency Disorders, 12,* 271–286.

Cross, D.E., & Olson, P. (1987). Interaction between jaw kinematics and voice onset for stutterers and nonstutterers in a URT task. *Journal of Fluency Disorders, 12,* 367–380.

Crosson, B. (1985). Subcortical functions in language: A working model. *Brain and Language, 25,* 257–292.

Crystal, D. (1973). Non-segmental phonology in language acquisition: A review of the issue. *Lingua, 32,* 1–45.

Crystal, D. (1976). Developmental intonology. In W. von Raffler-Engel & V. Lebrun (Eds.), *Baby talk and infant speech* (pp. 55–65). Amsterdam: Swets and Zeitlinger.

Curry, F. (1967). A comparison of left-handed and right-handed subjects on verbal and non-verbal dichotic listening tasks. *Cortex, 3,* 343–352.

Cutler, A. (Ed.). (1982). *Slips of the tongue and language production.* Amsterdam: Mouton.

Cutler, A., & Foss, D.J. (1977). On the role of sentence stress in sentence processing. *Language and Speech, 20,* 1–10.

Dalton, P., & Hardcastle, W.J. (1977). *Disorders of fluency.* New York: Elsevier.

Daniels, E.M. (1940). An analysis of the relation between handedness and stuttering with special reference to the Orton-Travis theory of cerebral dominance. *Journal of Speech Disorders, 5,* 309–326.

Danzger, M., & Halpern, H. (1973). Relation of stuttering to word abstraction, part of speech, word length and word frequency. *Perceptual and Motor Skills, 37,* 959-962.

Darley, F.L. (1955). The relationship of parental attitudes and adjustments to the development of stuttering. In W. Johnson (Ed.), *Stuttering in children and adults* (pp. 74-153). Minneapolis: University of Minnesota Press.

Daughtry, G.H. (1982). Click location in sentences: A test of the linguistic competence of seven-year-old fluent and disfluent males. *Journal of Fluency Disorders, 7,* 259-272.

Davis, D.M. (1939). The relation of repetitions in the speech of young children to certain measures of language maturity and situational factors: Part I. *Journal of Speech Disorders 4,* 303-318.

Davis, D.M. (1940). The relations of repetitions in the speech of young children to certain measures of language maturity and situational factors. *Journal of Speech Disorders, 5,* (pts. 2 & 3), 235-246.

Davis, G.A. (1983). *A survey of adult aphasia.* Englewood Cliffs, NJ: Prentice-Hall.

Day, E.J. (1932). The development of language in twins: I. A comparison of twins and single children. *Child Development, 3,* 179-199.

Day, M.E. (1964). An eye movement phenomenon relating to attention, thought and anxiety. *Perceptual and Motor Skills, 19,* 443-446.

Deese, J. (1962). Form class and the determinants of association. *Journal of Verbal Learning and Verbal Behavior, 1,* 79-84.

Deese, J. (1965). *The structure of associations in language and thought.* Baltimore, MD: Johns Hopkins Press.

Delattre, P. (1958). Acoustic cues in speech: a first report. *Phonetica, 2,* 108-118, 226-251.

Denes, P.B. (1963). On the statistics of spoken English. *Journal of the Acoustical Society of America, 35,* 892-904.

Dewey, G. (1923). *Relative frequency of English speech sounds.* Cambridge, MA: Harvard University Press.

Doyle, J.A. (1981). *Phrasal stress patterns in the fluent speech of stutterers and nonstutterers: A replication.* Masters thesis, Washington State University, Pullman.

Drieman, G.H.J. (1962). Differences between spoken and written language. *Acta Psychologica, 20,* 36-57.

Dudley, H. (1940). The carrier nature of speech. *Bell System Technical Journal, 19,* 495-515.

Duke, J.D. (1968). Lateral eye movement behavior. *Journal of General Psychology, 78,* 189-195.

Egland, G.O. (1938). *An analysis of repetitions and prolongations in the speech of young children.* Masters thesis, University of Iowa, Iowa City.

Eisenson, J. (1937a). A note on the perseverative tendency in stutterers. *Journal of Genetic Psychology, 50,* 195-198.

Eisenson, J. (1937b). Some characteristics of the written speech of stutterers. *Pedagogical Seminary and Journal of General Psychology, 50,* 457-458.

Eisenson, J. (1947). Aphasics: Observations and tentative conclusions. *Journal of Speech Disorders, 12,* 291-292.

Eisenson, J. (1954). *Examining for aphasia.* New York: Psychological Corp.

Eisenson, J. (1958). A perseverative theory of stuttering. In J. Eisenson (Ed.), *Stuttering: A symposium* (pp. 223-271). New York: Harper & Row.

Eisenson, J. (1971). Aphasia in adults: Basic considerations. In L.E. Travis (Ed.), *Handbook of Speech Pathology and Audiology* (pp. 1219–1240, Chapter 48). Englewood Cliffs, NJ: Prentice-Hall.

Eisenson, J. (1975). Stuttering as perseverative behavior. In J. Eisenson (Ed.), *Stuttering: A second symposium* (pp. 401–452). New York: Harper & Row.

Eisenson, J., & Horowitz, E. (1945). The influence of propositionality on stuttering. *Journal of Speech Disorders, 10,* 193–197.

Eisenson, J., & Pastel, E. (1936). A study of the perseverating tendency in stuttering. *Quarterly Journal of Speech, 22,* 626–631.

Eisenson, J., & Winslow, C. (1938). The perseverative tendency in stutterers in a perceptual function. *Journal of Speech Disorders, 3,* 195–198.

Emerick, L.L. (1963). A clinical observation on the "final" stuttering. *Journal of Speech and Hearing Disorders, 28,* 194–195.

Ervin, S. (1961). Changes with age in the verbal determinants of word association. *American Journal of Psychology, 74,* 361–372.

Examiner Manual for the SRA Primary Mental Abilities. (1949). Chicago: Science Research Associates.

Fagan, W.T. (1982). The relationship of the "maze" to language planning and production. *Research in the Teaching of English, 16,* 85–95.

Fairbanks, G. (1937). Some correlates of sound difficulty in stuttering. *Quarterly Journal of Speech, 23,* 67–69.

Fairbanks, H. (1944). The quantitative differentiation of samples of spoken language. *Psychological Monographs, 56,* 19–38.

Feuchtwanger, E. (1923). Die funktionen des stirnhirns [The functions of the frontal lobes]. In O. Forster & H. Willmanns (Eds.), *Monographen aus der gesamtgebiete der neurologie und psychiatrie.* Berlin: Springer.

Fiedler, P.A., & Standop, R. (1983). *Stuttering: Integrating theory and practice.* Rockville, MD: Aspen Systems.

Fisher, C.M. (1961). Clinical syndromes in cerebral hemorrhage. In W.S. Fields (Ed.), *Pathogenesis and treatment of cerebrovascular disease* (pp. 318–338). Springfield, IL: Thomas.

Fisher, M.S. (1932). Language patterns of preschool children. *Journal of Experimental Education, 1,* 70–85.

Fisher, M.S. (1934). Language patterns of preschool children. *Child Development Monographs, Whole* (15).

Fletcher, J.M. (1928). *The problem of stuttering.* New York: Longmans Green.

Floyd, S., & Perkins, W.H. (1974). Early syllable dysfluency in stutterers and nonstutterers: A preliminary report. *Journal of Communication Disorders, 7,* 279–282.

Fonagy, I. (1966). Electrophysiological and acoustic correlates of stress and stress perception. *Journal of Speech and Hearing Research, 9,* 231–244.

Font, M.M. (1955). A comparison of the free associations of stutterers and nonstutterers. In W. Johnson (Ed.), *Stuttering in children and adults* (pp. 389–390). Minneapolis: Univeristy of Minnesota Press.

Forrester, E. (1947). *Aristotle: Problemata,* (Vol. 10). (Translation). Oxford: Clarendon Press.

Foss, D.J., & Hakes, D.T. (1978). *Psycholinguistics.* Englewood Cliffs, NJ: Prentice-Hall.

Fowler, C. (1980). Coarticulation and theories of extrinsic timing. *Journal of Phonetics, 8,* 113-133.

Fraisse, P., & Breyton, M. (1959). Comparaisons entre les langages oral et ecrit [Comparisons between written and oral language]. *L'anne Psychologique, 59,* 61-71.

Francis, W.N. (1958). *The structure of American English.* New York: Ronald Press.

Freedman, J.L., & Loftus, E.F. (1971). Retrieval of words from long-term memory. *Journal of Verbal Learning and Verbal Behavior, 10,* 107-115.

Freeman, F.J. (1979). Phonation in stuttering: A review of current research. *Journal of Fluency Disorders, 4,* 79-89.

French, N.R., Carter C.W., & Koenig, W. (1930). The words and sounds of telephone conversations. *Bell System Technical Journal, 9,* 290-324.

Fries, C.C. (1952). *The structure of English.* New York: Harcourt-Brace.

Fries, C.C., & Traver, A.A. (1950). *English word lists.* Ann Arbor, MI: Wahr.

Froeschels, E. (1913-1914). Zur pathologie des stotterns. *Archiv fur Experimentelle und Kleine Phonetik [On the pathology of stuttering], 1,* 372-380.

Froeschels, E. (1921). A study of the symptomatology of stuttering. *Monatschrift fur Ohrenheilkunde, 55,* 1109-1112.

Froeschels, E. (1961). New viewpoints on stuttering. *Folia Phoniatrica, 13,* 187-201.

Fromkin, V.A. (1973a). Introduction. In V.A. Fromkin (Ed.), *Speech errors as linguistic evidence* (pp. 11-45). The Hague: Mouton.

Fromkin, V.A. (Ed.). (1973b). *Speech errors as linguistic evidence.* The Hague: Mouton.

Fromkin, V.A. (1980). *Errors in linguistic performance.* New York: Academic Press.

Fry, D.B. (1947). The frequency of occurrence of speech sounds in Southern English. *Archives Neerlandaises Phonetique Experimentale, 20,* 103-106.

Fry, D.B. (1955). Duration and intensity as physical correlates of linguistic stress. *Journal of the Acoustical Society of America, 27,* 765-768.

Fry, D.B., Abramson, A.S., Eimas, P.D., & Liberman, A.M. (1962). The identification and discrimination of synthetic vowels. *Language and Speech, 5,* 171-189.

Fudge, E.C. (1969). Syllables. *Journal of Linguistics, 5,* 253-286.

Gaddes, W.H., & Crockett, D.J. (1975). The Spreen-Benton Aphasia Tests: Normative data as a measure of normal language. *Brain and Language, 2,* 257-280.

Garnes, S., & Bond, Z.S. (1975). Slips of the ear: Errors in perception of casual speech. *Proceedings of the 11th Regular Meeting of the Chicago Linguistic Society,* 214-225.

Garrett, M.F. (1976). Syntactic processes in sentence production. In R.J. Wales & E. Walker (Eds.), *New approaches to language mechanisms* (pp. 231-256). New York: Elsevier North Holland.

Gay, T. (1978). Effect of speaking rate on vowel formant movements. *Journal of the Acoustical Society of America, 63,* 223-230.

Gerstman, H. (1964). A case of aphasia. *Journal of Speech and Hearing Disorders, 29,* 89-91.

Geschwind, N. (1967). The varieties of naming errors. *Cortex, 3,* 97-112.

Geschwind, N., & Galaburda, A.M. (1984). *Cerebral dominance: The biological foundations.* Cambridge, MA: Harvard University Press.

Gold, J. (1941). *A study of auditory perseveration tendencies in stutterers and normal speakers.* Masters thesis, University of Utah, Salt Lake City.

Goldman-Eisler, F. (1952). Individual differences between interviewers and their effects on interviewees' conversational behavior. *Journal of Mental Science, 98,* 660–671.

Goldman-Eisler, F. (1954a). A study of individual differences and of interaction in the behavior of some aspects of language in interviews. *Journal of Mental Science, 100,* 177–197.

Goldman-Eisler, F. (1954b). On the variability of the speed of talking and on its relation to the length of utterance in conversation. *British Journal of Psychology, General Section, 45,* 94–107.

Goldman-Eisler, F. (1955). Speech-breathing activity—a measure of tension and affect during interviews. *British Journal of Psychology, General Section, 46,* 53–63.

Goldman-Eisler, F. (1956). Speech-breathing activity and context in psychiatric interviews. *British Journal of Psychology, Medical Section, 29,* 35–48.

Goldman-Eisler, F. (1957). Speech production and language statistics. *Nature, 180,* 1497.

Goldman-Eisler, F. (1958a). Speech analysis and mental processes. *Language and Speech, 1,* 59–75.

Goldman-Eisler, F. (1958b). Speech production and the predictability of words in context. *Quarterly Journal of Experimental Psychology, 10,* 96–106.

Goldman-Eisler, F. (1958c). The predictability of words in context and the length of pauses in speech. *Language and Speech, 1,* 226–231.

Goldman-Eisler, F. (1961a). A comparative study of two hesitation phenomena. *Language and Speech, 4,* 18–26.

Goldman-Eisler, F. (1961b). The continuity of speech utterance, its determinance and its significance. *Language and Speech, 4,* 220–231.

Goldman-Eisler, F. (1964). Hesitation, information and levels of speech production. In A.V.S. de Reuck & M. O'Connor (Eds.), *Disorders of language* (pp. 96–111). Boston: Little-Brown.

Goldman-Eisler, F. (1968). *Psycholinguistics: Experiments in spontaneous speech.* New York: Academic Press.

Goldsand, J.G. (1944). Sensory perseveration in stutterers and nonstutterers. *Speech Abstracts., 31,* 40.

Goodglass, H., Kaplan, E., Weintraub, S., & Ackerman, N. (1976). The "Tip of the Tongue" phenomenon in aphasia. *Cortex, 12,* 145–153.

Goodglass, H., & Stuss, D.T. (1979). Naming to picture versus description in three aphasic subgroups. *Cortex, 15,* 199–211.

Gordon, H.W., & Bogen, J.E. (1974). Hemispheric lateralization of singing after intracarotid sodium amylobarbitone. *Journal of Neurology, Neurosurgery and Psychiatry, 37,* 727–738.

Gott, P.S. (1973). Language after dominant hemispherectomy. *Neurosurgery and Psychiatry, 36,* 1082–1088.

Gray, M. (1940). The "X" family: A clinical and laboratory study of a "stuttering" family. *Journal of Speech Disorders, 5,* 343–348.

Green, W.B. (1967). Differential diagnosis: Relationship of motor perseveration to expressive variables associated with stuttering. *Asha, 9,* 374 (Abstr.).

Griggs, S., & Still, A.W. (1979). An analysis of individual differences in words stuttered. *Journal of Speech and Hearing Research, 22,* 572–580.

Grossman, M.P.E. (1910). Danger signals in young children. *Addresses and Proceedings of the National Education Association, Boston,* 878.

Gur, R.E. (1975). Conjugate lateral eye movements as an index of hemispheric activation. *Journal of Personality and Social Psychology, 31,* 751–757.

Hahn, E.F. (1940). A study of the relationship between the social complexity of the oral reading situation and the severity of stuttering. *Journal of Speech Disorders, 5,* 5–14.

Hahn, E.F. (1942a). A study of the relationship between stuttering occurrence and grammatical factors in oral reading. *Journal of Speech Disorders, 7,* 329–335.

Hahn, E.F. (1942b). A study of the relationship between stuttering occurrence and phonetic factors in oral reading. *Journal of Speech Disorders, 7,* 143–151.

Hahn, E.F. (1956). *Stuttering: Significant theories and therapies.* Stanford, CA: Stanford University Press.

Halle, M., & Vergnaud, J.R. (1980). Three dimensional phonology. *Journal of Linguistic Research, 1,* 83–105.

Hanes, B. (1950). *A study of verbal associations in adult stutterers.* Masters thesis, Pennsylvania State University, University Park.

Hannah, E.P., & Gardner, J.G. (1968). A note on syntactic relationships in nonfluency. *Journal of Speech and Hearing Research, 11,* 853–860.

Harris, J.W. (1983). *Syllable structure and stress in Spanish: A nonlinear analysis.* Cambridge, MA: MIT Press.

Harvey-Fisher, C., & Brutten, G.J. (1977). Part-word repetitions in preschool stutterers and nonstutterers. *Asha, 19,* 652 (Abstr.).

Head, H. (1963). *Aphasia and kindred disorders of speech.* New York: Hafner.

Hegde, M.N. (1982). Antecedents of fluent and dysfluent oral reading: A descriptive analysis. *Journal of Fluency Disorders, 7,* 323–341.

Hejna, R.F. (1955). A study of the loci of stuttering in spontaneous speech. Doctoral dissertation, Northwestern University, Evanston, IL.

Hejna, R.F. (1963). Stuttering frequency in relation to word frequency usage. *Asha, 5,* 781 (Abstr.).

Hejna, R.F. (1968, November). *A study of stutterers' versus normal speakers' responses on a word association test.* Paper presented at the convention of the American Speech and Hearing Association, Denver, CO.

Helmreich, H.G., & Bloodstein, O. (1973). The grammatical factor in childhood disfluency in relation to the continuity hypothesis. *Journal of Speech and Hearing Research, 16,* 731–738.

Henderson, A., Goldman-Eisler, F., & Skarbek, A. (1965). Temporal patterns of cognitive activity and breath control in speech. *Language and Speech, 8,* 236–242.

Henrikson, E.H. (1948). An analysis of Wood's articulation index. *Journal of Speech and Hearing Disorders, 13,* 233–235.

Hill, A.A. (1973). A theory of speech errors. In V.A. Fromkin (Ed.), *Speech errors as linguistic evidence* (pp. 205–214). The Hague: Mouton.

Hill, H. (1942). *Perseveration in normal speakers and stutterers.* Masters thesis, University of Indiana, Bloomington.

Hockett, C.F. (1955). *A manual of phonology.* Baltimore, MD: Waverly Press.

Hockett, C.F. (1967). Where the tongue slitps, there slip I. *Janua Linguarum, 32,* 910–936.

Hooper, J.B. (1976). *An introduction to natural generative phonology.* New York: Academic Press.

Horn, E. (1926). *A basic writing vocabulary. University of Iowa Monographs in Education* (4).

Horovitz, L.J., Johnson, S.B., Pearlman, R.C., Schaffer, E.J., & Hedin, A.K. (1978). Stapedial reflex in fluent and disfluent speakers. *Journal of Speech and Hearing Research, 21,* 762-767.

Horowitz, M.W., & Newman, J.B. (1964). Spoken and written expression: An experimental analysis. *Journal of Abnormal and Social Psychology, 68,* 640-647.

Howes, D.J. (1957a). On the relation between intelligibility and frequency of occurrence of English words. *Journal of the Acoustical Society of America, 29,* 296-305.

Howes, D.J. (1957b). On the relation between the probability of a word as an association and in general linguistic usage. *Journal of Abnormal and Social Psychology, 54,* 75-85.

Howes, D.J. (1964). Application of the word-frequency concept to aphasia. In A.V.S. de Reuck & M. O'Connor (Eds.), *Disorders of language* (pp. 47-75). Boston: Little-Brown.

Howes, D.J., & Geschwind, N. (1969). Quantitative studies of aphasic language. In D.M. Rioch & E.A. Weinstein (Eds.), *Disorders of communication* (pp. 229-244). New York: Hafner.

Hughes, J. (1943). *A quantative study of repetition in the speech of two-year-old and four-year-old children.* Masters thesis, University of Iowa, Iowa City.

Hultzen, L.S., Allen, J.H.D. Jr., & Miron, M.S. (1964). *Tables of transitional frequencies of English phonemes.* Urbana, IL: University of Illinois Press.

Hunt, J. (1967). *Stammering and stuttering, their nature and treatment.* London: Hafner. (Original work published in 1870.)

Ingham, R.J., Montgomery, J., & Ulliana, L. (1983). The effect of manipulating phonation duration on stuttering. *Journal of Speech and Hearing Research, 26,* 579-587.

Jakobovits, L.A. (1966). Utilization of semantic satiation in stuttering: A theoretical analysis. *Journal of Speech and Hearing Disorders, 31,* 105-114.

Jamison, D.J. (1955). Spontaneous recovery of the stuttering response as a function of the time following adaptation. In W. Johnson & R.R. Leutenegger (Eds.), *Stuttering in children and adults* (pp. 245-248). Minneapolis: University of Minnesota Press.

Jasper, H.H. (1932). A laboratory study of diagnostic indices of bilateral neuromuscular organization in stutterers and normal speakers. *Psychological Monographs, 43,* 72-174.

Jasper, H.H., & Murray, E. (1932). A study of the eye movements of stutterers during oral reading. *Journal of Experimental Psychology, 15,* 528-538.

Jayaram, M. (1981). Grammatical factors in stuttering. *Journal of the Indian Institute of Science, 63,* 141-147.

Jayaram, M. (1984). Distribution of stuttering in sentences. Relationship to sentence length and clause position. *Journal of Speech and Hearing Research, 27,* 338-341.

Jesperson, O. (1960). Monosyllabism in English. In O. Jesperson (Ed), *Selected writings.* London: G. Allen and Unwin.

Johannsen, H.S., & Victor, C. (1986). Visual information processing in the left and right hemispheres during unilateral tachistoscopic stimulation of stutterers. *Journal of Fluency Disorders, 11,* 285–291.

Johnson, W. (1934). Stuttering in the preschool child. *University of Iowa Child Welfare Bulletin, No. 37.*

Johnson, W. (1937). The dominant thumb in relation to stuttering, eyedness and handedness. *American Journal of Psychology, 49,* 293–297.

Johnson, W. (1942). A study of the onset and development of stuttering. *Journal of Speech and Hearing Disorders, 7,* 251–257.

Johnson, W. (1944a). The Indians have no word for it: Stuttering in adults. *Quarterly Journal of Speech, 30,* 456–465.

Johnson, W. (1944b). The Indians have no word for it: Stuttering in children. *Quarterly Journal of Speech, 30,* 330–337.

Johnson, W. (1946). *People in quandaries: The semantics of personal adjustment.* New York: Harper.

Johnson, W. (1955). A study of the onset and development of stuttering. In W. Johnson & R.R. Leutenegger (Eds.), *Stuttering in children and adults* (pp. 37–73). Minneapolis: University of Minnesota Press.

Johnson, W. (1961a). Measurements of oral reading and speaking rate and disfluency of adult male and female stutterers and nonstutterers. *Journal of Speech and Hearing Disorders, Monograph Supplement 7,* 1–20.

Johnson, W. (1961b). *Stuttering and what you can do about it.* Minneapolis: University of Minnesota Press.

Johnson, W. (1963). The problem of stuttering. In W. Johnson, F.L. Darley, & D.C. Spriestersbach, *Diagnostic methods in speech pathology* (pp. 240–276). New York: Harper & Row.

Johnson, W., Boehmler, R.M., Dahlstrom, W.G., Darley, F.L., Goodstein, L.D., Kools, J.A., Neelley, J.N., Prather, W.F., Sherman, D., Thurman, C.G., Trotter, W.D., Williams, D., & Young, M. (1959). *The onset of stuttering.* Minneapolis: University of Minnesota Press.

Johnson, W., & Brown, S.F. (1935). Stuttering in relation to various speech sounds. *Quarterly Journal of Speech, 21,* 481–496.

Johnson, W., & Brown, S.F. (1939). Stuttering in relation to various speech sounds: A correction. *Quarterly Journal of Speech, 25,* 20–22.

Johnson, W., Brown, S.F., Curtis, J.F., Edney, C.W., & Keaster, J. (1956). *Speech handicapped school children.* New York: Harper & Row.

Johnson, W., & Duke, L. (1935). Changes in handedness associated with onset or disappearance of stuttering: sixteen cases. *Journal of Experimental Education, 4,* 112–132.

Johnson, W., & Knott, J.R. (1937). Studies in the psychology of stuttering: I. The distribution of moments of stuttering during successive readings of the same material. *Journal of Speech Disorders, 2,* 17–19.

Johnson, W., & Knott, J.R. (1955). A systematic approach to the psychology of stuttering. In W. Johnson & R.R. Leutenegger (Eds.), *Stuttering in children and adults* (pp. 25–33). Minneapolis: University of Minnesota Press.

Johnson, W., & Leutenegger, R.R. (Eds.). (1955). *Stuttering in children and adults.* Minneapolis: University of Minnesota Press.

Jonas, G. (1977). *Stuttering: The disorder of many theories.* New York: Farrar, Straus and Giroux.

Jonas, S. (1981). The supplementary motor region and speech emission. *Journal of Communication Disorders, 14,* 349–373.

Kaasin, K., & Bjerkan, B. (1982). Critical words and the locus of stuttering in speech. *Journal of Fluency Disorders, 7,* 433–446.

Kaczmarek, B.L.J. (1984). Neurolinguistic analysis of verbal utterances in patients with focal lesions of frontal lobes. *Brain and Language, 21,* 52–58.

Kapos, E., & Standlee, L.S. (1958). Behavioral rigidity in adult stutterers. *Journal of Speech and Hearing Research, 1,* 294–296.

Karlin, I.W. (1959). Stuttering: Basically an organic disorder. *Logos, 2,* 61–63.

Kendon, A. (1967). Some functions of gaze direction in social interaction. *Acta Psychologica, 26,* 22–63.

Kent, R.D., & Moll, K.L. (1969). Vocal tract characteristics of the stop consonants. *Journal of the Acoustical Society of America, 46,* 1549–1555.

Kent, G.H., & Rosanoff, A.J. (1910). A study of association in insanity. *American Journal of Insanity, 67,* 37–96, 317–390.

Kent, G.H., & Rosanoff, A.J. (1921). *Free association test.* Chicago: Stoelting.

Kidd, K.K. (1980). Genetic models of stuttering. *Journal of Fluency Disorders, 5,* 187–202.

Kidd, K.K. (1983). Recent progress on the genetics of stuttering. In E. Ludlow & J. Cooper (Eds.), *Genetic aspects of speech and language disorders* (pp. 197–213). New York: Academic Press.

Kidd, K.K. (1984). Stuttering as a genetic disorder. In R. Curlee & W. Perkins (Eds.), *Nature and treatment of stuttering: New directions* (pp. 149–169). San Diego: College-Hill.

Kidd, K.K. Heimbuch, R.C., & Records, M.A. (1981). Vertical transmission of stuttering: Support for a genetic etiology. *Proceedings of the National Academy of Science, 78,* 606–610.

Kimura, D. (1964). Left-right differences in the perception of melodies. *Quarterly Journal of Experimental Psychology, 16,* 355–358.

King, P.T. (1953). *Perseverative factors in a stuttering and non-stuttering population.* Doctoral dissertation, Pennsylvania State University, University Park.

King, P.T. (1961). Perseveration in stutterers and non-stutterers. *Journal of Speech and Hearing Research, 4,* 346–357.

Kinsbourne, M. (1972). Eye and head turning indicates cerebral lateralization. *Science, 176,* 539–541.

Klatt, D.H. (1974). The duration of [s] in English words. *Journal of Speech and Hearing Research, 17,* 51–63.

Kleist, K. (1928). *Gehirnpathologie.* Leipzig, GDR: Barth.

Kline, D. (1959). *An experimental study of the frequency of stuttering in relation to certain goal-activity drives in basic human behavior.* Doctoral dissertation, University of Missouri, Columbia.

Kline, M.L., & Starkweather, C.W. (1979). Receptive and expressive language performance in young stutterers. *Asha, 21,* 797 (Abstr.).

Klingbeil, G.M. (1939). The historical background of the modern speech clinic. *Journal of Speech Disorders, 4,* 115–132.

Knabe, J.M., Nelson, L.A., & Williams, F. (1966). Some general characteristics of linguistic output: Stutterers versus nonstutterers. *Journal of Speech and Hearing Disorders, 31,* 178–182.

Kools, J.A. (1956). *Speech nonfluencies of stuttering and nonstuttering children.* Masters thesis, University of Iowa, Iowa City.

Kools, J.A., & Berryman, J.D. (1971). Differences in disfluency behavior between male and female nonstuttering children. *Journal of Speech and Hearing Research, 14,* 125–130.

Kopp, H.G. (1963). Eye movements in reading as related to speech dysfunction in male stutterers. *Speech Monographs, 30,* 248 (Abstr.).

Kowal, S., O'Connell, D.C., & Sabin, E.J. (1975). Development of temporal patterning and vocal hesitations in spontaneous narratives. *Journal of Psycholinguistic Research, 4,* 195–207.

Kozhevnikov, V.A., & Chistovich, L.A. (1965). *Speech: Articulation and perception.* Springfield, VA: U.S. Department of Commerce, Joint Publications Research Service, Vol. 30.

Kussmaul, A. (1877). Disturbances of speech. *Ziemssen's Cyclopaedia of the Practice of Medicine, 14.*

Ladefoged, P. (1963). Some physiological parameters in speech. *Language and Speech, 6,* 109–119.

Ladefoged, P. (1968). Linguistic aspects of respiratory phenomena. *Annals of the New York Academy of Science, 155,* 1–381.

Lamendella, J.T. (1977). The limbic system in human communication. In H. Whitaker & H.A. Whitaker (Eds.), *Studies in neurolinguistics, vol. 3* (pp. 157–222). New York: Academic Press.

Lanyon, R.I. (1968). Some characteristics of nonfluency in normal speakers and stutterers. *Journal of Abnormal Psychology, 73,* 550–555.

Lanyon, R.I. (1969). Speech: Relation of nonfluency to information value. *Science, 164,* 451–452.

Lanyon, R.I., & Duprez, D.A. (1970). Nonfluency, information and word length. *Journal of Abnormal Psychology, 76,* 93–97.

Lashley, K.S. (1951). The problem of serial order in behavior. In L.A. Jeffress (Ed.), *Cerebral Mechanisms in Behavior* (pp. 112–136). New York: Wiley.

Lass, N.J., & Noll, J.D. (1970). A comparative study of rate characteristics in cleft palate and noncleft palate speakers. *Cleft Palate Journal, 7,* 275–283.

Leeson, R. (1979). *Fluency and language teaching.* London: Longman.

Levin, H., & Silverman, I. (1965). Hesitation phenomena in children's speech. *Language and Speech, 8,* 65–85.

Levin, H., Silverman, I., & Ford, B.L. (1967). Hesitations in children's speech during explanations and description. *Journal of Verbal Learning and Verbal Behavior, 6,* 560–564.

Levy, J., Nebes, R.D., & Sperry, R.W. (1971). Expressive language in the surgically separated minor hemisphere. *Cortex, 7,* 49–58.

Lewis, M.M. (1934). *Infant speech: A study of the beginnings of language.* New York: Harcourt-Brace.

Liberman, A.M. (1970). The grammars of speech and language. *Cognitive Psychology, 1,* 301–323.

Liberman, A.M., Harris, K.S., Kinney, J., & Lane, H. (1961). The discrimination of relative onset time of the components of certain speech and nonspeech patterns. *Journal of Experimental Psychology, 61,* 379–388.

Lieberman, P. (1960). Some acoustic correlates of word stress in American English. *Journal of the Acoustical Society of America, 32,* 451–453.

Lieberman, P. (1963). Some effects of semantic and grammatical context on the production and perception of speech. *Language and Speech, 6,* 172–187.

Lieberman, P. (1967). *Intonation, perception, and language.* Cambridge, MA: MIT Press.

Lieberman, P. (1972). Primate vocalizations and human linguistic ability. In S.L. Washburn & P. Dolhinov (Eds.), *Perspectives on Human Evolution* (pp. 444–467). New York: Holt, Rinehart and Winston.

Lieberman, P. (1975). *On the origins of language: An introduction to the evolution of human speech.* New York: Macmillan.

Lieberman, P. (1984). *The biology and evolution of language.* Cambridge, MA: Harvard University Press.

Loban, W.D. (1961). *Language ability in the middle grades of the elementary school.* Department of Health, Education and Welfare, Office of Education, Report No. CRP-324, Research Program. Berkeley, CA.

Loban, W.D. (1976). *The language of elementary school children.* Urbana, IL: National Council of Teachers of English.

Long, R. (1961). *The sentence and its parts.* Chicago: University of Chicago Press.

Love, L.R., & Jeffress, L.A. (1971). Identification of brief pauses in the fluent speech of stutterers and nonstutterers. *Journal of Speech and Hearing Research, 14,* 229–240.

Luessenhop, A.J., Boggs, J.S., Laborowit, L.J., & Walle, E.L. (1973). Cerebral dominance in stutterers determined by Wada testing. *Neurology, 23,* 1190–1192.

Luper, H.L., & Mulder, R.L. (1964). *Stuttering: Therapy for children.* Englewood Cliffs, NJ: Prentice-Hall.

Luria, A.R. (1966). *Higher cortical functions in man.* London: Tavistock.

Luria, A. R. (1970). *Traumatic aphasia.* The Hague: Mouton.

Luria, A.R. (1972). *The man with a shattered world.* New York: Basic.

MacDonald, J.D., & Martin, R.R. (1973). Stuttering and disfluency as two reliable and unambiguous response classes. *Journal of Speech and Hearing Research, 16,* 691–699.

MacKay, D.G. (1972). The structure of words and syllables: Evidence from errors in speech. *Cognitive Psychology, 3,* 210–227.

MacKay, D.G. (1974). Aspects of the syntax of behavior: Syllable structure and speech rate. *Quarterly Journal of Experimental Psychology, 26,* 642–657.

MacKay, D.G. (1978). Speech errors inside the syllable. In A. Bell & J.B. Hooper (Eds.), *Syllables and Segments* (pp. 201–212). Amsterdam: North Holland.

Maclay, H., & Osgood, C.E. (1959). Hesitation phenomena in spontaneous English speech. *Word, 15,* 19–44.

MacLean, P.D. (1978). The evolution of the three mentalities. In S.L. Washburn & E.R. McCown (Eds.), *Human evolution: Biosocial perspectives* (pp. 35–37). Menlo Park, CA: Cummings.

MacNeilage, P.F., & DeClerk, J.L. (1969). On the motor control of coarticulation in CVC syllables. *Journal of the Acoustical Society of America, 46,* 1217–1233.

MacNeilage, P.F., & Scholes, G.N. (1964). An electromyographic study of the tongue during vowel production. *Journal of Speech and Hearing Research, 7,* 209–232.

Mader, J.B. (1954). The relative frequency of occurrence of English consonant sounds in words in the speech of children in grades one, two and three. *Speech Monographs, 21,* 294–300.

Mahl, G.F. (1956a). Disturbances and silences in the patient's speech in psychotherapy. *Journal of Abnormal and Social Psychology, 53,* 1–15.

Mahl, G.F. (1956b). *Disturbances in the patient's speech as a function of anxiety.* Paper presented at the meeting of the Eastern Psychological Association, March 23–24, Atlantic City.

Mahl, G.F. (1956c, August 30–September 5). *"Normal" disturbances in spontaneous speech.* Paper presented at the meeting of the American Psychological Association, Chicago.

Mahl, G.F. (1958). On the use of "ah" in spontaneous speech: quantitative, developmental, characterological, situational and linguistic aspects. *American Psychologist, 13,* 349.

Mahl, G.F. (1959a). Exploring emotional states by content analysis. In I. Pool (Ed.), *Trends in content analysis* (pp. 89–130). Urbana, IL: University of Illinois Press.

Mahl, G.F. (1959b). Measuring the patient's anxiety during interviews from "expressive" aspects of his speech. *Transactions of the New York Academy of Sciences, 21* (Series 11), 249.

Mahl, G.F. (1960, December). The lexical and linguistic levels in the expression of the emotions. In *Expression of the Emotions in Man: A Symposium on the Methods of Study and the Psychological Classification of Emotional Phenomena* (Chapter 5). Meeting of the American Association for the Advancement of Science, New York.

Mahl, G.F. (1981). Normal disturbances in speech. In R.L. Russel (Ed.), *Spoken interaction in psychotherapy: Strategies of discovery.* New York: Irvington.

Malmberg, B. (1963). *Phonetics.* New York: Dover.

Mann, M.B. (1937). *Stuttering in relation to speech sounds for young children.* Masters thesis, University of Iowa, Iowa City.

Mann, M.B. (1944). Studies in language behavior: III. The quantitative differentiation of samples of written language. *Psychological Monographs, 56,* 41–74.

Markham, C.H., & Rand, R. (1963). Stereotaxic surgery in Parkinson's disease. *Neurology, 3,* 621–634.

Marler, P. (1975). On the origin of speech from animal sounds. In J.F. Kavanagh & J.E. Cutting (Eds.), *The role of speech in language* (pp. 11 to 37). Cambridge, MA: MIT Press.

Martin, J.G. (1972). Rhythmic (hierarchical) versus serial structure in speech and other behavior. *Psychological Review, 79,* 487–509.

Martin, J.G., & Strange, W. (1968). The perception of hesitation in spontaneous speech. *Perception and Psychophysics, 3,* 427–438.

Martin, R. (1962). Stuttering and perseveration in children. *Journal of Speech and Hearing Research, 5,* 332–339.

Mateer, C.A., & Ojemann, G.A. (1983). Thalamic mechanisms in language and memory. In S.J. Segalowitz (Ed.), *Language functions and brain organization* (pp. 171–191). New York: Academic Press.

McCarthy, D.A. (1930). The language development of the preschool child. University of Minnesota Institute of Child Welfare Monograph Series (4). Minneapolis: University of Minnesota Press.

McClean, M., Goldsmith, H., & Cerf, A. (1984). Lower-lip EMG and displacement during bilabial disfluencies in adult stutterers. *Journal of Speech and Hearing Research, 27,* 342–349.

McCormack, W.C. (1966). *Kannada: A cultural introduction to the spoken styles of the language.* Madison, WI: University of Wisconsin Press.

McDowell, E.D. (1928). Educational and emotional adjustments of stuttering children. Columbia University Teachers College, Contributions to Education, (314).

McFarling, D., Rothi, L.J., & Heilman, K.M. (1982). Transcortical aphasia from ischaemic infarcts of the thalamus: A report of two cases. *Journal of Neurology, Neurosurgery and Psychiatry, 45,* 107–112.

McNeill, D. (1966). A study of word association. *Journal of Verbal Learning and Verbal Behavior, 5,* 548–557.

McNeill, D. (1970). *The acquisition of language.* New York: Harper & Row.

McNeill, D., & Lindig, K. (1973). The perceptual reality of phonemes, syllables, words and sentences. *Journal of Verbal Learning and Verbal Behavior, 12,* 419–430.

Meissner, J.H. (1946). The relationship between voluntary non-fluency and stuttering. *Journal of Speech Disorders, 11,* 13–23.

Milisen, R.L. (1937). *Anticipation of stuttering as related to the frequency, type and point of occurrence of overt stuttering.* Doctoral dissertation, University of Iowa, Iowa City.

Milisen, R., & Johnson, W. (1936). A comparative study of stutterers, former stutters and normal speakers whose handedness has been changed. *Archives of Speech, 1,* 61–86.

Miller, G.A. (1951). *Language and communication*. New York: McGraw-Hill.

Miller, G.A. (1963). *Language and communication.* (2nd ed.). New York: McGraw-Hill.

Miller, G.A., Newman, E.B., & Friedman, E.A. (1958). Length-frequency statistics for written English. *Information and Control, 1,* 370–389.

Milner, B. (1962). Laterality effects in audition. In V.B. Mountcastle (Ed.), *Interhemispheric relations and cerebral dominance* (pp. 177–195). Baltimore, MD: Johns Hopkins Press.

Milner, B. (1964). Some effects of frontal lobectomy in man. In K.M. Warren & K. Akert (Eds.), *The frontal granular cortex and behavior* (pp. 313–334). New York: McGraw-Hill.

Milner, B. (1967). Brain mechanisms suggested by studies of temporal lobes. In F. Darley (Ed.), *Brain mechanisms underlying speech and language* (pp. 122–131). New York: Grune and Stratton.

Minifie, F.D., & Cooker, H.S. (1964). A disfluency index. *Journal of Speech and Hearing Disorders, 29,* 189–192.

Monrad-Krohn, G.H. (1947). Dysprosody or altered "melody of language." *Brain, 70,* 405–415.

Monrad-Krohn, G.H. (1963). The third element of speech: Prosody and its disor-

ders. In J. Halpern (Ed.), *Problems of dynamic neurology* (pp. 110–117). Jerusalem: Hebrew University Press.
Moscovici, S., & Humbert, C. (1960). Etudes sur le comportement verbal: Langage oral et langage ecrit [Studies of verbal behavior: Oral and written language]. *Psychologie Francaise, 5,* 175–186.
Moser, H.M. (1935). A photographic analysis of eye movements during stuttering. *Proceedings of the American Speech Correction Association, 5,* 71–74.
Moser, H.M. (1938). A qualitative analysis of eye movements during stuttering. *Journal of Speech Disorders, 3,* 131–139.
Moser, H., Dreher, J.J., & Oyer, H.J. (1957). *One Syllable Words.* Technical Report No. 41, Contract No. AF 19(604)-1577. Columbus, OH: Ohio State University Research Foundation.
Muma, J.R. (1971). Syntax of preschool fluent and disfluent speech: A transformational analysis. *Journal of Speech and Hearing Research, 14,* 428–441.
Murray, E. (1931). Dysintegration of breathing and eye movements in stutterers during silent reading and reasoning. *Psychological Monographs, 43,* 218–274.
Murray, H., & Reed, C. (1977). Language abilities of preschool stuttering children. *Journal of Fluency Disorders, 2,* 171–176.
Myers, R.E. (1978). Comparative neurology of vocalization and speech. In S.L. Washburn & E.R. McCown (Eds.), *Human evolution: Biosocial perspectives* (pp. 58–75). Menlo Park, CA: Cummings.
Newman, P.W., Fawcett, K.D., & Russon, K.V. (1986). Cognitive processing in stuttering as related to translating Slurvian. *Journal of Fluency Disorders, 11,* 251–256.
Nice, M. (1915). The speech of a left-handed child. *Psychological Clinic, 9,* 115–117.
Nicol, M.A., & Miller, R.M. (1959). Word redundancy in written English. *Australian Journal of Psychology, 11,* 81–91.
O'Connor, J.D. (1977). *Phonetics.* New York: Penguin.
Ohman, S.E.G. (1963). Coarticulation of stops with vowels. *Quarterly Progress and Status Report, 2/63,* 1–8. Speech Transmission Laboratory, Royal Institute of Technology, Stockholm.
Ohman, S.E.G. (1966). Coarticulation in VCV utterances: Spectrographic measurements. *Journal of the Acoustical Society of America, 39,* 151–168.
Ojemann, G.A., & Ward, A.A. Jr. (1971). Speech representation in ventrolateral thalamus. *Brain, 94,* 669–680.
Ojemann, G.A., Fedio, P., & Van Buren, J.M. (1968). Anomia from pulvinar and subcortical parietal stimulation. *Brain, 91,* 99–116.
Ojemann, G.A., Hoyenga, K., & Ward, A. Jr. (1971). Prediction of short term verbal memory disturbance after ventrolateral thalamotomy. *Journal of Neurosurgery, 35,* 203–210.
Okasha, A., Bishry, Z., Kamel, M., & Hassan, A.H. (1974). Psychosocial study of stammering in Egyptian children. *British Journal of Psychiatry, 124,* 531–533.
Oller, D.K. (1980). The emergence of the sounds of speech in infancy. In G.H. Yeni-Komshian, J.F. Kavanagh, & C.A. Ferguson (Eds.), *Child phonology, vol. 1: Production* (pp. 93–112). New York: Academic Press.
Ortleb, R. (1937). An objective study of emphasis in oral reading of emotional and unemotional material. *Speech Monographs, 4,* 56–68.
Orton, S.T. (1927). Studies in stuttering: Introduction. *Archives of Neurology and Psychiatry, 18,* 671–672.

Orton, S.T. (1929). A physiological theory of reading disability and stuttering in children. *New England Journal of Medicine, 199,* 1046–1052.

Osgood, C.E. (1971). Where do sentences come from? In D. Steinberg & L.A. Jakobovits (Eds.), *Semantics: An interdisciplinary reader in philosophy, linguistics and psychology* (pp. 497–529). London: Cambridge University Press.

Osgood, C.E., & Sebeok, T.A. (Eds.), (1954). *Psycholinguistics: A survey of theory and research problems.* Baltimore, MD: Waverly Press.

Oxtoby, E.T. (1943). *A quantitative study of repetition in the speech of three-year-old children.* Masters thesis, University of Iowa, Iowa City.

Oxtoby, E.T. (1946). *A quantitative study of certain phenomena related to expectancy of stuttering.* Doctoral dissertation, University of Iowa, Iowa City. (A condensation of this paper appears as Chapter 10 in W. Johnson, (Ed.). (1955). *Stuttering in children and adults.* Minneapolis: University of Minnesota Press.)

Palen, C., & Peterson, J.M. (1982). Word frequency and children's stuttering: The relationship to sentence structure. *Journal of Fluency Disorders, 7,* 55–67.

Palermo, D.S., & Jenkins, J.J. (1964). *Word association norms: Grade school through college.* Minneapolis: University of Minnesota Press.

Parker, H.T. (1932). Defects of speech in school children. *Educational Research Series No. 15.* Melbourne, Australia: University of Melbourne Press.

Pease, D.M., & Goodglass, H. (1978). The effects of cueing on picture naming in aphasia. *Cortex, 14,* 178–189.

Pelc, M.W., & Leeper, H.A. Jr. (1976). An aerodynamic investigation of syllable asymmetry during sentence production. *Central States Speech Journal, 27,* 109–112.

Penfield, W., & Roberts, L. (1959). *Speech and brain mechanisms.* Princeton, NJ: Princeton University Press.

Perkell, J.S. (1969). *Physiology of speech production: Results and implications of a quantitative cineradiographic study.* Research Monograph No 53. Cambridge, MA: MIT Press.

Perkins, W.H. (1983). The problem of definition: Commentary on "stuttering." *Journal of Speech and Hearing Disorders, 48,* 246–249.

Perozzi, J.A. (1970). Phonetic skill (sound mindedness) of stuttering children. *Journal of Communication Disorders, 3,* 207–210.

Perozzi, J.A., & Kunze, L.H. (1969). Language abilities of stuttering children. *Folia Phoniatrica, 2,* 386–392.

Perret, E. (1974). The left frontal lobe of man and the suppression of habitual responses in verbal categorical behavior. *Neuropsychologia, 12,* 323–330.

Peterson, G.E., & Lehiste, I. (1960). Duration of syllable nuclei in English. *Journal of the Acoustical Society of America, 32,* 693–703.

Peterson, H.A. (1969). Affective meaning of words as rated by stuttering and nonstuttering readers. *Journal of Speech and Hearing Research, 12,* 337–343.

Peterson, H.A., Rieck, M.B., & Hoff, R.K. (1969). A test of satiation as a function of adaptation in stuttering. *Journal of Speech and Hearing Research, 12,* 110–117.

Pinsky, S.D., & McAdam, D.W. (1980). Electroencephalographic and dichotic indices of cerebral laterality in stutterers. *Brain and Language, 11,* 374–397.

Pittenger, K. (1940). A study of the duration of temporal intervals between successive moments of stuttering. *Journal of Speech Disorders, 5,* 333–341.

Polyani, M. (1964). *Personal knowledge: Towards a post-critical philosophy.* New York: Harper & Row.

Porter, H. (1939). Studies in the psychology of stuttering: XIV. Stuttering phenomena in relation to size and personnel of audience. *Journal of Speech Disorders, 4,* 323–333.

Postman, L., & Keppel, G. (1970). *Norms of word association.* New York: Academic Press.

Potter, S.O.L. (1882). *Speech and its defects.* Philadelphia; Blakiston.

Preus, A., Gullikstad, L., Grotterod, H., Erlandson, O., & Halland, J. (1970). En undersokelse over forekomst av stamming i en lest tekst. *Norsk tidsskrift for logopedi, 16,* 11–18.

Primary mental abilities. (1949). Chicago: Science Research.

Prins, D., & Beaudet, R. (1980). Defense preference and stutterers' speech disfluencies: Implications for the nature of the disorder. *Journal of Speech and Hearing Research, 23,* 757–768.

Ptacek, P.H., & Sanders, E.K. (1966). Age recognition from voice. *Journal of Speech and Hearing Research, 9,* 273–277.

Quarrington, B. (1965). Stuttering as a function of the information value and sentence position of words. *Journal of Abnormal Psychology, 70,* 221–224.

Quarrington, B., Conway, J., & Siegel, N. (1962). An experimental study of some properties of stuttered words. *Journal of Speech and Hearing Research, 5,* 387–394.

Rapaport, D., Gill, M., & Schafer, R. (1946). *Diagnostic psychological testing* (Vol 2). Chicago: Year Book.

Razdol'skii, V.A. (1965). State of speech in stammerers when alone. *Zhurnal Nevropatologii i Psikhiatrii imeni S.S. Korsakova, 65,* 1717–1720.

Records, M.A., Heimbuch, R.C., & Kidd, K.K. (1977). Handedness and stuttering: A dead horse? *Journal of Fluency Disorders, 2,* 271–282.

Reich, A., Till, J., & Goldsmith, H. (1981). Laryngeal and manual reaction times of stuttering and nonstuttering adults. *Journal of Speech and Hearing Research, 24,* 192–196.

Reid, L. (1946). Some facts about stuttering. *Journal of Speech Disorders, 11,* 3–12.

Rieber, R.W., & Wollock, J. (1977). The historical roots of the theory and therapy of stuttering. In R.W. Rieber, (Ed.), *The problem of stuttering: Theory and therapy* (pp. 3–24). New York: Elsevier.

Riklan, M., & Levita, E. (1970). Psychological studies of thalamic lesions in humans. *Journal of Nervous and Mental Disease, 150,* 251–265.

Robbins, S.D. (1936). The relative attention paid to vowels and consonants by stammerers and normal speakers. *Proceedings of the American Speech Correction Association, 6,* 7–22.

Roberts, A.H. (1965). *A statistical linguistic analysis of American English.* The Hague: Mouton.

Robinson, B.W. (1972). Anatomical and physiological contrasts between human and other primate vocalizations. In S.L. Washburn & P. Dolhinov (Eds.), *Perspectives on human evolution.* New York: Holt, Rinehart and Winston.

Robinson, B.W. (1976). Limbic influences on human speech. *Annals of the New York Academy of Science, 280,* 761–771.

Ronson, I. (1976). Word frequency and stuttering: The relationship to sentence structure. *Journal of Speech and Hearing Research, 19,* 813–819.

Rosenbek, J., Messert, B., Collins, M., & Wertz, R.T. (1978). Stuttering following brain damage. *Brain and Language, 6,* 82–96.

Rosenfield, D.B. (1980). Cerebral dominance and stuttering. *Journal of Fluency Disorders, 5,* 171–185.

Ross, E.D. (1981). The aprosodias. *Archives of Neurology, 38,* 561–569.

Ross, E.D., & Mesulam, M-M. (1979). Dominant language functions of the right hemisphere? *Archives of Neurology, 36,* 144–148.

Runyan, C.M., & Adams, M.R. (1979). Unsophisticated judges' perceptual evaluations of the speech of "successfully treated" stutterers. *Journal of Fluency Disorders, 4,* 29–38.

Russell, W.A., & Jenkins, J.J. (1954). *The complete Minnesota norms for responses to 100 words from the Kent-Rosanoff word association test.* (Tech. Rep. No. 11). Minneapolis: University of Minnesota Press, Studies on the Role of Language Behavior.

Rylander, G. (1948). Personality analysis before and after frontal lobotomy. *Research Publications of the Association for Nervous and Mental Disease, 27,* 691–705.

Sachs, M.W. (1924). Zur aetiologie des Stottern [On the etiology of stuttering]. *Klinische Wochenschrift, 37,* 113–115.

Sachs, J., Brown, R., & Salerno, R. (1976). Adult speech to children. In W. Von Raffler-Engel & Y. Lebrun (Eds.), *Baby talk and infant speech* (pp. 240–245). Amsterdam: Swets and Zeitlinger.

St. Louis, K.O., & Martin, R.R. (1976). Motor speech awareness in stutterers: Reorganization of distinctive features. *Asha, 18,* 593. (Abstr.)

St. Onge, K.R. (1963). The stuttering syndrome. *Journal of Speech and Hearing Research, 6,* 195–197.

Samra, K., Riklan, M., Levita, E., Zimmerman, J., Waltz, J.M., Bergmann, L., & Cooper, I.S. (1969). Language and speech correlates of anatomically verified lesions in thalamic surgery for Parkinsonism. *Journal of Speech and Hearing Research, 12,* 510–540.

Samson, C.L., & Cooper, E.B. (1980). Motor perseverative behavior in adult stutterers and nonstutterers. *Journal of Fluency Disorders, 5,* 359–372.

Sanford, F. (1942). Speech and personality. *Psychological Bulletin, 39,* 811–845.

Sankoff, D., & Lessard, R. (1975). Vocabulary richness: A sociolinguistic analysis. *Science, 190,* 689–690.

Saporta, S. (1955). Linguistic structure as a factor and as a measure in word association. In J.J. Jenkins (Ed.), *Associative processes in verbal behavior* (pp. 210–214). Minneapolis: University of Minnesota Press.

Savin, H. (1963). The word frequency effect and errors in the perception of speech. *Journal of the Acoustical Society of America, 35,* 200–206.

Schaie, K.W. (1955). A test of behavioral rigidity. *Journal of Abnormal and Social Psychology, 51,* 604–610.

Schaie, K.W. (1960). *Test of behavioral rigidity, research edition.* Palo Alto, CA: Consulting Psychologists Press.

Schaie, K.W. (1970). A reinterpretation of age-related changes in cognitive structure and functioning. In L.R. Goulet & P.B. Baltes (Eds.), *Life-span developmental psychology: Research and theory* (pp. 486–507). New York: Academic Press.

Schaie, K.W., & Parham, I.A. (1975). *Test of behavioral rigidity.* Palo Alto, CA: Consulting Psychologists Press.

Schaltenbrand, G. (1965). The effects of stereotactic electrical stimulation in the depth of the brain. *Brain, 88,* 835–840.

Schaltenbrand, G., Spuer, H., Wahren, W., & Rummler, B. (1971). Electro-anatomy of the thalamic ventral-oral nucleus based on stereotactic stimulation in man. *Zeitschrift fur Neurologie, 199,* 259–276.

Schiffman, H.F. (1983). *A reference grammer of spoken Kannada.* Seattle: University of Washington Press.

Schlesinger, I.M., Forte, M., Fried, B., & Melkman, R. (1965). Stuttering, information load and response strength. *Journal of Speech and Hearing Disorders, 30,* 32–36.

Schlesinger, I.M., Melkman, R., & Levy, R. (1966). Word length and frequency as determinants of stuttering. *Psychonomic Science, 6,* 255–256.

Schramm, W.L. (1937). The acoustical nature of accent in American speech. *American Speech, 12,* 49–56.

Selby, G. (1967). Stereotactic surgery for the relief of Parkinson's disease: II. An analysis of the results of a series of 303 patients (413 operations). *Journal of Neurological Science, 5,* 343–375.

Self-Therapy for the Stutterer (4th ed.). Memphis, TN: Speech Foundation of America, Publication No. 12.

Selkirk, E. (1984). On the major class features and syllable theory. In M. Aronoff & R. T. Oehrle (Eds.), *Language sound and structure* (pp. 107–136). Cambridge, MA: MIT Press.

Shankweiler, D. (1966). Effects of temporal lobe damage on perception of dichotically presented melodies. *Journal of Comparative and Physiological Psychology, 62,* 115–119.

Shankweiler, D. (1971). An analysis of laterality effects in speech perception. In D.L. Horton & J.J. Jenkins (Eds.), *The perception of language* (pp. 185–200). Columbus, OH: Merrill.

Shannon, C.E., & Weaver, W. (1949). *The mathematical theory of communication.* Urbana, IL: University of Illinois Press.

Shapiro, B.E., & Danly, M. (1985). The role of the right hemisphere in the control of speech prosody in propositional and affective contexts. *Brain and Language, 25,* 19–36.

Shapiro, C.W. (1970). *Phrasal stress patterns of the fluent speech of stutterers and non-stutterers.* Masters thesis, State University of New York at Buffalo.

Shattuck-Hufnagel, S. (1981). Position constraints on segment exchange errors in production and memory. *Journal of the Acoustical Society of America, 70* (S 13. Suppl. 1).

Shattuck-Hufnagel, S. (1983). Sublexical units and suprasegmental structure in speech production and planning. In P.F. MacNeilage (Ed.), *The production of speech* (pp. 109–136). New York: Springer-Verlag.

Shattuck-Hufnagel, S. (1987). The role of word-onset consonants in speech production planning: New evidence from speech error patterns. In E. Keller & M. Gopnik (Eds.), *Motor and sensory processes of language* (pp. 17–51). Hillsdale, NJ: Erlbaum.

Shattuck-Hufnagel, S., & Klatt, D.H. (1975). An analysis of 1500 phonetic errors in spontaneous speech. *Journal of the Acoustical Society of America, 58,* (S62. Suppl. 1).

Shattuck-Hufnagel, S., & Klatt, D.H. (1979). The limited use of distinctive features and markedness in speech production: Evidence from speech error data. *Journal of Verbal Learning and Verbal Behavior, 18,* 41–55.

Sheehan, J.G. (1953). Theory and treatment of stuttering as an approach-avoidance conflict. *Journal of Psychology, 36,* 27–49.

Sheehan, J.G. (1958). Conflict theory of stuttering. In J. Eisenson (Ed.), *Stuttering: A symposium* (pp. 121–166). New York: Harper & Row.

Sheehan, J.G. (1969). Cyclic variation in stuttering: Comment on Taylor and Taylor's "Test of predictions from the conflict hypothesis of stuttering." *Journal of Abnormal Psychology, 74,* 452–453.

Sheehan, J.G. (1970). *Stuttering: Research and therapy.* New York: Harper & Row.

Sheehan, J.G. (1974). Stuttering behavior: A phonetic analysis. *Journal of Fluency Disorders, 7,* 193–212.

Sheehan, J.G. (1975). Conflict theory and avoidance-reduction therapy. In J. Eisenson (Ed.), *Stuttering: A second symposium* (pp. 99–198). New York: Harper & Row.

Sheets, B. (1941). *A study of visual perseverative tendencies of stutterers and normal speakers.* Masters thesis, University of Utah, Salt Lake City.

Silverman, E.M. (1972). Generality of disfluency data collected from preschoolers. *Journal of Speech and Hearing Research, 5,* 84–92.

Silverman, E.M. (1973). The influence of preschoolers' speech usage on their disfluency frequency. *Journal of Speech and Hearing Research, 16,* 474–481.

Silverman, E.M. (1974). Word position and grammatical function in relation to preschoolers' speech disfluency. *Perceptual and Motor Skills, 39,* 267–272.

Silverman, F.H. (1965). The loci of disfluencies in the speech of stutterers and nonstutterers during oral reading. *Asha, 7,* 381 (Abstr.).

Silverman, F.H. (1970). Course of nonstutterers' disfluency adaptation during 15 consecutive oral readings of the same material. *Journal of Speech and Hearing Research, 13,* 382–386.

Silverman, F.H. (1974). Disfluency behavior of elementary school stutterers and non-stutterers. *Language, Speech and Hearing Services in Schools, 5,* 32–37.

Silverman, F.H., & Williams, D.E. (1967a). Loci of disfluencies in the speech of nonstutterers during oral reading. *Journal of Speech and Hearing Research, 10,* 790–794.

Silverman, F.H., & Williams, D.E. (1967b). Loci of disfluencies in the speech of stutterers. *Perceptual and Motor Skills, 24,* 1085–1086.

Silverman, F.H., & Williams, D.E. (1971). The adaptation effect for six types of speech disfluency. *Journal of Speech and Hearing Research, 14,* 525–530.

Sitzman, B. (1968). *Stuttering as a function of word predictability.* Doctoral dissertation, University of California at Los Angeles.

Slobin, D. (1966). Grammatical transformations in childhood and adulthood. *Journal of Verbal Learning and Verbal Behavior, 5,* 219–227.

Smith, A. (1966). Speech and other functions following left (dominant) hemispherectomy. *Journal of Neurology, Neurosurgery and Psychiatry, 29,* 467–471.

Smith, H.L. (1959). Toward redefining English prosody. *Studies in Linguistics, 14,* (3 & 4). Buffalo, NY: University of Buffalo.

Smyth, G.E., & Stern, K. (1938). Tumours of the thalamus. *Brain, 61,* 339–360.

Snidecor, J.C. (1943). A comparative study of pitch and duration characteristics of impromptu speaking and oral reading. *Speech Monographs, 10,* 50–56.

Snidecor, J.C. (1944). An objective study of phrasing in impromptu speaking and oral reading. *Speech Monographs, 11,* 97–104.

Snow, C. (1972). Mothers' speech to children learning language. *Child Development, 43,* 549–565.

Soderberg, G.A. (1962a). Phonetic influences upon stuttering. *Journal of Speech and Hearing Research, 5,* 315–320.

Soderberg, G.A. (1962b). What is "average" stuttering? *Journal of Speech and Hearing Disorders, 27,* 85–86.

Soderberg, G.A. (1966). The relations of stuttering to word length and word frequency. *Journal of Speech and Hearing Research, 9,* 584–589.

Soderberg, G.A. (1967). Linguistic factors in stuttering. *Journal of Speech and Hearing Research, 10,* 801–810.

Soderberg, G.A. (1969). A comparison of adaptation trends in the oral reading of stutterers, inferior speakers and superior speakers. *Journal of Communication Disorders, 2,* 99–108.

Soderberg, G.A. (1971). Relations of word information and word length to stuttering disfluencies. *Journal of Communication Disorders, 4,* 9–14.

Soderberg, G.A. (1972, November). *Symposium on linguistic-motor determinants of stuttering.* Presented at the annual convention of the *American Speech and Hearing Association,* San Francisco.

Soderberg, G.A., & MacKay, D.G. (1972). The function relating stuttering to phoneme frequency and transition probability. *Journal of Verbal Learning and Verbal Behavior, 11,* 83–91.

Solomon, M. (1932). Stuttering as an emotional disorder. *Proceedings of the American Speech Correction Association, 2,* 118–121.

Solomon, N.D. (1951). *A comparison of rigidity of behavior manifested by a group of stutterers compared with "fluent" speakers in oral and other performances as measured by the Einstellung effect.* Masters thesis, University of Michigan, Ann Arbor.

Sparks, R., Helm, N., & Albert, M. (1974). Aphasia rehabilitation from Melodic Intonation Therapy. *Cortex, 10,* 303–316.

Spotting and stopping stuttering. (1983, October). *Changing Times,* pp. 64–67.

Stark, R.E. (1980). Stages of speech development in the first year of life. In G.H. Yeni-Komshian, J.F. Kavanagh, & C.A. Ferguson (Eds.), *Child phonology, vol. 1: Production* (pp. 73–92). New York: Academic Press.

Steer, M.D., & Tiffin, J. (1934). A photographic study of the use of intensity by superior speakers. *Speech Monographs, 1,* 72–78.

Stein, L. (1942). *Speech and voice.* London: Methuen.

Stemberger, J.P. (1983). Inflectional malapropisms: Form-based errors in English morphology. *Linguistics, 21,* 573–602.

Still, A.W., & Griggs, S. (1979). Changes in the probability of stuttering following a stutter: A test of some recent models. *Journal of Speech and Hearing Research, 22,* 565–571.

Still, A.W., & Sherrard, C.A. (1976). Formalizing theories of stuttering. *British Journal of Mathematical and Statistical Psychology, 29,* 129–138.

Strickland, R.G. (1962). The language of elementary school children: Its relation to the language of reading texts and the quality of reading of selected children. *Bulletin, School of Education, Indiana University, 38* (4).

Studdert-Kennedy, M. (1975). From continuous signal to discrete message: Syllable to phoneme. In J.F. Kavanagh & J.E. Cutting (Eds.), *The role of speech in language* (pp. 113–125). Cambridge, MA: MIT Press.

Sumby, W.H., & Pollack, I. (1954). *Short-time processing of information.* (Tech. Rep. No. 54–6.) Human Factors Operations Research Laboratories.

Sussman, H.M., & MacNeilage, P.F. (1975). Hemispheric specialization for speech production and perception in stutterers. *Neuropsychologia, 13,* 19–26.

Sweet, H. (1877). Handbook of phonetics. Oxford: Clarendon Press.

Taylor, I.K. (1966a). The properties of stuttered words. *Journal of Verbal Learning and Verbal Behavior, 5,* 112–118.

Taylor, I.K. (1966b). What words are stuttered? *Psychological Bulletin, 65,* 233–242.

Taylor, I.K. (1976). *Introduction to psycholinguistics* (p. 345). New York: Holt, Rinehart and Winston.

Taylor, I.K., & Taylor, M.M. (1967). Test of predictions from the conflict hypothesis of stuttering. *Journal of Abnormal Psychology, 72,* 431–433.

Telser, E.B. (1971). *An assessment of word-finding skills in stuttering and nonstuttering children.* Doctoral dissertation, Northwestern University, Evanston, IL.

Terman, L.M., & Merrill, M.A. (1937). *Measuring intelligence.* New York: Houghton Mifflin.

Thorndike, E.L., & Lorge, I. (1944). *The teacher's word book of 30,000 words.* New York: Teachers College, Columbia University Press.

Thurstone, L.L. (1938). *Primary mental abilities.* Chicago: University of Chicago Press.

Thurstone, L.L., & Thurstone, T.G. (1941). *Factorial studies of intelligence.* Chicago: University of Chicago Press.

Thurstone, T.G., Thurstone, L.L., & Strandskov, H.H. (1955). *A psychological study of twins.* Chapel Hill, NC: Psychometric Laboratory, University of North Carolina (Rep. No. 4).

Tiffany, W.R. (1963a). Slurvian translation as a speech research tool. *Speech Monographs, 30,* 23–30.

Tiffany, W.R. (1963b). Sound-mindedness: Studies in the measurement of "phonetic ability." *Western Speech, 27,* 5–15.

Tiffin, J., & Steer, M.D. (1937). An experimental analysis of emphasis. *Speech Monographs, 4,* 69–74.

Tornick, G.B., & Bloodstein, O. (1976). Stuttering and sentence length. *Journal of Speech and Hearing Research, 19,* 651–654.

Trager, G.L., & Smith, H.L. (1962). *An outline of English structure.* Washington, DC: American Council of Learned Societies.

Travis, L.E. (1928). The influence of the group upon the stutterer's speech in free association. *Journal of Abnormal and Social Psychology, 23,* 45–51.

Travis, L.E. (1933a). A neurological consideration of stuttering. *Spoken Word, 1,* 8–11.

Travis, L.E. (1933b). Speech pathology. In C. Murchison (Ed.), *A Handbook of*

Child Psychology, (2nd ed.). (pp. 650–698). Worcester, MA: Clark University Press.
Travis, L.E. (1971). *Handbook of speech pathology and audiology.* Englewood Cliffs, NJ: Prentice-Hall.
Travis, L.E. (1978a). Cerebral dominance theory of stuttering: 1931–1978. *Journal of Speech and Hearing Disorders, 43,* 278–281.
Travis, L.E. (1978b). Neurophysiological dominance. *Journal of Speech and Hearing Disorders, 43,* 275–277.
Travis, L.E., & Johnson, W. (1934). Stuttering and the concept of handedness. *Psychological Review, 41,* 534–562.
Treiman, R. (1983). The structure of spoken syllables: Evidence from novel word games. *Cognition, 15,* 49–74.
Treiman, R. (1985). Onsets and rimes as units of spoken syllables: Evidence from children. *Journal of Experimental Child Psychology, 39,* 161–181.
Trnka, B. (1968). *A phonological analysis of present day standard English.* University, AL: University of Alabama Press.
Trotter, W.D. (1956). Relationship between severity of stuttering and word conspicuousness. *Journal of Speech and Hearing Disorders, 21,* 198–201.
Tweney, R.D., Tkacz, S., & Zaruba, S. (1975). Slips of the tongue and lexical storage. *Language and Speech, 18,* 388–396.
Ustvedt, H. (1937). Über die Untersuchung der musikalischen Functionen bei Patienten mit Aphasie. *Acta Otolaryngolica,* Supplement.
Vandenberg, S.G. (1962). The hereditary abilities study: Hereditary components in a psychological test battery. *American Journal of Human Genetics, 14,* 220–237.
Vandenberg, S.G. (1964). The developmental study of twins. *American Psychologist, 19,* 537.
Vandenberg, S.G. (1967). Hereditary factors in psychological variables in man, with a special emphasis on cognition. In J.N. Spuhler (Ed.), *Genetic diversity and human behavior* (pp. 99–133). Chicago: Aldine.
Van Dusen, C.R. (1939). A laterality study of nonstutterers and stutterers. *Journal of Speech Disorders, 4,* 261–265.
Van Riper, C. (1937). The effect of devices for minimizing stuttering on the creation of symptoms. *Journal of Abnormal and Social Psychology, 32,* 185–192.
Van Riper, C. (1954). *Speech correction: Principles and methods* (3rd ed.). Englewood Cliffs, NJ: Prentice-Hall.
Van Riper, C. (1963). *Speech correction: Principles and methods* (4th ed.). Englewood Cliffs, NJ: Prentice-Hall.
Van Riper, C. (1971). *The nature of stuttering.* Englewood Cliffs, NJ: Prentice-Hall.
Van Riper, C. (1973). *The treatment of stuttering.* Englewood Cliffs, NJ: Prentice-Hall.
Van Riper, C., & Hull, C.J. (1955). The quantitative measurement of the effect of certain situations on stuttering. In W. Johnson & R.R. Leutenegger (Eds.), *Stuttering in children and adults* (pp. 199–206). Minneapolis: University of Minnesota Press.
Venneman, T. (1972a). On the theory of syllabic phonology. *Linguistische Berichte, 18,* 1–18.

Venneman, T. (1972b). Phonological uniqueness in natural generative grammar. *Glossa, 6,* 105–116.

Vilkki, J., & Laitinen, L.V. (1974). Differential effects of left and right ventrolateral thalamotomy on receptive and expressive verbal performances and face-matching. *Neuropsychologia, 12,* 11–19.

Vilkki, J., & Laitinen, L.V. (1976). Effects of pulvinotomy and ventrolateral thalamotomy on some cognitive functions. *Neuropsychologia, 14,* 67–78.

Voelker, C.H. (1937). A comparative study of investigations of phonetic dispersion in connected American English. *Archives Neerlandises de Phonetique Experimentale, 13,* 138–152.

Voelker, C.H. (1944). A preliminary investigation for a normative study of fluency, a clinical index to the severity of stuttering. *American Journal of Orthopsychiatry, 14,* 285–294.

Wall, M.J. (1980). A comparison of syntax in young stutterers and non-stutterers. *Journal of Fluency Disorders, 5,* 321–326.

Wall, M.J., Starkweather, C.W., & Cairns, H.S. (1981). Syntactic influences on stuttering in young child stutterers. *Journal of Fluency Disorders, 6,* 283–298.

Wang, W. S-Y. (1965). Review of *Tables of Transitional Frequencies of English Phonemes,* by L.S. Hultzen, J.H.D. Allen, Jr., and M.S. Miron. *Language, 41,* 525–529.

Wang, W. S-Y., & Crawford, J. (1960). Frequency studies of English consonants. *Language and Speech, 3,* 131–139.

Wechsler Adult Intelligence Scale. (1955). New York: Psychological Corp.

Weintraub, S., Mesulam, M-M., & Kramer, L. (1981). Disturbances in prosody: A right hemisphere contribution to language. *Neurology, 23,* 130–135.

Weisenberg, T., & McBride, K.F. (1964). Aphasia. New York: Hafner.

Wells, G.B. (1979). Effect of sentence structure on stuttering. *Journal of Fluency Disorders, 4,* 123–129.

Wells, G.B. (1983). A feature analysis of stuttered phonemes. *Journal of Fluency Disorders, 8,* 119–124.

Wertz, R.T., & Lemme, M.L. (1974). Input and output measures with aphasic adults. *Research and Training Center 10* (Final Rep.). Washington, DC: Social and Rehabilitation Services.

West, R. (1943). The pathology of stuttering. *Nervous Child, 2,* 96–106.

West, R. (1958). An agnostic's speculations about stuttering. In J. Eisenson (Ed.), *Stuttering: A symposium* (pp. 167–222). New York: Harper & Row.

West, R., & Ansberry, M. (1968). *The rehabilitation of speech.* New York: Harper & Row.

West, R., Ansberry, M., & Carr, A. (1957). *The rehabilitation of speech.* New York: Harper.

West, R., Kennedy, L., & Carr, A. (1937). *The rehabilitation of speech.* New York: Harper.

Westby, C.E. (1979). Language performance of stuttering and nonstuttering children. *Journal of Communication Disorders, 12,* 133–145.

Weuffen, V.M. (1961). An investigation of the word-finding of normal and stuttering school-age children from eight to sixteen. *Folia Phoniatrica, 13,* 255–268.

Wexler, K.B., & Mysak, E.D. (1982). Disfluency characteristics of 2-, 4-, and 6-year-old males. *Journal of Fluency Disorders, 7,* 37–46.

Whipple, G.M. (1911). The left-handed child. *Journal of Educational Psychology, 2,* 1-78, 574-575.
Williams, D.E. (1955). Intensive clinical case studies of stuttering therapy. In W. Johnson & R.R. Leutenegger (Eds.), *Stuttering in children and adults* (pp. 405-414). Minneapolis: University of Minnesota Press.
Williams, R.M. (1960). *Phonetic spelling for college students.* New York: Oxford University Press.
Williams, D.E., Silverman, F.H., & Kools, J.A. (1968). Disfluency behavior of elementary school stutterers and nonstutterers: The adaptation effect. *Journal of Speech and Hearing Research, 11,* 622-630.
Williams, D.E., Silverman, F.H., & Kools, J.A. (1969a). Disfluency behavior of elementary school stutterers and nonstutterers: The consistency effect. *Journal of Speech and Hearing Research, 12,* 301-307.
Williams, D.E., Silverman, F.H., & Kools, J.A. (1969b). Disfluency behavior of elementary school stutterers and nonsutterers: Loci of instances of disfluency. *Journal of Speech and Hearing Research, 12,* 308-318.
Williams, D.E., Wark, M., & Minifie, F. (1963). Ratings of stuttering by audio, visual and audiovisual cues. *Journal of Speech and Hearing Research, 6,* 91-100.
Wingate, M.E. (1962). Evaluation and stuttering: I. Speech characteristics of young children. *Journal of Speech and Hearing Disorders, 27,* 106-115.
Wingate, M.E. (1964). A standard definition of stuttering. *Journal of Speech and Hearing Disorders, 29,* 484-489.
Wingate, M.E. (1966a). Behavioral rigidity in stutterers. *Journal of Speech and Hearing Research, 9,* 626-629.
Wingate, M.E. (1966b). Prosody in stuttering adaptation. *Journal of Speech and Hearing Research, 9,* 550-556.
Wingate, M.E. (1966c). Stuttering adaptation and learning: I. The relevance of adaptation studies to stuttering as "learned behavior." *Journal of Speech and Hearing Disorders, 31,* 148-156.
Wingate, M.E. (1966d). Stuttering adaptation and learning: II. The adequacy of learning principles in the interpretation of stuttering. *Journal of Speech and Hearing Disorder, 31,* 211-218.
Wingate, M.E. (1967a). Slurvian skill of stutterers. *Journal of Speech and Hearing Research, 10,* 844-848.
Wingate, M.E. (1967b). Stuttering and word length. *Journal of Speech and Hearing Research, 10,*146-152.
Wingate, M.E. (1968). *Thurstone's word-fluency factor in stuttering.* Unpublished manuscript.
Wingate, M.E. (1969a). Sound and pattern in "artificial" fluency. *Journal of Speech and Hearing Research, 12,* 677-686.
Wingate, M.E. (1969b). Stuttering as phonetic transition defect. *Journal of Speech and Hearing Disorders, 34,* 107-108.
Wingate, M.E. (1970a). *Balanced forms of the "Slurvians" test.* Unpublished manuscript.
Wingate, M.E. (1970b). Effect on stuttering of changes in audition. *Journal of Speech and Hearing Research, 13,* 861-873.
Wingate, M.E. (1971). Phonetic ability in stuttering. *Journal of Speech and Hearing Research, 14,* 189-194.

Wingate, M.E. (1976). *Stuttering: Theory and treatment.* New York: Irvington-Wiley.

Wingate, M.E. (1977a). Criteria for stuttering. *Journal of Speech and Hearing Research, 20,* 596–607.

Wingate, M.E. (1977b). The immediate source of stuttering: An integration of evidence. *Journal of Communciation Disorders, 10,* 45–52.

Wingate, M.E. (1977c). The relationship of theory to therapy in stuttering. *Journal of Communication Disorders, 10,* 37–44.

Wingate, M.E. (1979a). The first three words. *Journal of Speech and Hearing Research, 22,* 604–612.

Wingate, M.E. (1979b). The loci of stuttering: Grammar or prosody. *Journal of Communication Disorders, 12,* 283–290.

Wingate, M.E. (1979c). Vocalization≠phonation. *Journal of Speech and Hearing Research, 22,* 657–658.

Wingate, M.E. (1981). Knowing what to look for: Comments on "Stuttering identification—Standard definition and moment of stuttering." *Journal of Speech and Hearing Research, 24,* 622.

Wingate, M.E. (1983). Speaking unassisted: Comments on a paper by Andrews et al. *Journal of Speech and Hearing Disorders, 48,* 255–263.

Wingate, M.E. (1984a). Fluency, disfluency, dysfluency and stuttering. *Journal of Fluency Disorders, 9,* 163–168.

Wingate, M.E. (1984b). Pause loci in stuttered and normal speech. *Journal of Fluency Disorders, 9,* 227–235.

Wingate, M.E. (1984c). Stutter events and linguistic stress. *Journal of Fluency Disorders, 9,* 295–300.

Wingate, M.E. (1985). *Structural characteristics of words in use: Data from various samples.* Unpublished manuscript.

Wingate, M.E. (1986a). Adaptation, consistency and beyond: I. Limitations and contradictions. *Journal of Fluency Disorders, 11,* 1–36.

Wingate, ME. (1986b). Adaptation, consistency and beyond: II. An integral account. *Journal of Fluency Disorders, 11,* 37–53.

Wingate, M.E. (1986c). Physiological and genetic factors. In G.H. Shames & H. Rubin (Eds.), *Stuttering: Then and now* (pp. 49–69). Columbus, OH: Merrill.

Wode, H. (1980). Grammatical intonation in child language. In L.R. Waugh & C.H. van Schooneveld (Eds.), *The melody of language* (pp. 331–345). Baltimore, MD: University Park Press.

Wood, F., Stump, D., McKeehan, A., Sheldon, S., & Proctor, J. (1980). Patterns of regional cerebral blood flow during attempted reading aloud by stutterers both on and off haloperidol medication: Evidence for inadequate left frontal activation during stuttering. *Brain and Language, 9,* 141–144.

Wyrick, D.R. (1949). *A study of normal nonfluency in conversation.* Masters thesis, University of Missouri, Columbia.

Yairi, E. (1972). Disfluency rates and patterns of stutterers and nonstutterers. *Journal of Communication Disordes, 5,* 225–231.

Yairi, E., & Clifton, N. (1972). Disfluent speech behavior of preschool children, high school seniors, and geriatric persons. *Journal of Speech and Hearing Research, 4,* 714–719.

Yairi, E., & Jennings, S.M. (1974). Relationships between the disfluent speech behavior of normal-speaking preschool boys and their parents. *Journal of Speech and Hearing Research, 17,* 94–98.

Yairi, E., & Lewis, B. (1984). Disfluencies at the onset of stuttering. *Journal of Speech and Hearing Research, 27,* 154–159.

Yamadori, A., Osumi, Y., Masuhara, L., & Okubo, M. (1977). Preservation of singing in Broca's aphasia. *Journal of Neurology, Neurosurgery and Psychiatry, 40,* 221–224.

Zangwill, O.L. (1966). Psychological deficits associated with frontal lobe lesions. *International Journal of Neurology, 5,* 395–402.

Zangwill, O.L. (1967). Speech and the minor hemisphere. *Acta Neuropsychiatrica, 67,* 1013–1020.

Zangwill, O.L. (1975). Excision of Broca's area without persistent aphasia. In K.J. Zulch, O. Creutzfeld, & G.C. Galbraith (Eds.), *Cerebral localization* (pp. 258–263). New York: Springer-Verlag.

Zangwill, O.L. (1978). Aphasia and the concept of brain centers. In G.A. Miller & E. Lenneberg (Eds.), *Psychology and biology of language and thought* (pp. 119–132). New York: Academic Press.

Zerbin, W. (1973). Erfassung der symptomatik stoternder [Inventory of stuttering symptoms]. *Die Sprachheilarbeit, 18,* 174–185.

Zimbardo, P.G., Mahl, G.F., & Barnard, J.W. (1963). The measurement of speech disturbances in anxious children. *Journal of Speech and Hearing Disorders, 28,* 362–370.

Zimmerman, G. (1980a). Articulatory dynamics of "fluent" utterances of stutterers and nonstutterers. *Journal of Speech and Hearing Research, 23,* 95–107.

Zimmerman, G. (1980b). Articulatory behaviors associated with stuttering: A cinefluorographic analysis. *Journal of Speech and Hearing Research, 23,* 108–121.

Zimmerman, G. (1980c). Stuttering: A disorder of movement. *Journal of Speech and Hearing Research, 23,* 122–136.

Zipf, G.K. (1935). *The psycho-biology of language.* New York: Houghton-Mifflin.

Zipf, G.K. (1949). *Human behavior and the principle of least effort.* Cambridge, MA: Addison-Wesley.

Zwitman, D.H. (1978). *The disfluent child.* Baltimore, MD: University Park Press.

Author Index

Subject Index

MIX
Papier aus verantwortungsvollen Quellen
Paper from responsible sources
FSC® C105338

If you have any concerns about our products,
you can contact us on
ProductSafety@springernature.com

In case Publisher is established outside the EU,
the EU authorized representative is:
Springer Nature Customer Service Center GmbH
Europaplatz 3, 69115 Heidelberg, Germany

Printed by Libri Plureos GmbH
in Hamburg, Germany